Coronary Physiology in Contemporary Clinical Practice

Editor

ALLEN JEREMIAS

CARDIOLOGY CLINICS

www.cardiology.theclinics.com

February 2024 • Volume 42 • Number 1

ELSEVIER

1600 John F. Kennedy Boulevard • Suite 1800 • Philadelphia, Pennsylvania, 19103-2899

http://www.theclinics.com

CARDIOLOGY CLINICS Volume 42, Number 1
February 2024 ISSN 0733-8651, ISBN-13: 978-0-443-29480-8

Editor: Joanna Gascoine
Developmental Editor: Isha Singh

Cardiology Clinics (ISSN 0733-8651) is published quarterly by Elsevier Inc., 360 Park Avenue South, New York, NY 10010-1710. Months of issue are February, May, August, and November. Business and Editorial Offices: 1600 John F. Kennedy Blvd., Ste. 1800, Philadelphia, PA 19103-2899. Customer Service Office: 3251 Riverport Lane, Maryland Heights, MO 63043. Periodicals post-age paid at New York, NY and additional mailing offices. Subscription prices are $396.00 per year for US individuals, $100.00 per year for US students and residents, $472.00 per year for Canadian individuals, $495.00 per year for international individuals, $100.00 per year for Canadian students/residents and $220.00 per year for international students/residents. To receive student/resident rate, orders must be accompanied by name of affiliated institution, data of term, and the *signature* of program/residency coordinator on institution letterhead. Orders will be billed at individual rate until proof of status is received. Foreign air speed delivery is included in all *Clinics* subscription prices. All prices are subject to change without notice. **POSTMASTER:** Send address changes to *Cardiology Clinics*, Elsevier Health Sciences Division, Subscription Customer Service, 3251 Riverport Lane, Maryland Heights, MO 63043. **Customer Service: 1-800-654-2452 (U.S. and Canada); 314-447-8871 (outside U.S. and Canada). Fax: 314-447-8029. E-mail: journalscustomerservice-usa@elsevier.com (for print support); journalsonlinesupport-usa@elsevier.com (for online support).**

Reprints. For copies of 100 or more, of articles in this publication, please contact the Commercial Reprints Department, Elsevier Inc., 360 Park Avenue South, New York, NY 10010-1710. Tel.: 212-633-3874; Fax: 212-633-3820; E-mail: reprints@elsevier.com.

Cardiology Clinics is also published in Spanish by McGraw-Hill Interamericana Editores S. A., P.O. Box 5-237, 06500, Mexico D. F., Mexico; in Portuguese by Reichmann and Alfonso Editores Rio de Janeiro, Brazil; and in Greek by Dimitrios P. Lagos, 8 Pondon Street, GR115-28 Ilissia, Greece.

Cardiology Clinics is covered in *MEDLINE/PubMed (Index Medicus), Excerpta Medica, The Cumulative Index to Nursing and Allied Health Literature* (CINAHL).

Contributors

EDITORIAL BOARD

JAMIL A. ABOULHOSN, MD, FACC, FSCAI
Director, Ahmanson/UCLA Adult Congenital
Heart Center, Streisand/American Heart
Association Endowed Chair, Divisions of
Cardiology and Pediatric Cardiology, David
Geffen School of Medicine at UCLA, Los
Angeles, California, USA

DAVID M. SHAVELLE, MD, FACC, FSCAI
Director, Department of Cardiology Director,
Interventional Cardiology MemorialCare Heart
and Vascular Institute (MHVI), Long Beach
Medical Center, Long Beach, California, USA

AUDREY H. WU, MD, MPH
Associate Professor, Advanced Heart Failure
and Transplant Program, Division of
Cardiovascular Medicine, Department of
Medicine, University of Michigan, Ann Arbor,
Michigan, USA

EDITOR

ALLEN JEREMIAS, MD, MSc
Associate Director, Cardiac Catheterization
Laboratory, St. Francis Hospital & Heart
Center, Roslyn, New York, USA

AUTHORS

RASHA AL-LAMEE, MA, MBBS, PhD
National Heart and Lung Institute,
Imperial College London, Imperial College
Healthcare NHS Trust, Hammersmith
Hospital, Du Cane Road, London, United
Kingdom

ADRIAN P. BANNING, MD
Heart Centre, John Radcliffe Hospital, Oxford
University Hospitals NHS Foundation Trust,
Oxford, United Kingdom

ADAM BLAND, MBBS
Department of Cardiology, Gosford
Hospital - Central Coast LHD, The University
of Newcastle - Central Coast Clinical
School, Gosford, New South Wales,
Australia

KI HONG CHOI, MD
Division of Cardiology, Department of Internal
Medicine, Heart Vascular Stroke Institute,
Samsung Medical Center, Sungkyunkwan
University School of Medicine, Seoul, Republic of
Korea

EUNICE CHUAH, MBBS
Department of Cardiology, Gosford Hospital -
Central Coast LHD, The University of
Newcastle - Central Coast Clinical School,
Gosford, New South Wales, Australia

CHRISTOPHER M. COOK, MBBS, PhD
Essex Cardiothoracic Centre, Mid and South
Essex NHS Hospitals Trust, Basildon, United
Kingdom; Anglia Ruskin University,
Chelmsford, Essex, United Kingdom

JOOST DAEMEN, MD, PhD
Department of Cardiology, Thoraxcenter, Erasmus University Medical Center, Rotterdam, the Netherlands

JAVIER ESCANED, MD, PhD
Interventional Cardiology Unit, Hospital Clínico San Carlos IDISCC, Complutense University of Madrid, Madrid, Spain

CAROLINA ESPEJO-PAERES, MD
Interventional Cardiology Unit, Hospital Clínico San Carlos IDISCC, Complutense University of Madrid, Madrid, Spain

SAMER FAWAZ, BMBS
Essex Cardiothoracic Centre, Mid and South Essex NHS Hospitals Trust, Basildon, United Kingdom; Anglia Ruskin University, Chelmsford, Essex, United Kingdom

MICHAEL FOLEY, MBBS, BSc
National Heart and Lung Institute, Imperial College London, Imperial College Healthcare NHS Trust, London, United Kingdom

THOMAS J. FORD, MBChB (Hons), PhD
Department of Cardiology, Gosford Hospital - Central Coast LHD, The University of Newcastle - Central Coast Clinical School, Gosford, New South Wales, Australia; University of Glasgow, ICAMS, Glasgow, United Kingdom

FRANK GIJSEN, PhD
Department of Biomedical Engineering, Erasmus University Medical Center, Rotterdam, the Netherlands

NIEVES GONZALO, MD, PhD
Interventional Cardiology Unit, Hospital Clínico San Carlos IDISCC, Complutense University of Madrid, Madrid, Spain

DAVID HONG, MD
Division of Cardiology, Department of Internal Medicine, Heart Vascular Stroke Institute, Samsung Medical Center, Sungkyunkwan University School of Medicine, Seoul, Republic of Korea

NILS P. JOHNSON, MD, MS
Weatherhead PET Center, Division of Cardiology, Department of Medicine, McGovern Medical School at UTHealth, Memorial Hermann Hospital, Houston, Texas, USA

TOBIN JOSEPH, MBBS, BSc
National Heart and Lung Institute, Imperial College London, Imperial College Healthcare NHS Trust, London, United Kingdom

YUHEI KOBAYASHI, MD
Division of Cardiology, NewYork-Presbyterian Brooklyn Methodist Hospital, Assistant Professor of Clinical Medicine, Weill Cornell Medical College, Brooklyn, New York, USA

JOO MYUNG LEE, MD, MPH, PhD
Division of Cardiology, Department of Internal Medicine, Heart Vascular Stroke Institute, Samsung Medical Center, Sungkyunkwan University School of Medicine, Seoul, Republic of Korea

SEUNG HUN LEE, MD, PhD
Department of Internal Medicine and Cardiovascular Center, Chonnam National University Hospital, Gwangju, Republic of Korea

WEIJIA LI, MD
Department of Medicine, Jacobi Medical Center, Albert Einstein College of Medicine, Bronx, New York, USA

WILLIAM MEERE, MBBS
Department of Cardiology, Gosford Hospital - Central Coast LHD, The University of Newcastle - Central Coast Clinical School, Gosford, New South Wales, Australia

HERNÁN MEJÍA-RENTERÍA, MD, PhD
Interventional Cardiology Unit, Hospital Clínico San Carlos IDISCC, Complutense University of Madrid, Madrid, Spain

SUKHJINDER SINGH NIJJER, BSc, MB ChB, FRCP, PhD
Consultant Cardiologist and Honorary Senior Clinical Lecturer, Imperial College London, Hammersmith Hospital, London, United Kingdom

MANISH A. PARIKH, MD
Division of Cardiology, NewYork-Presbyterian Brooklyn Methodist Hospital, Weill Cornell Medical College, Brooklyn, New York, USA

SONAL PRUTHI, MD
Division of Cardiology, Department of
Medicine, NYU Langone Health, New York,
New York, USA

**ROBERT D. SAFIAN, MD, MSCAI, FACC,
FSCCT**
The Lucia Zurkowski Endowed Chair, Center
for Innovation and Research in Cardiovascular
Diseases (CIRC), Department of
Cardiovascular Medicine, Professor of
Medicine, Oakland University, William
Beaumont School of Medicine, Beaumont
Hospital-Royal Oak, Royal Oak, Michigan,
USA

ALESSANDRA SCOCCIA, MD
Department of Cardiology, Thoraxcenter,
Erasmus University Medical Center,
Rotterdam, the Netherlands

SAMINEH SEHATBAKHSH, MD
Division of Cardiology, Montefiore Medical
Center, Albert Einstein College of Medicine,
Bronx, New York, USA

PATRICK W. SERRUYS, MD, PhD
Department of Cardiology, National University
of Ireland, Galway, Ireland; National Heart and
Lung Institute, Imperial College London,
London, United Kingdom

ARNOLD H. SETO, MD, MPA, FSCAI, FACC
Long Beach Veterans Administration Medical
Center, Long Beach, California, USA

ASAD SHABBIR, MD
Interventional Cardiology Unit, Hospital Clínico
San Carlos IDISCC, Complutense University of
Madrid, Madrid, Spain

DOOSUP SHIN, MD
Division of Cardiology, Duke University
Medical Center, Durham, North Carolina, USA

EMAAD SIDDIQUI, MD
Division of Cardiology, Department of
Medicine, NYU Langone Health, New York,
New York, USA

NATHANIEL R. SMILOWITZ, MD, MS
Assistant Professor of Medicine, The Leon H.
Charney Division of Cardiology, NYU Langone
Health, NYU School of Medicine, Cardiology
Section, Department of Medicine, VA New York
Harbor Healthcare System, New York, New
York, USA

KAYO TAKAHASHI, MD
Department of Cardiology, Ehime University
Graduate School of Medicine, Toon, Ehime,
Japan

TATSUNORI TAKAHASHI, MD
Department of Medicine, Jacobi Medical
Center, Albert Einstein College of Medicine,
Bronx, New York, USA

DAVID M. TEHRANI, MD, MS
Ronald Reagan UCLA Medical Center, Los
Angeles, California, USA

ALEJANDRO TRAVIESO, MD
Interventional Cardiology Unit, Hospital Clínico
San Carlos IDISCC, Complutense University of
Madrid, Madrid, Spain

GIJS VAN SOEST, PhD
Department of Biomedical Engineering,
Erasmus University Medical Center,
Rotterdam, the Netherlands

**ANNEMIEKE C. ZIEDSES DES PLANTES,
BSC**
Department of Cardiology, Thoraxcenter,
Erasmus University Medical Center,
Rotterdam, the Netherlands

Contents

Despite the now routine integration of invasive physiologic systems into coronary catheter laboratories worldwide, it remains critical that all operators maintain a sound understanding of the fundamental physiologic basis for coronary pressure assessment. More specifically, performing operators should be well informed regarding the basis for hyperemic (ie, fractional flow reserve) and nonhyperemic (ie, instantaneous wave-free ratio and other nonhyperemic pressure ratio) coronary pressure assessment. In this article, we provide readers a comprehensive history charting the inception, development, and validation of hyperemic and nonhyperemic coronary pressure assessment.

Fractional flow reserve (FFR) has become the gold standard for invasively assessing the functional significance of coronary artery disease (CAD) to guide revascularization. The amount of evidence supporting the role of FFR in the cardiac catheterization laboratory is large and still growing. However, FFR uptake in the daily practice is limited by a variety of factors such as invasive instrumentation of the coronary artery that requires extra time and need for vasodilator medications for hyperemia. In this review, we describe the details of wire-based alternatives to FFR, providing insights as to their development, clinical evidence, and limitations.

Fractional flow reserve (FFR) and nonhyperemic pressure ratios (NHPRs) provide an important clinical tool to evaluate the hemodynamic significance of coronary lesions. However, these indices have major limitations. As these indices are meant to be surrogates of coronary flow, clinical scenarios such as aortic stenosis (with increased end-systolic and end-diastolic pressures) or atrial fibrillation (with significant beat-to-beat cardiac output variability) can have significant effect on the accuracy and reliability of these hemodynamic indices. Here, we provide a comprehensive evaluation of the pitfalls, limitations, and strengths of FFR and NHPRs in common clinical scenarios paired with coronary artery disease.

During the past 30 years, fractional flow reserve (FFR) has moved from animal models to class IA recommendations in guidelines. However, the FLOWER-MI, RIPCORD-2, FUTURE, and FAME 3 trials in 2021 were "negative"—has FFR exceeded its expiration date? We critically examine these randomized trials in order to draw insights not

Coronary computed tomography angiography (CCTA) and CCTA-derived fractional flow reserve (FFRCT) are the best non-invasive techniques to assess coronary artery disease (CAD) and myocardial ischemia. Advances in these technologies allow a paradigm shift to the use of CCTA and FFRCT for advanced plaque characterization and planning myocardial revascularization.

Ischemic heart disease (IHD) affects more than 20 million adults in the United States. Although classically attributed to atherosclerosis of the epicardial coronary arteries, nearly half of patients with stable angina and IHD who undergo invasive coronary angiography do not have obstructive epicardial coronary artery disease. Ischemia with nonobstructive coronary arteries is frequently caused by microvascular angina with underlying coronary microvascular dysfunction (CMD). Greater understanding the pathophysiology, diagnosis, and treatment of CMD holds promise to improve clinical outcomes of patients with ischemic heart disease.

Coronary microvascular dysfunction (CMD) is a common cause of ischemia but no obstructive coronary artery disease that results in an inability of the coronary microvasculature to meet myocardial oxygen demand. CMD is challenging to diagnose and manage due to a lack of mechanistic research and targeted therapy. Recent evidence suggests we can improved patient outcomes by stratifying antianginal therapies according to the diagnosis revealed by invasive assessment of the coronary microcirculation. This review article appraises the evidence for management of CMD, which includes treatment of cardiovascular risk, antianginal therapy and therapy for atherosclerosis.

The use of coronary physiology allows for rational decision making at the time of PCI, contributing to better patient outcomes. Yet, coronary physiology is only one aspect of optimal revascularization. State-of-the-art PCI must also consider other important aspects such as intracoronary imaging guidance and specific procedural expertise, as tested in the SYNTAX II study. In this review, we highlight the technical aspects pertaining to the use of physiology as used in that trial and offer a glimpse into the future with emerging physiologic metrics, including functional coronary angiography, which have already established themselves as useful indices to guide decision making.

CARDIOLOGY CLINICS

Preface

Coronary Physiology to Optimize Percutaneous Coronary Intervention

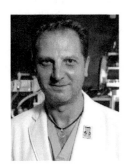

Allen Jeremias, MD, MSc
Editor

Since the original description by Pijls and colleagues in 1993, Fractional Flow Reserve (FFR) has established itself as the key diagnostic tool to determine lesion severity during coronary angiography and the deciding factor whether a percutaneous coronary intervention (PCI) is indicated and necessary. Since the original publication of the "Physiology" issue in *Interventional Cardiology Clinics* in 2015, the routine use of physiology during PCI in the United States has more than doubled to ~25%. Importantly, the clinical applications of coronary physiology measurements have also increased substantially over the past few years. The addition of resting indices to determine lesion severity instead of FFR led to increased procedure efficiency and patient comfort. The advent of a physiology pullback allows the colocalization of pressure gradients to the angiogram and creates a "coronary physiology map" that ultimately allows the treating physician to identify the hemodynamically important lesions that may require PCI. Finally, the importance of post-PCI physiology has been increasingly recognized as a prognostic indicator for long-term clinical outcomes, and multiple randomized trials are underway to assess whether the routine use of this technology will lead to a reduction in major adverse events.

This issue of *Cardiology Clinics* is therefore dedicated to the recent advances in the area of coronary physiology, building on the prior issue that covered the basic concepts, clinical trial evidence, and practical applications. Once again, the new issue includes international experts in coronary physiology that have significant scientific contributions in this space. The first three articles provide a nuanced overview of resting indices, including their scientific basis, individual differences, and their use in special circumstances, such as aortic stenosis or atrial fibrillation. There is a dedicated article discussing more recent literature comparing FFR with angiographic guidance for PCI that (seemingly) did not demonstrate any benefits for an FFR-based strategy. An important addition to the prior issue has been a thorough description of the utility of physiology for PCI guidance and post-PCI assessment as well as its coutilization with intravascular imaging. This issue also includes advances in intravascular imaging and CT-derived physiology assessment, two modalities that will likely dominate the diagnostic coronary physiology space in the future. Two articles address the diagnosis and treatment of microvascular disease, a condition that is increasingly recognized to be responsible for anginal chest pain among patients with normal or nonobstructive coronary artery disease. Finally, there is a summary article addressing the use of coronary physiology as a state-of the-art PCI strategy.

Cardiol Clin 42 (2024) xi–xii
https://doi.org/10.1016/j.ccl.2023.08.002
0733-8651/24/© 2023 Published by Elsevier Inc.

cardiology.theclinics.com

The authors are part of the SYNTAX study group and share their experience from the large data sets of the original SYNTAX trial as well as SYNTAX II.

It is my hope that this issue will contribute to a deeper understanding of the versatile use of coronary physiology applications and will lead to an expanded use of this technology beyond a simple assessment of lesion severity. I would like to extend my gratitude to all the authors who graciously contributed their time and expertise to this issue of *Cardiology Clinics*. I am confident that this issue provides a relevant and up-to-date overview of coronary physiology and will help implement some of these concepts into daily clinical practice.

Allen Jeremias, MD, MSc
Cardiac Catheterization Laboratory
St. Francis Hospital & Heart Center
100 Port Washington Boulevard
Suite #105
Roslyn, NY 11576, USA

E-mail address:
allen.jeremias@chsli.org

Understanding the Basis for Hyperemic and Nonhyperemic Coronary Pressure Assessment

Samer Fawaz, BMBS[a,b], Christopher M. Cook, MBBS, PhD[a,b,*]

KEYWORDS

- Hyperemia • NHPR • iFR • FFR • Coronary flow

KEY POINTS

- Hyperemic and nonhyperemic pressure ratios are both developed using the principles of Ohm's law.
- Both can be used safely to guide treatment and deferral at their respective cutoff points.
- Discordance between hyperemic and nonhyperemic occurs in around 20% of cases.
- Several nonhyperemic pressure ratios have been developed in recent years that have similar results to instantaneous wave-free ratio.

INTRODUCTION

Since the inception of the fractional flow reserve (FFR) almost 30 years ago[1] (and the subsequent introduction and validation of the instantaneous wave-free ratio [iFR]), physiology-guided revascularization in symptomatic patients despite optimal medical therapy has become an integral part of the contemporary management of stable coronary artery disease. Invasive physiologic assessment facilitates the in-depth functional assessment of coronary stenosis severity, the quantification of epicardial coronary-related ischemia and, more recently, has implications for the planning[2] and optimizing of percutaneous coronary interventions.[3,4]

Both FFR and iFR utilize coronary pressure ratios to provide an estimation of the limitation of coronary blood flow imposed by an epicardial stenosis. The rationale for using coronary pressure (rather than a direct measurement of coronary flow) for this purpose relates to the ease, reproducibility, and robustness of performing coronary pressure measurements in routine clinical practice. Crucial for the widespread clinical adoption of coronary physiology, both indices are supported by randomized controlled clinical trial data[5–8] and international treatment guidelines.[9,10]

Prefractional Flow Reserve Era

In the early days of coronary angiography, the assessment of coronary stenosis severity during angiography was limited to the two-dimensional projections achieved during standard fluoroscopy. Gould and colleagues began the study of attempting to quantify stenosis severity based on more than just visual stenosis percentage. In early explorative studies, experiments were conducted on living animals, whereby flowmeters and vessel constrictive devices were implanted into canine subjects to examine the effects of a stenosis on epicardial coronary flow.[11] Gould and colleagues demonstrated that resting coronary flow measurements did not reduce until there was an 85% epicardial stenosis. Furthermore, gamma cameras

This article originally appeared in *Interventional Cardiology Clinics*, Volume 12 Issue 1, January 2023.
[a] Essex Cardiothoracic Centre, Mid and South Essex NHS Hospitals Trust, Basildon SS16 5NL, United Kingdom;
[b] Anglia Ruskin University, Chelmsford, Essex CM1 1SQ, United Kingdom
* Corresponding author. Dr. Christopher M. Cook, Research Office, Roding Ward, Essex Cardiothoracic Centre, Basildon Hospital, Nethermayne SS16 5NL, United Kingdom.
E-mail address: Christopher.cook@nhs.net

Cardiol Clin 42 (2024) 1–11
https://doi.org/10.1016/j.ccl.2023.07.012

demonstrated that myocardial blood flow distribution was uniform during left atrial injection of [131]Iodine-macroaggregated albumin despite a severe coronary stenosis. Distribution, however, did decrease after administration of an intracoronary hyperemic stimulus (**Fig. 1**). This represented the first documented demonstration of using a hyperemic stimulus to elucidate and quantify an ischemic response secondary to a coronary stenosis.[11] This also led to the first efforts at quantification of the coronary flow reserve (CFR), defined as the ratio of maximal hyperemic coronary flow to coronary flow in the resting state.[11]

During the next 15 years, the validity of CFR was confirmed with noninvasive imaging,[12–17] thermodilution-derived coronary sinus flow[18] and Doppler-tipped catheters.[19] By the early 1990s, the CFR evolved into an accepted physiologic measure of coronary stenosis severity.[20]

Quantification of the Intra-Coronary Pressure-Gradient

The pressure-sensor coronary guidewires used in modern practice are the result of decades of technological advancement and miniaturization of equipment. In the pioneering days of percutaneous transluminal coronary angioplasty (PTCA), such equipment was not available. At the time, the quantification of pressure gradients across peripheral arterial stenoses was commonplace, as was the measurement of gradients across cardiac valves. Grüntzig and colleagues recognized the potential importance of recording pressure gradients across coronary stenoses before and after treatment with PTCA.[21] This trans-stenotic pressure drop was measured using fluid-filled 3F PTCA balloon dilatation catheters. This method, however, was often unreliable due to significant damping and the impediment of antegrade flow caused by the bulky balloon catheter.[22] Owing to these limitations, this method did not achieve widespread clinical adoption.

In the early 1990s, however, intracoronary pressure and Doppler-flow pressure wires became sufficiently miniaturized to be used with accuracy in the human epicardial coronary circulation.[23] This led to the proposal of several coronary physiology measurements.[24] Additionally, the concept of measuring intracoronary pressure gradients during hyperemia was trialled. At this stage, focus was centered around quantifying coronary flow in response to a stenosis, with pressure gradients considered merely supportive of why flow may or may not increase in response to hyperemic stimulus.[24]

The Fractional Flow Reserve Era

In 1993, Pijls and colleagues first published study on the FFR.[1] FFR sought to quantify the physiologic significance of a coronary stenosis using only pressure gradients during hyperemia. Pijls described a theoretic model that followed on from the study of Gould and colleagues, whereby the coronary system was described as a circuit with several components of varying resistances positioned in series, of which the epicardial artery was a single component.[15,25] Pijls applied the principle of Ohm's law ($V = IR$) to rationalize that when resistance is minimal and stable, a directly proportional relationship can be assumed between coronary pressure and flow as is the case during maximal arterial vasodilatation.[20] Accordingly, FFR was devised to estimate the ratio of maximum flow in the presence of an epicardial stenosis, to normal maximum flow without the presence of an epicardial stenosis.[26]

Following on from this, Pijls further devised a theoretic model for the differing components of the coronary circulation and suggested a series of equations to describe the FFR in both the stenotic coronary artery as well as the myocardial vascular bed, further subdividing it into the proportional contributing flows of the epicardial coronary and collateral circulations (**Table 1**).[1] The theory was tested in anesthetized dogs, in which FFR was compared with invasive coronary artery flow reserve in surgically dissected left circumflex coronary arteries with surgically implanted Doppler flowmeters and balloon inflatable ligation devices. This experiment confirmed a strong correlation

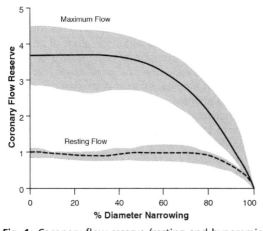

Fig. 1. Coronary flow reserve (resting and hyperemic coronary flow) plotted against angiographic %Diameter narrowing in canine model. (Adapted with permissions from K. Lance Gould, et al. "Does Coronary Flow Trump Coronary Anatomy" JACC: Cardiovascular Imaging, Volume 2, Issue 8, 2009, Pages 1009-1023. DOI: https://doi.org/10.1016/j.jcmg.2009.06.004.)

Table 1
Fractional flow reserve calculations

Coronary Circulation component	Abbreviation	Derivation
FFR myocardium	FFR_{myo}	$\dfrac{Pd - Pv}{Pa - Pv}$ (Under hyperemic conditions)
FFR coronary	FFR_{Cor}	$\dfrac{Pd - Pw}{Pa - Pw}$ (Under hyperemic conditions)
FFR collateral	FFR_{coll}	$FFRmyo - - FFRcor$ (Under hyperemic conditions)

between pressure-derived FFR and Doppler-derived flow in the idealized animal model.[1]

Fractional Flow Reserve Validation in Humans

Following the successful demonstration of FFR in canines, Pijls and colleagues conducted the first-in-man study that focused on identifying a physiologically significant cutoff point.[26] The first study group consisted of 60 consecutive patients with stable angina pectoris who were due to undergo PTCA. Ischemia was confirmed with exercise testing (ET) on a bicycle ergometer where ischemia was considered to be present if there was 1 mm or greater ST depression in at least 2 adjacent leads. FFR was then measured in the stenotic artery before and after PTCA. Following PTCA, the ET was repeated to demonstrate resolution of ischemia. The pre-PTCA FFR was only considered to be consistent with ischemia if the post-PTCA ET showed resolution of ischemic changes. The key findings from this first group of patients demonstrated that an FFR_{myo} cutoff point of less than 0.75 accurately distinguished between ischemic and nonischemic coronary disease.[26] The second group in the study consisted of 5 patients with angiographically normal coronary arteries. Calculation of FFR_{myo} in this group resulted in a mean of 0.98 ± 0.03, thereby supporting the hypothesis that a normal FFR_{myo} should be equal to 1. In modern practice, FFR is now calculated as distal coronary pressure (Pd)/aortic pressure (Pa) during hyperemia, without any correction for venous pressure.

Fractional Flow Reserve Clinical Outcome Studies

Deferral versus performance of percutaneous transluminal coronary angioplasty in patients without documented ischemia trial

Following on from the successful validation of FFR in humans and the identification of an appropriate ischemic FFR cutoff, clinical outcome studies commenced. The Deferral versus Performance of PTCA in Patients Without Documented Ischemia (DEFER) trial was the first landmark clinical outcome study comparing the outcomes of patients with coronary lesions with an FFR of 0.75 or greater randomized to either PTCA or deferral of treatment with optimal medical treatment (OMT).[27] A total of 303 patients were enrolled. Those with an FFR less than 0.75 underwent PTCA (n = 144), serving as the "reference" group. Cases with an FFR of 0.75 or greater were randomized 1:1 to either "perform" with PTCA (n = 90), or "defer" with OMT (n = 91). At 5-year follow-up, the event-free survival (freedom from myocardial infarction, coronary angioplasty, coronary artery bypass grafting, all-cause mortality) was not different between the "perform" and "defer" groups (73% and 80% respectively, $P = .52$) but was significantly worse in the "reference" group (63%, $P = .03$). The composite rate of acute myocardial infarction and cardiac death in the "defer" and "perform" cohorts was not significantly different (3.3% to 7.9% respectively, $P = .21$). This outcome was significantly higher in the "reference" group (15.7%, $P = .003$).[27] The 15-year follow-up data from DEFER is also available, confirming that deferral of PTCA in vessels with an FFR of 0.75 or greater is safe, with similar rates of all-cause mortality between the "defer" and "perform" groups (33% and 31% respectively, $P = .789$). Furthermore, the rates of myocardial infarction were higher in the "perform" group than the "defer" group (10% and 2.2% respectively, $P = .033$), further highlighting that deferring PTCA with an FFR of 0.75 or greater is associated with a favorable outcome.[28]

The Fractional Flow Reserve versus Angiography for Guiding Percutaneous Coronary Intervention trials

The DEFER study supported that deferral of PTCA in angiographically intermediate severity lesions with an FFR of 0.75 or greater was at least as effective as PTCA, prompting the next stage in clinical trials. The Fractional Flow Reserve versus Angiography for Guiding Percutaneous Coronary Intervention (FAME) study was conducted to compare the outcome of FFR-guided versus an angiography-only guided PTCA in patients with multivessel coronary artery disease.[6] This was a prospective, multicenter, randomized controlled trial with 1005 patients included. Patients were randomly assigned to FFR-guided PTCA, versus an angiography-only guided approach. In contrast to previous studies, a cutoff point of an FFR of 0.80 or lesser was used, the rationale being that this cutoff point identified ischemic lesions with an accuracy of 90%,[29–31] thereby reducing the number of ischemic lesions that were missed.[6]

The results of the trial were supportive of the use of FFR. The composite endpoint of death, myocardial infarction, and repeat revascularization at 1-year was significantly lower in the FFR group versus the angiography-only group (13.2% vs 18.3% respectively, $P = .02$). Furthermore, FFR usage decreased the number of stents deployed (1.9 $\pm$ 1.2 in FFR group, 2.7 $\pm$ 1.2 in angiography-only group, $P < .001$), the total length of stenting (37.9 $\pm$ 27.8 mm in FFR group, 51.9 $\pm$ 24.6 mm in angiography-only group, $P < .001$), and the volume of contrast agent used (272 $\pm$ 133 mL in FFR group, 302 $\pm$ 127 mL in angiography-only group, $P < .001$), highlighting the value of FFR-guided revascularization.

The Fractional Flow Reserve-Guided PCI versus Medical Therapy in Stable Coronary disease (FAME II) study sought to test the hypothesis that for hemodynamically significant stenoses, PTCA with OMT was superior to OMT alone.[5] FAME II was a prospective, multicenter randomized trial randomizing patients with at least one functionally significant stenosis (FFR $\leq$0.80) to FFR-guided PTCA plus the best available medical therapy (PTCA group), or the best medical therapy alone (medical-therapy group). Recruitment was halted prematurely after enrollment of 1220 patients, of which 888 underwent randomization, due a significant between-group difference in the percentage of patients who had a primary endpoint of a composite of death, myocardial infarction, or urgent revascularization (4.3% in the PCI group and 12.7% in the medical-therapy group, hazard ratio 0.32; 95% confidence interval [CI], 0.19 to 0.53, $P < .001$). This difference was driven by a lower rate of urgent revascularization in the PTCA versus medical therapy group in an open label trial design.[5]

In 2021, the most recent study in the FAME series of trials reported its findings. The Fractional Flow Reserve-Guided PCI as Compared with Coronary Bypass Surgery (CABG; FAME III) study was a multicenter, international, randomized, noninferiority trial for patients with 3-vessel coronary artery disease.[32] A total of 1500 patients underwent 1:1 randomization to CABG or FFR-guided PTCA with current-generation zotarolimus-eluting stents. FFR-guided PTCA was found to be *not* noninferior to CABG with respect to the incidence of a composite of death, myocardial infarction, stroke, or repeat revascularization at 1 year (10.6% vs 6.9% for PCI and CABG, respectively, hazard ratio 1.5, 95% confidence interval 1.1–2.2, $P = .35$ for noninferiority).[32] Although beyond the scope of this article, one of the principal critiques of the FAME III study has been the low usage of intravascular imaging techniques (12%) in the FFR-guided PTCA group.

Nonhyperemic pressure indices
Following the successful application of FFR as a pressure-derived surrogate of coronary flow, clinical attention turned to the possibility of using coronary pressure gradients in the nonhyperemic or "resting" state. Such an approach was considered clinically attractive because it circumvented the need for vasodilatory agents. Specifically, adenosine, the most frequently used hyperemic agent, which often induces transient side effects in patients characterized by angina-like chest discomfort, dyspnea, and transient AV block.[33]

Whole cycle Pd/Pa was one of the earliest nonhyperemic coronary pressure ratios to be considered for this purpose. However, as the name suggests, whole-cycle Pd/Pa includes both systole and diastole when determining the transstenotic pressure ratio. Because of this, whole-cycle Pd/Pa lacks the discriminatory ability to determine physiologically significant from physiologically nonsignificant in moderate angiographic severity stenoses—the so-called narrow dynamic range.[34] To circumvent this limitation of nonhyperemic pressure assessment, the concept of selective sampling of the trans-stenotic pressure ratio during diastole only (where myocardial resistance is stable and where coronary flow is highest without the need for hyperemia[35]) emerged.

Instantaneous wave-free ratio
As described earlier, in accordance with Ohm's law (and subsequently FFR theory), pressure can be used as a surrogate for flow when resistance is constant and stable.[1] Building on this shared concept, and informed by wave intensity analysis,[36] the iFR was developed following identification of a period during diastole where microvascular resistance is naturally stable[35]—

the so-called wave-free period (WFP). Accordingly, iFR measures the ratio of Pd during the WFP versus the Pa during the WFP of diastole (**Fig. 2**).

Instantaneous wave-free ratio development and validation

The Adenosine Vasodilator Independent Stenosis Evaluation study was a multicenter, international nonrandomized proof of concept study involving 131 patients awaiting coronary angiography or PTCA.[35] All patients underwent initial pressure and flow recordings using a combined pressure and Doppler wire placed distally in the coronary. Following this, adenosine was administered to induce hyperemia and an FFR was calculated for all. In a post hoc fashion, WIA was performed to identify a period of maximal flow and stable resistance within the cardiac cycle, this was named the WFP. Using this period, iFR was calculated using the equation, $iFR = \frac{Pd\ during\ wave-free\ period}{Pa\ during\ wave-free\ period}$. The iFR value was found to be closely correlated with FFR (r = 0.90, y = 1x + 0.03), despite being inherently nonhyperemic. Furthermore, iFR was found to have excellent reproducibility (r = 0.996).[35]

The CLARIFY study assessed the diagnostic performance of iFR and FFR against another, independent reference standard—the hyperemic stenosis resistance (HSR).[37] The HSR is an index of combined intracoronary pressure and flow velocity.[38] In turn, this circumvents the limitations of a pressure-only index and is true to the initial pressure-flow curves as described by Gould.[39] HSR has been found to be a better independent predictor of reversible perfusion defects than CFR and FFR.[38] The study compared the diagnostic performance of iFR and FFR, as well as adenosine-mediated iFR (iFRa) to HSR as a reference standard. The study found equal agreement with the classification of stenosis severity as determined by HSR. Additionally, there was no diagnostic benefit to administering adenosine with iFR,[37] thereby further emphasizing an independence from the need for hyperemia. Another study[40] evaluated the diagnostic performance of FFR, iFR, and Pd/Pa with respect to ^{13}N-ammonia positron emission tomography (PET)-derived CFR. This study found that their diagnostic accuracies to be similar for CFR less than 2.0 (FFR 69.6%, iFR 73.9%, and Pd/Pa 70.4%). Similarly, de Waard and colleagues demonstrated that iFR and FFR had equivalent diagnostic accuracy with regards to myocardial blood flow (MBF) as determined by [150]H$_2$O PET imaging (FFR AUROC 0.85, iFR

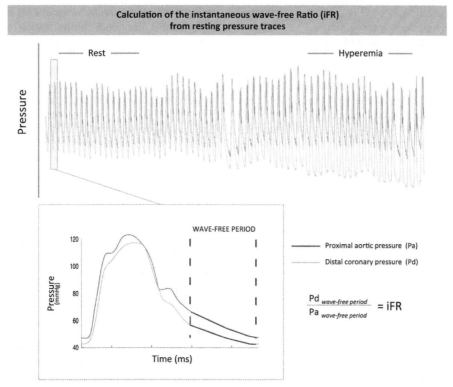

Fig. 2. iFR wave-free period. Reproduced under Creative Commons license CC-BY 3.0. (*From* Nijjer SS, Sen S, Petraco R, et al. Improvement in coronary haemodynamics after percutaneous coronary intervention: assessment using instantaneous wave-free ratio Heart 2013;99:1740-1748.)

AUROC 0.86, $P = .71$).[41] The larger JUSTIFY-CFR study investigated the diagnostic performance of iFR and FFR with regards to invasive coronary flow-velocity reserve in 216 stenoses in 186 patients.[42] Diagnostic agreements were assessed for both pressure indices against multiple cutoff points of CFR. Interestingly, nonhyperemic iFR performed better than hyperemic FFR, across all cutoff points of CFR.

Instantaneous wave-free ratio clinical outcome studies

Following on from the aforementioned validation studies, 2 landmark clinical iFR outcome trials have since been conducted. The "Use of Instantaneous Wave-Free Ratio or Fractional Flow Reserve" (DEFINE-FLAIR) and "Instantaneous Wave-free Ratio versus Fractional Flow Reserve to Guide PCI" (IFR-SWEDEHEART) trials, were simultaneously published in May 2017. Both trials assessed whether an iFR-guided approach to revascularization was noninferior to FFR-guidance. IFR-SWEDEHEART was a multicenter, randomized, controlled, open-label trial involving patients from the Swedish Coronary Angiography and Angioplasty Registry.[7] A total of 2037 patients with stable angina and non-ST elevation myocardial infarction were enrolled. Patients were randomly assigned to FFR-guided intervention versus iFR-guided intervention. The primary endpoint was a composite of all-cause mortality, unplanned revascularization, and nonfatal myocardial infarction at 12 months postprocedure. This composite endpoint occurred in 6.7% of the iFR group, and 6.1% of the FFR group ($P = .007$ for noninferiority), indicating that iFR was noninferior to FFR. DEFINE-FLAIR was a multicenter, international, randomized, blinded trial initially recruiting 2492 patients.[8] As with IFR-SWEDEHEART, patients were randomized 1:1 to an FFR-guided PTCA versus an iFR-guided PTCA. The primary outcome measure was a composite endpoint identical to that of IFR-SWEDEHEART. Once again, noninferiority was met as the primary endpoint occurred in 6.8% of the iFR group, and 7.0% of the FFR group ($P < .001$ for noninferiority). Additionally, the number of patients who had adverse procedural side effects and symptoms of angina and dyspnea was significantly lower in the iFR group (3.1% vs 30.8%, $P < .001$).

The emergence of several nonhyperemic pressure ratios

Following the conception, validation, and clinical adoption of iFR, several alternative nonhyperemic pressure ratios (NHPRs) have since been devised and studied. Using the VERIFY2 population, a comparative study investigating the differences between resting Pd/Pa, iFR and FFR.[43] Van't Veer and colleagues demonstrated that several periods during diastole could be used to derive a pressure ratio that was numerically similar to iFR.[44] Using the diastolic period (diastolic pressure ratio [dPR]), 25% to 75% of the diastolic period (dPR_{25-75}), the midpoint of diastole (dPR_{mid}), and shortened sections of the WFP (iFR_{-50ms} and iFR_{-100ms}), the authors reported near identical numerical results to iFR.[44–46] Subsequently, several other NHPRs have been proposed, each sampling differing sections of the cardiac cycle (**Table 2**). Comparative studies have shown them to be near identical numerical alternatives to iFR.[47] However, it is of note that none have been validated in prospective clinical outcome studies in the manner that iFR has.

Discordance between hyperemic and nonhyperemic coronary pressure assessment

A frequently encountered clinical dilemma is how to interpret discordance between the functional categorization of FFR versus an NHPR (ie, FFR+/NHPR− or vice versa). As iFR is the most widely studied and recognized NHPR, this section will focus on physiologic mechanism underlying the discordance between hyperemic FFR and nonhyperemic iFR functional categorization.

From the VERIFY2 study (and representative of clinical practice) approximately 20% of iFR measurements were diagnostically discordant with FFR.[43] Several studies have investigated the possible factors influencing discordance between iFR and FFR functional categorization. Demiray and colleagues conducted a multivariate analysis investigating clinical, hemodynamic, and angiographic factors that may influence discordance.[51] A total of 587 patients were included, of which 466 (79.4%) showed concordance between FFR and iFR. Compared with FFR, iFR was said to be negatively concordant (FFR+/iFR−) in 69 (11.8%) patients, and positively concordant (FFR−/iFR+) in 52 patients (8.9%). Predictors of a negatively concordant iFR were stenosis location (left main or proximal left anterior descending), increasing stenosis severity, younger age, and slower heart rate. Predictors of a positively concordant iFR were absence of a beta-blocker, older age, and less severe stenosis.

A study by Cook and colleagues sought to investigate the physiologic mechanism underpinning discordance between FFR and iFR.[52] A total of 366 stenosed arteries and 201 unobstructed arteries were assessed with combined coronary pressure and Doppler flow velocity

Table 2
Nonhyperemic pressure ratios

NHPR	Name	Definition	Cutoff Point	Company	Key Evidence
Pd/Pa	Resting whole-cycle Pd/Pa	Average Pd/Pa across the entire cardiac cycle (average of 3 beats)	≤0.91	Generic	
iFR	Instantaneous wave-free ratio	Average Pd/Pa during wave-free period (average of 5 beats)	≤0.89	Phillips	DEFLINE-FLAIR and IFR SWEDEHEART,[7,8] IFR-GRADIENT,[48] DEFINE PCI[4]
DPR	Diastolic pressure ratio	Pd/Pa across the entire diastolic period. (average more than 5 beats)	≤0.89	Generic/OpSens/ ACIST	Van't Veer et al[44]
dPR	Diastolic pressure ratio	Pd/Pa during flat period on the dP/dt of aortic pressure when the resistance is constant and low (Average of 5 beats)[49]	≤0.89	Generic/Erasmus MC	The dPR study[50]
RFR	Resting full cycle ratio	Minimum Pd/Pa ratio across entire cardiac cycle	≤0.89	Abbott	VALIDATE RFR[46]
DFR	Diastolic hyperemia free	Average Pd/Pa during the period where Pa < mean Pa and Pa is downsloping (Average of 5 beats)	≤0.89	Boston Scientific	Analysis from the VERIFY2 and CONTRAST studies[45]

measurements. Overall, FFR agreed with iFR in 86% (316 of 366) of stenosed vessels. Stenoses discordantly classified as FFR+/iFR− demonstrated no significant difference in hyperemic coronary flow velocity or CFR compared with FFR−/iFR− and angiographically unobstructed vessels. Similarly, for stenoses discordantly classified as FFR−/iFR+, the hyperemic coronary flow velocity and CFR were similar to the FFR+/iFR + group.

Therefore, in summary, this study demonstrated that when FFR and iFR disagreed, the difference in stenosis classification was explained by differences in hyperemic coronary flow velocity. This finding is explained by the physiologic relationship between pressure loss due to a stenosis (ΔP) and arterial flow velocity (V) being related by the equation, $\Delta P = FV + SV2$ (where F is the coefficient of pressure loss due to viscous friction in the stenotic segment and S is the coefficient of pressure loss due to flow separation at the diverging end of the stenosis. As demonstrated by Cook and colleagues,[52] if arterial flow velocity (V) increases by a large amount during hyperemia, the transstenotic pressure gradient (ΔP) also increases. In this scenario, the Pd value falls and the resultant FFR value is low; categorizing the stenosis as functionally significant despite demonstrably high coronary flow conditions. For clinical purposes, this finding suggests that when FFR/iFR discordance occurs, the true hyperemic flow-limiting potential of a stenosis is more accurately discernible by the iFR rather than the FFR measurement (**Fig. 3**).

Building on these earlier studies, in another study, by Warisawa and colleagues, sought to investigate whether the physiologic pattern of coronary disease was a significant influencing factor in determining FFR/iFR discordance.[53] A total of 360 intermediate coronary lesions were assessed with both iFR and FFR, as well as accompanying

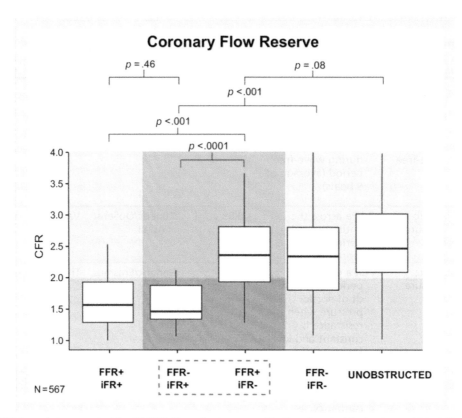

Fig. 3. CFR Box plots separated by FFR/iFR discordant groups. Median denoted by horizontal black line. IQR denoted by box. Whiskers is the range of values. CFR > 2 in green. CFR < 2 in pink. CFR was significantly higher in the FFR+/iFR– group versus the FFR–/iFR+ group. (Reproduced under Creative Commons License CC-BY, from Cook, C.M. et al. "Fractional Flow Reserve/Instantaneous Wave-Free Ratio Discordance in Angiographically Intermediate Coronary Stenoses: An Analysis Using Doppler-Derived Coronary Flow Measurements" J Am Coll Cardiol Intv.2017;10(24):2514-24.)

iFR pullback recordings. From these iFR pullback recordings the physiologic pattern of disease for each coronary artery was classified as "focal" or "diffuse." Overall, FFR disagreed with iFR in 22% of vessels. A physiologically focal pattern of disease was significantly associated with FFR+/iFR– disease, and a physiologically diffuse pattern was significantly associated with FFR–/iFR+ disease. The explanations for these findings were as follows: first, in physiologically diffuse patterns of disease, frictional losses along the length of the vessel account for the pressure energy loss, which is evident at rest (iFR+) with only minimal increase during hyperemia. Second, in focal disease, separation losses near the focal stenosis itself would be the primary mode of pressure energy loss which is minimally present at rest (iFR–) but more evident in hyperemia (FFR+).[53]

Although no randomized data exists, a few studies have investigated the clinical outcomes of patients that showed discordance between FFR and iFR. A study by Hun Lee and colleagues evaluated the physiologic characteristics of vessels showing discordance between iFR and FFR, as well as patient-oriented composite outcomes (POCO) of all-cause mortality, any myocardial infarction, and any revascularization at 5 years.[54] A total of 840 vessels from 596 patients were classified according to iFR and FFR (combinations of high or low iFR, and high or low FFR). PTCA was recommended for those with a low FFR (≤0.80); however, the final decision was left at the discretion of the operator. In concordance with the study by Cook and colleagues,[52] the study found significant differences in CFR as well as resistance reserve ratio between groups classified by iFR and FFR, particularly among the FFR–/iFR+ and FFR–/iFR+ groups. There was no significant difference in the index of microcirculatory dysfunction between the groups. Discordance of FFR/iFR, however, was not related to an increased risk of POCO at 5 years, suggesting the safety of using either index to guide revascularization decision-making.

CLINICS CARE POINTS

- Hyperemic and nonhyperemic coronary pressure ratios can both provide an estimate to the limitation of coronary flow imposed by an epicardial stenosis.

- Clinical outcome studies have demonstrated safety regarding the deferral of revascularization of epicardial coronary stenoses when using fractional flow reserve (FFR) and instantaneous wave-free ratio (iFR) at their respective cutoff values.

- Several nonhyperemic pressure ratios have emerged in recent years that sample different segments of the cardiac cycle. They have been shown to be almost numerically identical to iFR.

- In approximately 20% of cases, FFR and iFR demonstrate physiologic diagnostic discordance when classifying epicardial stenosis severity. These instances of discordance can be rationalized by differences in hyperemic coronary flow velocity, as well as the physiologic pattern of disease.

- No randomized controlled studies have been conducted to investigate the clinical outcome when treating FFR/iFR discordant lesions; however, small observational study data has not shown any difference in outcome.

SUMMARY

Within this article, we have provided readers a comprehensive overview of the physiologic basis for hyperemic and nonhyperemic coronary pressure assessment. We have detailed the conceptual framework (and subsequent validation, verification, and clinical outcome studies) that emphasize the integral role invasive physiologic assessment plays in the contemporary management of coronary artery disease.

Although there are physiologic and clinical differences between these 2 broad groups of pressure-based physiologic tools, both hyperemic and nonhyperemic indices are commonly rooted in the fundamental use of trans-stenotic coronary pressure ratios to estimate the limitation to coronary flow imposed by an epicardial stenosis. Cognizant of the evolving landscape of clinical practice, specifically the increasing requirement to offer combined epicardial and microcirculatory functional assessment, both the hyperemic and resting physiologic state will continue to coexist and occupy critical roles in invasive physiologic assessment.

DISCLOSURE

Dr Cook is a consultant for Philips Healthcare, Viz.ai. He receives speaker's fees from Boston Scientific and has equity in Cerebria.ai. Dr Keeble has received honoraria and institutional research funding from Abbott Vascular, Medtronic, Terumo, Zoll, and Shockwave. He has received consulting fees from BD and has received speaker fees from Cardionovum, Abbott Vascular, and Astra Zeneca. Dr Davies has received research grants from Abbott Vascular and Medtronic, and has received speaker fees from Boston Scientific. The remaining authors have no disclosures.

REFERENCES

1. Pijls NHJ, van Son JAM, Kirkeeide RL, et al. Experimental basis of determining maximum coronary, myocardial, and collateral blood flow by pressure measurements for assessing functional stenosis severity before and after percutaneous transluminal coronary angioplasty. Circulation 1993;87(4):1354–67.

2. Kikuta Y, Cook CM, Sharp ASP, et al. Pre-Angioplasty Instantaneous Wave-Free Ratio Pullback Predicts Hemodynamic Outcome In Humans With Coronary Artery Disease. JACC: Cardiovasc Interventions 2018;11(8):757–67.

3. Diletti R, Masdjedi K, Daemen J, et al. Impact of Poststenting Fractional Flow Reserve on Long-Term Clinical Outcomes: The FFR-SEARCH Study. Circ Cardiovasc interventions 2021;14(3). https://doi.org/10.1161/CIRCINTERVENTIONS.120.009681.

4. Jeremias A, Davies JE, Maehara A, et al. Blinded Physiological Assessment of Residual Ischemia After Successful Angiographic Percutaneous Coronary Intervention: The DEFINE PCI Study. JACC Cardiovasc interventions 2019;12(20):1991–2001.

5. de Bruyne B, Pijls NHJ, Kalesan B, et al. Fractional Flow Reserve–Guided PCI versus Medical Therapy in Stable Coronary Disease. N Engl J Med 2012; 367(11):991–1001.

6. Tonino PAL, de Bruyne B, Pijls NHJ, et al. Fractional Flow Reserve versus Angiography for Guiding Percutaneous Coronary Intervention. N Engl J Med 2009;360(3):213–24.

7. Götberg M, Christiansen EH, Gudmundsdottir IJ, et al. Instantaneous Wave-free Ratio versus Fractional Flow Reserve to Guide PCI. N Engl J Med 2017;376(19):1813–23.

8. Davies JE, Sen S, Dehbi HM, et al. Use of the Instantaneous Wave-free Ratio or Fractional Flow Reserve in PCI. N Engl J Med 2017;376(19):1824–34.

9. Neumann FJ, Sechtem U, Banning AP, et al. 2019 ESC Guidelines for the diagnosis and management of chronic coronary syndromes. Eur Heart J 2020; 41(3):407–77.

10. Lawton JS, Tamis-Holland JE, Bangalore S, et al. 2021 ACC/AHA/SCAI Guideline for Coronary Artery Revascularization: A Report of the American College of Cardiology/American Heart Association Joint Committee on Clinical Practice Guidelines. Circulation 2022;145(3). https://doi.org/10.1161/CIR.0000000000001038.

11. Gould KL, Lipscomb K, Hamilton GW. Physiologic basis for assessing critical coronary stenosis. The Am J Cardiol 1974;33(1):87–94.

12. Schelbert HR, Wisenberg G, Phelps ME, et al. Noninvasive assessment of coronary stenoses by myocardial imaging during pharmacologic coronary vasodilation. The Am J Cardiol 1982;49(5):1197–207.

13. Gould KL. Noninvasive assessment of coronary stenoses by myocardial perfusion imaging during pharmacologie coronary vasodilatation. I. Physiologic basis and experimental validation. The Am J Cardiol 1978;41(2):267–78.

14. Gould KL, Goldstein RA, Mullani NA, et al. Noninvasive assessment of coronary stenoses by myocardial perfusion imaging during pharmacologic coronary vasodilation. VIII. Clinical feasibility of positron cardiac imaging without a cyclotron using generator-produced Rubidium-82. J Am Coll Cardiol 1986;7(4):775–89.

15. Kirkeeide RL, Gould KL, Parsel L. Assessment of coronary stenoses by myocardial perfusion imaging during pharmacologic coronary vasodilation. VII. Validation of coronary flow reserve as a single integrated functional measure of stenosis severity reflecting all its geometric dimensions. J Am Coll Cardiol 1986;7(1):103–13.

16. Gould KL, Schelbert HR, Phelps ME, et al. Noninvasive assessment of coronary stenoses with myocardial perfusion imaging during pharmacologic coronary vasodilatation. The Am J Cardiol 1979;43(2):200–8.

17. Gould KL. Assessment of coronary stenoses with myocardial perfusion imaging during pharmacologic coronary vasodilatation. IV. Limits of detection of stenosis with idealized experimental cross-sectional myocardial imaging. The Am J Cardiol 1978;42(5):761–8.

18. Brown BG, Josephson MA, Petersen RB, et al. Intravenous dipyridamole combined with isometric handgrip for near maximal acute increase in coronary flow in patients with coronary artery disease. The Am J Cardiol 1981;48(6):1077–85.

19. Wilson RF, Laughlin DE, Ackell PH, et al. Transluminal, subselective measurement of coronary artery blood flow velocity and vasodilator reserve in man. Circulation 1985;72(1):82–92.

20. Gould KL, Kirkeeide RL, Buchi M. Coronary flow reserve as a physiologic measure of stenosis severity. J Am Coll Cardiol 1990;15(2):459–74.

21. Grüntzig AR, Å Senning, Siegenthaler WE. Nonoperative Dilatation of Coronary-Artery Stenosis:percutaneous transluminal coronary angioplasty. N Engl J Med 2010;301(2):61–8.

22. Serruys PW, Wijns W, Reiber JH, et al. Values and limitations of transstenotic pressure gradients measured during percutaneous coronary angioplasty. Herz 1985;10(6):337–42.

23. Emanuelsson H, Dohnal M, Lamm C, et al. Initial experiences with a miniaturized pressure transducer during coronary angioplasty. Cathet Cardiovasc Diagn 1991;24(2):137–43.

24. Serruys PW, di Mario C, Meneveau N, et al. Intracoronary pressure and flow velocity with sensor-tip guidewires: A new methodologic approach for assessment of coronary hemodynamics before and after coronary interventions. The Am J Cardiol 1993;71(14):D41–53.

25. Gould KL. Identifying and measuring severity of coronary artery stenosis. Quantitative coronary arteriography and positron emission tomography. Circulation 1988;78(2):237–45.

26. Pijls NHJ, van Gelder B, van der Voort P, et al. Fractional Flow Reserve. Circulation 1995;92(11):3183–93.

27. Pijls NHJ, van Schaardenburgh P, Manoharan G, et al. Percutaneous Coronary Intervention of Functionally Nonsignificant Stenosis. J Am Coll Cardiol 2007;49(21):2105–11.

28. Zimmermann FM, Ferrara A, Johnson NP, et al. Deferral vs. performance of percutaneous coronary intervention of functionally non-significant coronary stenosis: 15-year follow-up of the DEFER trial. Eur Heart J 2015;36(45):3182–8.

29. Pijls NHJ, van Gelder B, van der Voort P, et al. Fractional flow reserve. A useful index to evaluate the influence of an epicardial coronary stenosis on myocardial blood flow. Circulation 1995;92(11):3183–93.

30. de Bruyne B, Pijls NHJ, Bartunek J, et al. Fractional flow reserve in patients with prior myocardial infarction. Circulation 2001;104(2):157–62.

31. Pijls NHJ, de Bruyne B, Peels K, et al. Measurement of fractional flow reserve to assess the functional severity of coronary-artery stenoses. N Engl J Med 1996;334(26):1703–8.

32. Fearon WF, Zimmermann FM, de Bruyne B, et al. Fractional Flow Reserve–Guided PCI as Compared with Coronary Bypass Surgery. N Engl J Med 2022;386(2):128–37.

33. Jacobson KA, Gao ZG. Adenosine. The Curated Reference Collection Neurosci Biobehavioral Psychol 2021;83–95. https://doi.org/10.1016/B978-0-12-809324-5.01791-0. Published online October 19.

34. Cook CM, Ahmad Y, Shun-Shin MJ, et al. Quantification of the Effect of Pressure Wire Drift on the Diagnostic Performance of Fractional Flow Reserve,

Instantaneous Wave-Free Ratio, and Whole-Cycle Pd/Pa. Circ Cardiovasc interventions 2016;9(4). https://doi.org/10.1161/CIRCINTERVENTIONS.115. 002988.

35. Sen S, Escaned J, Malik IS, et al. Development and Validation of a New Adenosine-Independent Index of Stenosis Severity From Coronary Wave–Intensity Analysis: Results of the ADVISE (ADenosine Vasodilator Independent Stenosis Evaluation) Study. J Am Coll Cardiol 2012;59(15):1392–402.

36. Sen S, Petraco R, Mayet J, et al. Wave Intensity Analysis in the Human Coronary Circulation in Health and Disease. Curr Cardiol Rev 2014;10(1): 17–23.

37. Sen S, Asrress KN, Nijjer S, et al. Diagnostic classification of the instantaneous wave-free ratio is equivalent to fractional flow reserve and is not improved with adenosine administration. Results of CLARIFY (Classification Accuracy of Pressure-Only Ratios Against Indices Using Flow Study). J Am Coll Cardiol 2013;61(13):1409–20.

38. Meuwissen M, Siebes M, Chamuleau SAJ, et al. Hyperemic stenosis resistance index for evaluation of functional coronary lesion severity. Circulation 2002;106(4):441–6.

39. Gould KL. Pressure-flow characteristics of coronary stenoses in unsedated dogs at rest and during coronary vasodilation. Circ Res 1978;43(2):242–53.

40. Hwang D, Jeon KH, Lee JM, et al. Diagnostic Performance of Resting and Hyperemic Invasive Physiological Indices to Define Myocardial Ischemia: Validation With 13N-Ammonia Positron Emission Tomography. JACC: Cardiovasc Interventions 2017; 10(8):751–60.

41. de Waard G, Danad I, Petraco R, et al. Hyperemic FFR and basal iFR have a similar diagnostic accuracy when compared to [15O]H2O PET perfusion imaging defined myocardial blood flow. J Nucl Med 2014;55(supplement 1).

42. Petraco R, van de Hoef TP, Nijjer S, et al. Baseline Instantaneous Wave-Free Ratio as a Pressure-Only Estimation of Underlying Coronary Flow Reserve. Circ Cardiovasc Interventions 2014;7(4):492–502.

43. Hennigan B, Oldroyd KG, Berry C, et al. Discordance Between Resting and Hyperemic Indices of Coronary Stenosis Severity. Circ Cardiovasc Interventions 2016;9(11). https://doi.org/10.1161/ CIRCINTERVENTIONS.116.004016.

44. van't Veer M, Pijls NHJ, Hennigan B, et al. Comparison of Different Diastolic Resting Indexes to iFR. J Am Coll Cardiol 2017;70(25):3088–96.

45. Johnson NP, Li W, Chen X, et al. Diastolic pressure ratio: new approach and validation vs. the instantaneous wave-free ratio. Eur Heart J 2019; 40(31):2585–94.

46. Svanerud J, Ahn JM, Jeremias A, et al. Validation of a novel non-hyperaemic index of coronary artery stenosis severity: the Resting Full-cycle Ratio (VALIDATE RFR) study. EuroIntervention : J EuroPCR collaboration Working Group Interv Cardiol Eur Soc Cardiol 2018;14(7):806–14.

47. Lee JM, Choi KH, Park J, et al. Physiological and Clinical Assessment of Resting Physiological Indexes: Resting Full-Cycle Ratio, Diastolic Pressure Ratio, and Instantaneous Wave-Free Ratio. Circulation 2019;139(7):889–900.

48. Kikuta Y, Cook CM, Sharp ASP, et al. Pre-Angioplasty Instantaneous Wave-Free Ratio Pullback Predicts Hemodynamic Outcome In Humans With Coronary Artery Disease: Primary Results of the International Multicenter iFR GRADIENT Registry. JACC Cardiovasc interventions 2018;11(8):757–67.

49. Kern MJ, Seto AH. DPR, another diastolic resting pressure ratio: Refinements and nuances with identical results. Circ Cardiovasc Interventions. 2018;11(12). https://doi.org/10.1161/CIRCINTERVENTIONS.118. 007540.

50. Ligthart J, Masdjedi K, Witberg K, et al. Validation of Resting Diastolic Pressure Ratio Calculated by a Novel Algorithm and Its Correlation With Distal Coronary Artery Pressure to Aortic Pressure, Instantaneous Wave–Free Ratio, and Fractional Flow Reserve. Circ Cardiovasc Interventions 2018;11(12). https://doi.org/10.1161/CIRCINTERVENTIONS.118. 006911.

51. Dérimay F, Johnson NP, Zimmermann FM, et al. Predictive factors of discordance between the instantaneous wave-free ratio and fractional flow reserve. Catheterization Cardiovasc Interventions 2019; 94(3):356–63.

52. Cook CM, Jeremias A, Petraco R, et al. Fractional Flow Reserve/Instantaneous Wave-Free Ratio Discordance in Angiographically Intermediate Coronary Stenoses. JACC: Cardiovasc Interventions 2017;10(24):2514–24.

53. Warisawa T, Cook CM, Howard JP, et al. Physiological Pattern of Disease Assessed by Pressure-Wire Pullback Has an Influence on Fractional Flow Reserve/Instantaneous Wave-Free Ratio Discordance. Circ Cardiovasc Interventions. 2019;12(5). https://doi.org/10.1161/CIRCINTERVENTIONS.118. 007494.

54. Hun Lee S, Hong Choi K, Myung Lee J, et al. Physiologic characteristics and clinical outcomes of patients with discordance between FFR and iFR. JACC Cardiovasc Interv 2019;12(20):2018–31.

Nonhyperemic Pressure Ratios—All the Same or Nuanced Differences?

Samineh Sehatbakhsh, MD[a], Weijia Li, MD[b], Tatsunori Takahashi, MD[b],
Kayo Takahashi, MD[c], Manish A. Parikh, MD[d], Yuhei Kobayashi, MD[d],*

KEYWORDS

- Nonhyperemic pressure ratios • Fractional flow reserve • Coronary artery disease

KEY POINTS

- Variety of guide-wire based coronary physiologic assessment methodology available in the cardiac catheterization laboratory materials-methods.
- Resting indices, which do not require adenosine, are mainly used these days to streamline the workflow.
- All resting indices yield very similar diagnostic performance against fractional flow reserve.
- Among resting indices, only instantaneous wave-free ratio is supported by the clinical outcome trial.

BACKGROUND

Fractional flow reserve (FFR) has become the gold standard for invasively assessing the functional significance of coronary artery disease (CAD) to guide revascularization in patients with CAD and is endorsed by the guideline.[1] FFR is derived from the ratio between the mean distal coronary artery pressure (Pd) to the mean aortic pressure (Pa) under maximum hyperemia and is considered to be significant with a threshold of 0.80 or lesser.[2] Several landmark trials supporting the role of FFR in the cardiac catheterization laboratory such as DEFER (Deferral of Percutaneous Coronary Intervention),[3] FAME (Fractional Flow Reserve vs Angiography for Multivessel Evaluation),[4] and FAME 2.[5]

However, FFR uptake in daily clinical practice is limited by a variety of factors such as need for a specialized guidewire and software, invasive instrumentation of the coronary artery, and vasodilator medications for hyperemia, which is typically adenosine. Furthermore, the use of adenosine can cause discomfort to our patients and can be costly/time consuming. Therefore, utilization of FFR remains relatively low and heterogeneous between different hospitals and health-care settings.

In this context, instantaneous wave-free ratio (iFR) was developed to avoid the use of adenosine and to assess the functional significance of obstructive CAD during resting status.[6] iFR is based on the hypothesis that during a part of resting period called "wave-free period," coronary microvascular resistance is minimal and thereby mimics hyperemic status. However, iFR requires a specific guidewire by Volcano Inc and its software is proprietary, which leads to the development of multiple similar nonhyperemic indices

This article originally appeared in *Interventional Cardiology Clinics*, Volume 12 Issue 1, January 2023.
Funding sources: None.
Ethical Approval: N/A.

[a] Division of Cardiology, Montefiore Medical Center, Albert Einstein College of Medicine, 111 210th Street, Bronx, NY 10467, USA; [b] Department of Medicine, Jacobi Medical Center, Albert Einstein College of Medicine, 1400 Pelham Parkway South, The Bronx, NY 10461, USA; [c] Department of Cardiology, Ehime University Graduate School of Medicine, Shitsukawa, Toon, Ehime 791-0295, Japan; [d] Division of Cardiology, New York-Presbyterian Brooklyn Methodist Hospital, Weill Cornell Medical College, 506 6th Street, Brooklyn, NY 11215, USA
* Corresponding author.
E-mail address: dxl9003@med.cornell.edu

cardiology.theclinics.com

from various vendors. These indices are called nonhyperemic pressure ratios (NHPRs).

DEVELOPMENT OF NEWER INDICES

Because adenosine can be expensive depending on the health-care settings and can cause side effects and discomfort to the patient, one of the options to induce hyperemia was to use radiographic contrast medium. Because contrast medium is readily available in the cardiac catheterization laboratory and known to cause some degree of hyperemia, the use of contrast-based FFR (cFFR) with a standard dose for coronary angiogram is tested prospectively in the multicenter registry fashion.[7] In this registry, the diagnostic accuracy of cFFR against FFR was 85.8% and that of iFR against FFR was 79.9%, demonstrating better diagnostic accuracy of cFFR than iFR against FFR. Importantly, cFFR does not require specific wire or software because this is purely based on the whole cardiac cycle. From this registry, diagnostic accuracy of cFFR, iFR, and Pd/Pa in the left main or proximal left anterior descending artery are reported to be lower compared with other lesion locations, likely related to the larger amount of myocardium supplied by these lesions and raised a concern for these indices.[8]

After iFR and cFFR were invented, 2 articles that are looking at the diagnostic accuracy of Pd/Pa against iFR were simultaneously published.[9,10] Kobayashi and colleagues reported resting Pd/Pa and iFR were highly correlated ($R^2 = 0.93$; $P < .001$). According to the receiver-operating characteristic curve analysis, Pd/Pa showed excellent agreement against iFR (area under the curve: 0.98; $P < .001$) with a best cutoff value of Pd/Pa 0.91 or lesser.[9] Lee and colleagues reported very similar results that resting Pd/Pa and iFR were highly correlated ($R = 0.97$; $P < .001$).[10] These 2 articles suggested even resting Pd/Pa based on the whole cardiac cycle can be interchangeably used instead of iFR, which is based on a specific diastolic cardiac cycle. Further supporting evidence is that Pd/Pa and iFR had similar diagnostic ability in defining intravascular imaging-defined stenosis severity and in diagnosing ^{13}N-ammonia positron emission tomography defined coronary flow reserve or relative flow reserve.[10,11]

Subsequently, van't Veer and colleagues reported the correlation of multiple diastolic indices and iFR. They looked at diastolic pressure ratio (dPR), which is a Pd/Pa ratio during whole diastole and also looked at 25% to 75% of diastole (dPR$_{25-75}$), and midpoint of diastole (dPR$_{mid}$), along with Matlab calculated iFR (iFR$_{matlab}$) and iFR-like indices by shortening the length of the wave free

period by 50 and 100 ms (iFR$_{-50ms}$ and iFR$_{-100ms}$), respectively. Their results showed correlations for all indices with the original iFR were greater than 0.99 ($P < .001$ for all; **Fig. 1**). Area under the curve values for predicting iFR were greater than 0.99 for all indexes as well.[12]

The above-mentioned study led to the development of various newer resting indices from all vendors as shown in **Fig. 2** and **Table 1**. Resting full-cycle ratio (RFR) is based on the lowest filtered Pd/Pa irrespective of a cardiac cycle and was tested in the VALIDATE-RFR study. RFR showed an excellent correlation with iFR ($R^2 = 0.99$; $P < .001$) with a diagnostic accuracy of 97.4% against iFR. Notably, the RFR was detected outside the diastole in 12.2% and especially in 32.4% of the right coronary artery lesions.[13] Another one not discussed yet is diastolic hyperemia-free ratio (DFR), which is based on Pd/Pa during the period between Pa less than

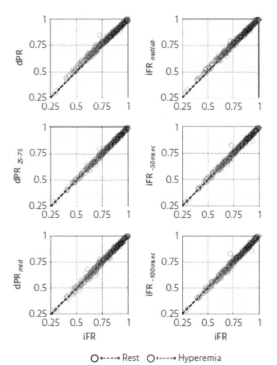

Fig. 1. Correlations between slightly different diastolic indices. When varying lengths of diastolic indices are compared with iFR that uses wave-free period, all correlations showed greater than 0.99, suggesting linear relationship. Above was repeated during hyperemia and results were similar. Blue and red circles represent rest and hyperemia, respectively. (Marcel van't Veer et al. Comparison of Different Diastolic Resting Indices to iFR: Are They All Equal?, Journal of the American College of Cardiology, 70 (25), 2017, 3088-3096. https://doi.org/10.1016/j.jacc.2017.10.066.)

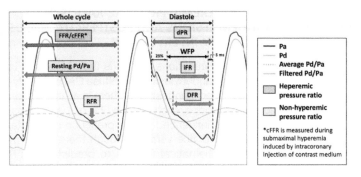

Fig. 2. NHPRs based on the cardiac cycle. Major hyperemic and nonhyperemic indices are shown in this figure to help understand the differences in their concept. FFR is essentially a whole cycle Pd/Pa ratio during maximal hyperemia with adenosine, whereas cFFR is a whole cycle Pd/Pa ratio during submaximal hyperemia with contrast medium. RFR is measured as an instantaneous maximal difference of Pd and Pa irrespective of systole or diastole. dPR, iFR, and DFR are based on solely a difference of Pd and Pa during diastole but different duration. cFFR, contrast fractional flow reserve; FFR, fractional flow reserve; Pd/Pa, distal coronary pressure to aortic pressure ratio.

mean Pa and down-sloping Pa. Again DFR showed an excellent correlation with iFR ($R^2 = 0.99$; $P < .001$) and high diagnostic performance with an area-under the curve of 0.99 against iFR.[14] Although all vendors named their resting index slightly differently (dPR, iFR, DFR, RFR), the key point to remember is that all indices will be highly correlated with each other and all share the same cutoff value of 0.89 or lesser as functionally significant.

The advantage of NHPRs is elimination of hyperemic medications, with the potential for reduction in time, side effects, and cost, which led to the significant increase in the adoption of coronary physiology in the cardiac catheterization laboratory. Specific to iFR, its software from the vendor allows for an overlay of the iFR values onto the angiogram during pullback, thereby facilitating physiological-angiographic fusion. Furthermore, this feature can be used to predict the physiology after percutaneous coronary intervention (PCI).[15] Drawbacks to some of these NHPRs include smaller gradients than FFR, thereby making them more sensitive to noise, hydrostatic effects,[16] and wire drift during pullback. Moreover, they could be more sensitive to variation of hemodynamic conditions (systemic blood pressure and heart rate) that affect baseline coronary flow,[17]

Table 1
Comparisons of wire-based coronary physiologic indices

Index	Vendor Specific	Definition	Hyperemia Required	Cutoff	RCT Available
FFR	Generic	Mean Pd/Pa during the whole cardiac cycle	Yes	≤0.80	Yes
cFFR	Generic	Lowest mean Pd/Pa after injection of contrast medium	Yes[a]	≤0.83	No
Resting Pd/Pa	Generic	Mean Pd/Pa over the whole cardiac cycle	No	≤0.91	No
iFR	Philips	Mean Pd/Pa during the wave-free period	No	≤0.89	Yes
DFR	Boston Scientific	Mean Pd/Pa when Pa < mean Pa and downsloping Pa	No	≤0.89	No
dPR	ACIST	Pd/Pa at the peak-to-peak midpoint	No	≤0.89	No
	OpSens	Mean Pd/Pa during the entire diastole	No	≤0.89	No
RFR	Abbott	Lowest filtered Pd/Pa during the whole cardiac cycle	No	≤0.89	No

Commonly available wire-based coronary physiologic indices are summarized in this table. Of note, only FFR and iFR are tested in the RCT settings, whereas other indices are tested in the observational studies.
Abbreviations: cFFR, contrast fractional flow reserve; dPR, diastolic pressure ratio; FFR, fractional flow reserve; Pd/Pa, distal coronary pressure to aortic pressure ratio; RCT, randomized clinical trial; RFR, resting full-cycle ratio.
[a] cFFR requires hyperemia with contrast medium, which is submaximal hyperemic compared with FFR with adenosine.

whereas induced maximal vasodilation saturates the intrinsic coronary autoregulation making FFR less exposed to hemodynamic status fluctuations.

RESTING INDICES AND OUTCOME

As discussed above, multiple studies have investigated the correlation between resting indices and iFR because iFR is the only resting index that has been tested in the randomized controlled trials. Based on the results of the 2 randomized controlled trials (DEFINE-FLAIR and iFR-SWEDEHEART) iFR is noninferior to FFR when used to guide PCI in terms of death, MI and unplanned revascularization in patients with relatively simple CAD.[18,19] No other indices such as Pd/Pa, RFR, dPR, and DFR were tested in the large randomized controlled trial setting but in the registry setting. However, practically speaking, it is impossible to detect a meaningful difference between iFR and other indices, given excellent correlations and diagnostic performances; and clinical outcomes will be very similar irrespective of which indices were used.

For example, Lee and colleagues reported that both resting Pd/Pa and iFR were significantly associated with the risk of 2-year adverse cardiovascular events in deferred patients (resting Pd/Pa hazard ratio per 0.10 increase: 0.48 [95% confidence interval: 0.25–0.92, P = .027]; iFR hazard ratio per 0.10 increase: 0.59 [0.37–0.92]; P = .020).[10]

Prognostic implications and clinical outcome of NHPRs including iFR, RFR, and dPR have been evaluated in a post hoc analysis of 3V FFR-FRIENDS study and the ^{13}N-ammonia PET registry. The association between NHPRs and the risk of 5-year vessel-oriented composite outcomes (Composite of cardiac death, vessel-related myocardial infarction, and ischemia-driven revascularization) were analyzed among 864 deferred vessels. Lesions with positive NHPRs (iFR, RFR, and dPR 0.89 or lesser) or FFR (0.80 or lesser) showed significantly higher risk of vessel-related myocardial infarction at 5 years than those with negative NHPRs or FFR, respectively. The cumulative incidence of vessel-oriented outcome among the groups with deferred concordant negative (NHPRs−/FFR−), deferred discordant (NHPRs+/FFR− or NHPRs−/FFR+), and revascularized vessels were 7.5%, 14.4%, and 14.8% (log-rank P < .001), respectively. The deferred discordant group showed similar risk of vessel-oriented outcome compared with the revascularized vessel group (hazard ratio, 0.98; 95% CI 0.43–2.22, P = .96), suggesting discordant physiologic lesions may require intervention or further medical management.[20]

NON-HYPEREMIC PRESSURE RATIOS IN TANDEM LESIONS AND POSTPERCUTANEOUS CORONARY INTERVENTION

One of the limitations of FFR is the complexity in assessing tandem lesions or diffuse CAD. Fluid dynamics theory suggests that there is an interaction between lesions, such that the FFR of the proximal stenosis is influenced by the presence of a distal stenosis and vice versa. Although there is a proposed mathematical formula to predict the FFR of each individual stenosis,[21] the interaction between lesions is complex and not easily calculated during routine PCI, impeding the assessment of the FFR value for each individual lesion. In the iFR gradient registry study by Kikuta and colleagues, the investigators postulated that because iFR uses a resting gradient, where coronary blood flow is more stable across most coronary stenoses (with the exception of a critical stenosis), it is possible to create a physiologic map of lesion severity along the length of the vessel and predict the change in iFR, after correction, for that specific stenosis.[15] In that study, iFR post-PCI (predicted) compared with the observed iFR value had a mean difference of 0.01 ± 0.004 and a 1.4% ± 0.5% error, clearly demonstrating that iFR is potentially useful in the assessment of tandem lesions with minimal interaction between individual coronary stenoses.

Despite advances in PCI technologies, 1 in 5 patients still has recurrent angina within the first year after successful PCI.[22] Multiple studies including meta-analysis have investigated the potential of post-PCI FFR measurements on improved clinical outcomes.[23–26] All studies noted that lower post-PCI FFR values have been associated with an increased risk of myocardial infarction (MI), revascularization, and death, illustrating the utility of post-PCI FFR in detecting clinical consequences of residual ischemia. However, FFR has been mostly used to guide clinical decision-making regarding the utility of performing PCI. When used to direct revascularization, FFR has been shown to improve clinical outcomes, including a reduction in the combined endpoint of MI, repeat revascularization, and potentially death. Despite increasing evidence for the utility of FFR in the post-PCI setting, clinical adoption remains limited.

One of the reasons post-PCI physiologic assessment utilization is limited is the cumbersome nature of its assessment. In this regard, NHPRs has an advantage in time and cost effectiveness compared with FFR by eliminating the need for hyperemia. DEFINE-PCI (Physiologic Assessment of Coronary Stenosis Following PCI) is the first study to use iFR to assess physiologic changes post-PCI.[27] This multicenter, prospective, single-arm, blinded study sought to evaluate the incidence and mechanisms of residual ischemia after angiographically successful PCI by using iFR. After PCI was performed, iFR and iFR pullback post-PCI was performed. Of the 500 patients enrolled in the study, 24% had an abnormal postprocedure iFR of 0.89 or lesser and demonstrated that angiographic diameter stenosis had poor correlation with post-PCI iFR. Moreover, the use of iFR instead of hyperemic physiology omits the use of a vasodilator, allowing the physician to perform multiple physiology assessments in less time and improving patient experience as discussed before.

FUTURE DIRECTIONS

The International Study of Comparative Health Effectiveness with Medical and Invasive Approaches (ISCHEMIA) trial has reemphasized the value of optimal medical treatment in patients with stable ischemic heart disease. However, the use of physiology-guided revascularization in the ISCHEMIA trial was relatively low (20.3% of initial invasive strategy arm and 9.3% of the total trial population).[28,29] Because part of the relative superiority of optimal medical treatment resulted from higher periprocedural myocardial infarction rates in the revascularization arm, better planning and guidance of PCI with physiologic assessment might have resulted in lower rates of that endpoint. This hypothesis is supported by the marked reduction in periprocedural myocardial infarction noted in SYNTAX II, physiology-based and imaging-guided revascularization trial, compared with the original SYNTAX study in which revascularization was mostly performed by angiographic planning.[30]

Furthermore, it should be noted that no previous study, including the ISCHEMIA trial, evaluated comparative prognosis between functionally optimized revascularization/functionally complete revascularization and optimal medical treatment.[31,32] As discussed previously, angiographically successful PCI does not necessarily result in functionally optimized PCI, which was consistently shown to have significantly better prognosis than functionally suboptimal PCI. Whether "ischemia-resolving PCI" would enhance patient prognosis still needs further clarification through future trials.

There are a few studies currently evaluating clinical relevance of physiology-based preprocedural planning. DEFINE-GPS study will compare target vessel failure at 2 years between iFR-guided PCI (iFR pullback and iFR-angiography coregistration system) versus angiography-guided PCI (NCT04451044). PICIO (Pullback with Resting Full-Cycle Flow ratio or Fractional Flow Reserve for the Prediction of Post-PCI Hemodynamic Outcomes) study will compare the capacity of preprocedural resting full-cycle ratio gradients versus FFR gradients to predict the hemodynamic outcomes after PCI (NCT04417634).

Furthermore, new "wireless" technology, which completely eliminated guide wire-based coronary physiologic assessment, is being invented such as coronary angiography-based FFR, intravascular ultrasound-based FFR, and optical coherence tomography-based FFR.[33] These new technologies estimate FFR based on invasive imaging and streamline the flow of coronary physiologic assessment in the cardiac catheterization laboratory. A recent meta-analysis confirmed these new technologies have an excellent diagnostic performance against invasive wire-based FFR irrespective of technologies, supporting its wider adoption in the future.[34]

SUMMARY

The very high correlation between iFR and other NHPRs implies that any pressure-derived nonhyperemic physiologic indices can be interchangeably used in the cardiac catheterization laboratory under the same clinical indications. At the same time, iFR is supported by 2 large-scale randomized controlled trials, and its software allows operators to plan their PCI procedures in a more sophisticated way. Although treatment decision-making to revascularize or defer can be made based on one physiologic index, simultaneous measurement of both NHPRs and FFR would provide better risk stratification when revascularization is deferred.

It is important to consider that the purpose of revascularization is not just to alleviate angiographic stenosis but to resolve myocardial ischemia and to potentially improve prognosis. Post-PCI physiologic assessment provides information about the functional results of revascularization and prognosis after PCI. In suboptimal post-PCI physiologic results, further investigations with FFR or NHPRs and interventions aimed to find potential reasons can improve the patient prognosis. Especially in this repeated setting, NHPRs may have an edge due to the reduced procedural time and cost. Whether procedural planning guided by pre-PCI pullback analysis or further intervention guided by post-PCI physiologic assessment will lead to improved clinical outcomes awaits the results of randomized clinical trials.

CLINICS CARE POINTS

- In the cardiac catheterization laboratory, we can use any resting physiologic indices interchangeably.
- Instantaneous wave-free ratio has a capability of coregistration with an angiogram and a virtual stenting.

ACKNOWLEDGMENTS

None.

DISCLOSURE

M.A. Parikh serves on the advisory boards of Abbott Vascular, Boston Scientific, and Medtronic. Y. Kobayashi serves as a consultant for Abbott Vascular. Others have no conflict of interest to disclose.

REFERENCES

1. Neumann F-J, Sousa-Uva M, Ahlsson A, et al. 2018 ESC/EACTS Guidelines on myocardial revascularization. EuroIntervention 2019;14:1435–534.
2. Pijls NHJ, de Bruyne B, Peels K, et al. Measurement of Fractional Flow Reserve to Assess the Functional Severity of Coronary-Artery Stenoses. N Engl J Med 1996;334:1703–8.
3. Pijls NHJ, van Schaardenburgh P, Manoharan G, et al. Percutaneous coronary intervention of functionally nonsignificant stenosis: 5-year follow-up of the DEFER Study. J Am Coll Cardiol 2007;49:2105–11.
4. Tonino PAL, De Bruyne B, Pijls NHJ, et al. Fractional flow reserve versus angiography for guiding percutaneous coronary intervention. N Engl J Med 2009;360:213–24.
5. De Bruyne B, Pijls NHJ, Kalesan B, et al. Fractional flow reserve-guided PCI versus medical therapy in stable coronary disease. N Engl J Med 2012;367:991–1001.
6. Sen S, Escaned J, Malik IS, et al. Development and validation of a new adenosine-independent index of stenosis severity from coronary wave-intensity analysis: results of the ADVISE (ADenosine Vasodilator Independent Stenosis Evaluation) study. J Am Coll Cardiol 2012;59:1392–402.
7. Johnson NP, Jeremias A, Zimmermann FM, et al. Continuum of Vasodilator Stress From Rest to Contrast Medium to Adenosine Hyperemia for Fractional Flow Reserve Assessment. JACC Cardiovasc Interv 2016;9:757–67.
8. Kobayashi Y, Johnson NP, Berry C, et al. The Influence of Lesion Location on the Diagnostic Accuracy of Adenosine-Free Coronary Pressure Wire Measurements. JACC Cardiovasc Interv 2016;9:2390–9.
9. Kobayashi Y, Johnson NP, Zimmermann FM, et al. Agreement of the Resting Distal to Aortic Coronary Pressure With the Instantaneous Wave-Free Ratio. J Am Coll Cardiol 2017;70:2105–13.
10. Lee JM, Park J, Hwang D, et al. Similarity and Difference of Resting Distal to Aortic Coronary Pressure and Instantaneous Wave-Free Ratio. J Am Coll Cardiol 2017;70:2114–23.
11. Hwang D, Jeon K-H, Lee JM, et al. Diagnostic Performance of Resting and Hyperemic Invasive Physiological Indices to Define Myocardial Ischemia: Validation With N-Ammonia Positron Emission Tomography. JACC Cardiovasc Interv 2017;10:751–60.
12. Van't Veer M, Pijls NHJ, Hennigan B, et al. Comparison of Different Diastolic Resting Indexes to iFR: Are They All Equal? J Am Coll Cardiol 2017;70:3088–96.
13. Svanerud J, Ahn J-M, Jeremias A, et al. Validation of a novel non-hyperaemic index of coronary artery stenosis severity: the Resting Full-cycle Ratio (VALIDATE RFR) study. EuroIntervention 2018;14:806–14.
14. Johnson NP, Li W, Chen X, et al. Diastolic pressure ratio: new approach and validation vs. the instantaneous wave-free ratio. Eur Heart J 2019;40:2585–94.
15. Kikuta Y, Cook CM, Sharp ASP, et al. Pre-Angioplasty Instantaneous Wave-Free Ratio Pullback Predicts Hemodynamic Outcome In Humans With Coronary Artery Disease: Primary Results of the International Multicenter iFR GRADIENT Registry. JACC Cardiovasc Interv 2018;11:757–67.
16. Johnson NP, Kirkeeide RL, Lance Gould K. Hydrostatic Forces. JACC: Cardiovasc Interventions 2017;10:1596–7.
17. de Waard GA, Di Mario C, Lerman A, et al. Instantaneous wave-free ratio to guide coronary revascularisation: physiological framework, validation and differences from fractional flow reserve. EuroIntervention 2017;13:450–8.
18. Davies JE, Sen S, Dehbi H-M, et al. Use of the Instantaneous Wave-free Ratio or Fractional Flow Reserve in PCI. N Engl J Med 2017;376:1824–34.
19. Götberg M, Christiansen EH, Gudmundsdottir IJ, et al. Instantaneous Wave-free Ratio versus Fractional Flow Reserve to Guide PCI. N Engl J Med 2017;376:1813–23.
20. Lee JM, Lee SH, Hwang D, et al. Long-Term Clinical Outcomes of Nonhyperemic Pressure Ratios: Resting Full-Cycle Ratio, Diastolic Pressure Ratio, and Instantaneous Wave-Free Ratio. J Am Heart Assoc 2020;9. https://doi.org/10.1161/jaha.120.016818.
21. De Bruyne B, Pijls NH, Heyndrickx GR, et al. Pressure-derived fractional flow reserve to assess serial

epicardial stenoses: theoretical basis and animal validation. Circulation 2000;101:1840–7.

22. Stone GW, Ellis SG, Gori T, et al. Blinded outcomes and angina assessment of coronary bioresorbable scaffolds: 30-day and 1-year results from the ABSORB IV randomised trial. Lancet 2018;392: 1530–40.

23. Li S-J, Ge Z, Kan J, et al. Cutoff Value and Long-Term Prediction of Clinical Events by FFR Measured Immediately After Implantation of a Drug-Eluting Stent in Patients With Coronary Artery Disease: 1- to 3-Year Results From the DKCRUSH VII Registry Study. JACC Cardiovasc Interv 2017;10:986–95.

24. Piroth Z, Toth GG, Tonino PAL, et al. Prognostic Value of Fractional Flow Reserve Measured Immediately After Drug-Eluting Stent Implantation. Circ Cardiovasc Interv 2017;10. https://doi.org/10.1161/CIRCINTERVENTIONS.116.005233.

25. Rimac G, Fearon WF, De Bruyne B, et al. Clinical value of post-percutaneous coronary intervention fractional flow reserve value: A systematic review and meta-analysis. Am Heart J 2017;183:1–9.

26. Agarwal SK, Kasula S, Hacioglu Y, et al. Utilizing Post-Intervention Fractional Flow Reserve to Optimize Acute Results and the Relationship to Long-Term Outcomes. JACC Cardiovasc Interv 2016;9: 1022–31.

27. Jeremias A, Davies JE, Maehara A, et al. Blinded Physiological Assessment of Residual Ischemia After Successful Angiographic Percutaneous Coronary Intervention: The DEFINE PCI Study. JACC Cardiovasc Interv 2019;12:1991–2001.

28. Maron DJ, Hochman JS, Reynolds HR, et al. Initial Invasive or Conservative Strategy for Stable Coronary Disease. N Engl J Med 2020;382:1395–407.

29. Spertus JA, Jones PG, Maron DJ, et al. Health-Status Outcomes with Invasive or Conservative Care in Coronary Disease. N Engl J Med 2020;382: 1408–19.

30. Escaned J, Collet C, Ryan N, et al. Clinical outcomes of state-of-the-art percutaneous coronary revascularization in patients with de novo three vessel disease: 1-year results of the SYNTAX II study. Eur Heart J 2017;38:3124–34.

31. Kobayashi Y, Nam C-W, Tonino PAL, et al. The Prognostic Value of Residual Coronary Stenoses After Functionally Complete Revascularization. J Am Coll Cardiol 2016;67:1701–11.

32. Kobayashi Y, Lønborg J, Jong A, et al. Prognostic Value of the Residual SYNTAX Score After Functionally Complete Revascularization in. ACS J Am Coll Cardiol 2018;72:1321–9.

33. Takahashi T, Theodoropoulos K, Latib A, et al. Coronary physiologic assessment based on angiography and intracoronary imaging. J Cardiol 2022;79:71–8.

34. Takahashi T, Shin D, Kuno T, et al. Diagnostic performance of fractional flow reserve derived from coronary angiography, intravascular ultrasound, and optical coherence tomography; a meta-analysis. J Cardiol 2022. https://doi.org/10.1016/j.jjcc.2022.02.015.

Is Coronary Physiology Assessment Valid in Special Circumstances?
Aortic Stenosis, Atrial Fibrillation, Left Ventricular Hypertrophy, and Other

David M. Tehrani, MD MS[a],*, Arnold H. Seto, MD, MPA, FSCAI, FACC[b]

KEYWORDS

- Fractional flow reserve • Nonhyperemic pressure ratios • Atrial fibrillation • Aortic stenosis
- Left ventricular hypertrophy • Serial lesions

KEY POINTS

- Although fractional flow reserve (FFR) and nonhyperemic pressure ratios (NHPRs) such as instantaneous wave-free ratio (iFR) are widely used to evaluate the hemodynamic significance of coronary lesions, both have important limitations in a variety of clinical scenarios that operators should be cognizant of.
- Aortic stenosis leads to increased left ventricular systolic and diastolic filling pressures, which seems to affect NHPR to a greater degree than FFR.
- Atrial fibrillation can have significant variability in beat-to-beat cardiac output, which leads to a significant reduction in reproducibility of iFR, although FFR evaluation remains largely reproducible and reliable.
- FFR has limitations for evaluating the hemodynamic significance of individual lesions in series, whereas NHPRs may be a more clinically relevant alternative for procedural planning.

INTRODUCTION

Fractional flow reserve (FFR) is defined as the ratio of the measured pressure distal of coronary stenosis (Pd) in relation to the pressure proximal to the stenosis (Pa). Although a direct comparison of flow in the presence and absence of a lesion would be ideal, pressure measurements are correlated with blood flow when coronary resistance is minimal and provide a useful surrogate. Although hyperemic agents are excellent tools to achieve minimal resistance, there are clinical scenarios in which they can be unreliable.

As the more recent introduction of nonhyperemic pressure ratios (NHPRs) such as relative flow reserve (RFR) and instantaneous wave-free ratio (iFR), there has been debate over the benefits or shortcomings of these techniques compared to FFR. FFR has greater than 20 years of data in well-conduced randomized trials showing clinical benefit for greater than 10 years,[1] something that NHPR overall lack. Nonetheless, NHPR indices have the benefit of simpler protocols, quicker evaluations, and the ability to exclude hyperemic medications that have potential side effects on patients. NHPRs are now integrated within most

This article originally appeared in *Interventional Cardiology Clinics*, Volume 12 Issue 1, January 2023.
[a] Ronald Reagan UCLA Medical Center, 650 Charles East Young Drive South, CHS A2-237, Los Angeles, CA 90095-1679, USA; [b] Long Beach Veterans Administration Medical Center, 5901 East 7th Street, 111C, Long Beach, CA 90822, USA
* Corresponding author.
E-mail address: Dtehrani@mednet.ucla.edu
Twitter: @DavidTehrani3 (D.M.T.); @arnoldseto (A.H.S.)

Cardiol Clin 42 (2024) 21–29
https://doi.org/10.1016/j.ccl.2023.07.010

cardiology.theclinics.com

current pressure wire systems and are widely available in cath laboratories. When deciding to use one index over another, not only procedural and patient-level risk versus benefits have to be weighed, but also reliability and accuracy. We discuss clinical scenarios outside of isolated stable coronary artery disease (CAD) where FFR and NHPR have been evaluated, to help clinicians understand the limitations and benefits of different coronary physiology assessment tools.

Aortic Stenosis

CAD is a common comorbidity in many patients with severe calcific stenosis. The prevalence of CAD is high not only in those with high- and intermediate-risk patients undergoing transcatheter aortic valve replacement (TAVR) at approximately 66%,[2,3] but also in those considered low-risk at nearly 30%.[4] Thus, oftentimes the assessment of significant CAD can play a role not only in the decision between surgical aortic valve replacement (SAVR) with coronary versus TAVR with PCI, but also the decisions regarding whether to proceed with PCI before TAVR. However, PCI before TAVR has not been associated with lower in-hospital or 1 year mortality.[5] These findings suggest that there is some ambiguity regarding identifying lesions that are hemodynamically significant before aortic valve intervention.

Evaluation of coronary physiology remains a commonly used tool when assessing the need for revascularization before either SAVR or TAVR. The hemodynamics associated with aortic stenosis (AS) is increased left ventricular systolic and diastolic filling pressures with impaired diastolic dysfunction. Similar to those with heart failure (HF), patients with severe AS will have increased left ventricular end-diastolic pressures (LVEDPs) and elevated venous pressures, with effects on coronary pressure and flow. Increased systolic myocardial compressive forces associated with severe AS may also affect physiological indices.

When evaluating FFR pre-TAVR versus post-TAVR in those with CAD, an initial observational study suggested that there were changes in FFR values although minimal and most notably in those with hemodynamically significant stenoses to start, which subsequently worsened after TAVR (0.71 ± 0.11 vs. 0.66 ± 0.14).[6] The postulated reason was that reduction of aortic outflow gradient post-TAVR leads to increased coronary flow, which may decrease post-TAVR FFR values. Overall, there was no difference in average FFR values pre-TAVR and post-TAVR and importantly only a small proportion (6%) crossed the 0.80 threshold. The effects of TAVR on iFR seem to

be more dramatic than on FFR. Scarsini and colleagues[7] showed that individual-level differences in pre-iFR versus post-iFR varied significantly, and that the increased variation in iFR values correlated well with the degree of post-TAVR gradient drop. Further, 15% of coronary lesions crossed the 0.89 threshold.

One of the first studies evaluating coronary physiology showed that patients with severe AS and post-TAVR had improvement in coronary flow reserve (CFR) at 12 month follow-up (**Fig. 1**).[8] In addition, immediate reductions in afterload post-TAVR may improve microvascular function.[9] Comparing patients without CAD, Wiegerinck and colleagues found that CFR was lower (1.9 ± 0.5 vs. 2.7 ± 0.7, $P < 0.001$) and hyperemic microvascular resistance was higher (2.10 ± 0.69 vs. 1.80 ± 0.60 mm Hg·cm·s^{-1}, $P = 0.096$) in the presence of AS. Among the 27 patients with AS, immediate post-TAVR hyperemic microvascular resistance decreased resulting in an increased CFR (1.9 ± 0.4 to 2.2 ± 0.6, P = 0.009) compared with pre-TAVR. This improved CFR, in turn, may explain why post-TAVR FFR values generally decrease in patients with CAD. The direction of change in NHPR in patients with TAVR is not completely clear, although a likely increase in basal flow would affect the values.

Most recently, a substudy of the randomized Nordic Aortic Valve Intervention trial revisited the effects of TAVR in intermediate coronary lesions pre-TAVR and post-TAVR at 6 months.[10] After ensuring no significant change in percent stenosis from baseline to 6 months in 50 lesions, they found that FFR did not significantly change from baseline to follow-up, while RFR (evaluated in 36 lesions) did significantly improve baseline to follow-up (0.88 vs. 0.92, $P = 0.003$). There were 8% (4) lesions that became positive after TAVR, whereas there were 31% (11) lesions that were initially RFR positive that became RFR negative after TAVR.

These findings suggest that FFR and NHPRs should be used with caution by making definitive decisions for revascularization before aortic valve interventions with AS. Fortunately, the risk of a particular lesion crossing the ischemic threshold is small, especially when using FFR. Also reassuring is that FFR guidance, as compared with angiographic guidance, was associated with fewer MACE events despite whatever changes occur around TAVR.[11] This was in the setting of a high deferral rate in most of the lesions (78.2%) in view of a preserved FFR greater than 0.80. Overall, these findings suggest that even if there is a small change in FFR after TAVR, it may only rarely be clinically relevant.

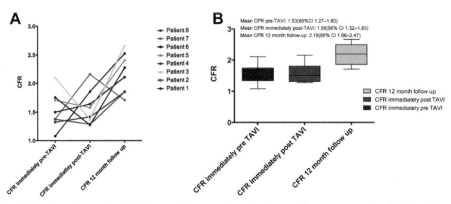

Fig. 1. (*A*) Individual patient serial CFR data with all patients having an improvement in CFR from baseline to 12 month assessment after transaortic valve implantation. (*B*) Serial mean CFR recordings (with 95% CI and ranges). The improvement in CFR from baseline to follow-up was statistically significant using a repeated-measures analysis of variance ($p = 0.0055$). (*From* Camuglia AC, Syed J, Garg P, et al. Invasively assessed coronary flow dynamics improve following relief of aortic stenosis with transcatheter aortic valve implantation. *J Am Coll Cardiol.* 2014;63(17):1808-1809. https://doi.org/10.1016/j.jacc.2013.11.040.)

Atrial Fibrillation

Atrial fibrillation (AF) is one of the most common arrhythmias seen concomitantly in those with CAD. Despite the use of FFR and NHPRs in these patients, there is a paucity of evidence regarding their reliability in AF given the variability in beat-to-beat cardiac output. Not surprisingly, this is of particular importance when patients with AF have rapid ventricular rates (RVRs), as myocardial oxygen demand increases inducing a pseudo-hyperemic state that could adversely affect baseline Pd/Pa documentation and iFR measurements.[12] However, even in non-RVR states, patients with AF have microvascular dysfunction that could affect the assessment of these baseline indices.[13] As shown in the verification of iFR and FFR for the Assessment of Coronary Artery Stenosis Severity in Everyday Practice study, NHPRs such as iFR are particularly susceptible to resting (nonhyperemic) heart rate and blood pressure variations with 2.5 to 4.4 times larger variance than FFR differences.[14]

Recently, Bentea and colleagues[15] conducted a small retrospective study comparing patients with AF undergoing FFR and iFR to those in sinus rhythm (SR) without a history of AF. The coefficient of variation was calculated for iFR based on dividing the area under the Pd curve by the area under the corresponding Pa curve for the number of beats considered in the analysis. FFR values were analyzed based on calculating seven beats centered around the minimum Pd/Pa during hyperemia. The coefficient of variation of beat-to-beat measurements for FFR was not significantly different between those in AF versus SR; however, there was significant beat-to-beat variability in iFR measurements in the AF versus SR groups (2.65

95% confidence interval [CI]: 1.33–4.04 vs. 0.69 95% CI: 0.24–1.98, <0.01) (**Fig. 2**). The coefficient of variation of iFR correlated positively with the variability of heart rate. Furthermore, when evaluating the reproducibility of FFR and iFR at test–retest in AF and SR, FFR was reproducible in both groups, whereas iFR was only reproducible in the SR group. Two replicated iFR measures did not correlate in the AF group ($p = 0.1352$, $p > 0.05$; Spearman correlation) and led to the reclassification of 53.8% of patients using an iFR cut-off of 0.89. When analyzed per each vessel, the quantitate assessment of coronary stenosis correlated with the corresponding FFR values in both AF and SR rhythm groups (see **Fig. 2**). The degree of stenosis also correlated with the corresponding iFR measurement in the AF and SR groups, but there was a significant difference in the slopes of these two regression lines with the SR group showing a more pronounced decrease of iFR values with increasing stenosis severity as compared with the AF group.

Ultimately, it seems that FFR evaluation remains reproducible and reliable in patients with AF, whereas the reproducibility of iFR in patients with AF is far less. These findings are likely related to the fact that coronary blood flow occurs primarily in diastole and drops significantly during systole.[16] Although the duration of systole remains nearly constant regardless of heart rate, the duration of diastole is highly dependent on heart rate, thus affecting NHPRs disproportionately compared with FFR.

Left main coronary artery disease and serial coronary lesions

Left main coronary artery (LMCA) disease is often seen in those undergoing coronary angiography.

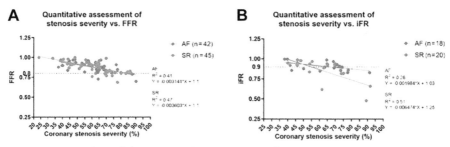

Fig. 2. Linear regression analysis of the quantitative assessment of coronary stenosis severity versus FFR (*A*) and versus iFR (*B*). For iFR, the slopes of the regressions are significantly different between AF and SR groups ($p < 0.05$), but not for FFR ($p = 0.58$). (*From* Pintea Bentea G, Berdaoui B, Samyn S, Morissens M, Rodriguez JC. Reliability of Fractional Flow Reserve and Instantaneous Wave-Free Ratio in Assessing Intermediate Coronary Stenosis in Patients With Atrial Fibrillation. *Am J Cardiol.* 2022;162:105-110. https://doi.org/10.1016/j.amjcard.2021.09.028.)

Studies have demonstrated the usefulness and benefit of FFR to guide the revascularization of the intermediate left main (LM) disease.[17] Hamilos and colleagues showed that among those with intermediate LMCA disease, deferring CABG based on an FFR greater than 0.80 led to similar 5 year mortality as compared with those who underwent bypass grafting based on an FFR less than 0.80. Event-free survival rates at 5 years were 74.2% and 82.8% in the nonsurgical and surgical groups, respectively ($P = 0.50$). However, LMCA stenosis in isolation is rare, with the downstream disease being the norm.[18]

Given that downstream disease in a vessel such as the left anterior descending coronary artery (LAD) will affect the assessment of LM disease severity by FFR when the pressure-sensor wire is in the LAD,[19,20] it is recommended to place the pressure-sensor in an artery that is free of stenosis. However, given blood flow across the LM is dependent on the outflow of branch vessels (in this case both the LAD and left circumflex artery [LCx]), disease in either vessel could alter the FFR value even if the pressure sensor is in the nondiseased vessel. To further elucidate the possibility of this phenomenon, Yong and colleagues[21] created a sheep model for various scenarios of downstream epicardial disease with variable degrees of stenosis created in the LM. LM stenosis was evaluated by having a pressure wire in a nonstenosed vessel and then doing pre-FFR (true FFR) and post-FFR (apparent FFR) evaluations after producing stenosis in the other branch vessel. The results of the study showed that LMCA FFR measurement may be overestimated in the presence of downstream epicardial disease despite measuring FFR in a nondiseased epicardial vessel (true FFR) and apparent FFR correlated with composite FFR of the LM plus stenosed artery ($r = -0.31$; $P < 0.001$). This

difference in the true and apparent FFR was most pronounced with increasing branch vessel epicardial stenosis. Fearon and colleagues[22] further confirmed these findings in humans after creating a model in which an intermediate LMCA stenosis was artificially created by balloon inflation in patients undergoing PCI in the LAD, LCx, or both to evaluate true versus apparent FFR in 91 pairs of measurements in 25 patients. True FFR of the LMCA was found to be significantly lower than apparent FFR (0.81 ± 0.08 vs. 0.83 ± 0.08, $p < 0.001$). A case example of the effect of variable downstream disease creation in a branch vessel on LM FFR is shown in **Fig. 3**. Similarly, in the animal model, the difference correlated with the severity of the downstream disease ($r = 0.35$, $p < 0.001$). Importantly, this FFR difference was found to be small, and in all cases in which apparent FFR was greater than 0.85, FFR, the true FFR was greater than 0.80. Because of these differences in LM FFR values in the setting of downstream disease, NHPR has been suggested as an alternative. Although little data correlating FFR and NHPR indices exist for the LM, the ongoing iLITRO study will aim to evaluate the concordance of FFR and iFR in LMCA lesions, while also evaluating a composite major adverse cardiac events outcome at 30 days, 1 year, and 5 years.[23]

Beyond evaluating LM stenosis in those with additional epicardial CAD, FFR generally has limitations for evaluating individual lesions in series. To calculate an accurate FFR, maximal hyperemia must be achieved, which is not possible when the first stenosis limits maximal flow across a downstream lesion. A commonly used technique to circumvent this is to do a pressure pull back during continuous hyperemia if the summed FFR is less than 0.80, allowing for the evaluation of which lesion has the largest effect on the Pd/Pa value.

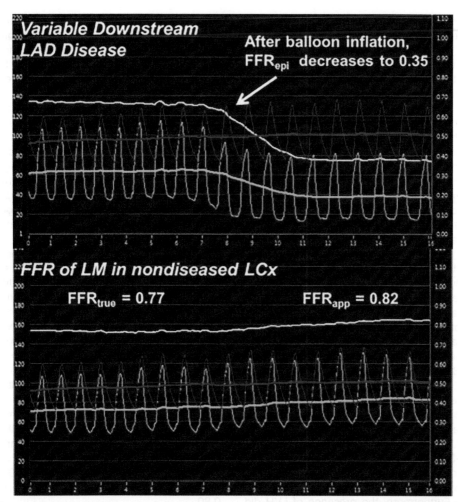

Fig. 3. Case example of LM FFR by use of simultaneous coronary pressure recordings during the creation of variable downstream stenosis using balloon inflation. (*Top panel*) The coronary pressure is recorded from the LAD pressure wire before and after balloon inflation within a newly placed LAD stent (the *green line* is distal coronary pressure, the *red line* is aortic pressure, and the *yellow line* is FFR value). (*Bottom panel*) The coronary pressure is recorded simultaneously from the LCx pressure wire (FFR$_{true}$ and FFR$_{app}$) before and after inflation of the balloon in the LAD, ultimately leading to complete occlusion (the *green line* is distal coronary pressure, the *red line* is aortic pressure, and the *yellow line* is the FFR value). (*From* Fearon WF, Yong AS, Lenders G, et al. The impact of downstream coronary stenosis on fractional flow reserve assessment of intermediate left main coronary artery disease: human validation. *JACC Cardiovasc Interv.* 2015;8(3):398-403. https://doi.org/10.1016/j.jcin.2014.09.027.)

Although not completely accurate, pullbacks are less complicated procedurally and mathematically than evaluating individual FFR for serial lesions with balloon occlusion.[19] IFR is noninferior in large clinical outcome trials,[24,25] and more recently has been of interest in evaluating the hemodynamic significance of individual lesions in series. Kikuta and colleagues[26] showed that iFR pullback was not only accurate in predicting physiological outcomes of PCI, but changed revascularization procedural planning in about one-third of the patients when compared with those making angiographic guidance-based decisions. Such a method has particular utility to differentiate the hemodynamic significance of a long lesion with the diffuse disease compared with a focal lesion that is amenable to PCI. The importance of defining the lesion of hemodynamic significance was brought to light in the DEFINE PCI study. In this multicenter, prospective, observational study, blinded iFR pullback was done in 562 vessels (500 patients) with angiographically successful PCI.[27] Residual ischemia (defined as iFR<0.90) was present in 24% of patients with a mean iFR in that population of 0.84 ± 0.06 (range 0.60–0.89). Importantly, among those patients with impaired post-PCI iFRs, 81.6% had untreated focal stenoses that were angiographically inapparent, suggesting they could be amenable to further optimization. Although these findings are interesting, it is unclear whether PCI optimization based on iFR translates to improved clinical outcomes. The currently enrolling, DEFINE GPS study will address whether iFR pullback guided PCI of lesions post-PCI will improve clinical outcomes.[28]

Left ventricular hypertrophy

The relationship between left ventricular hypertrophy (LVH) with FFR is complex. In general, there is an inverse relationship between the degree of territory, or in this case, myocardial mass, that a vessel with stenosis supplies and the FFR value. Essentially, similar stenosis would have a lower FFR value in the presence of a larger jeopardized myocardial mass. For example, an angiographically stenotic lesion in the proximal LAD will have a significantly lower FFR value compared with a similar one in the distal LAD, LCx, or right coronary artery (0.80 ± 0.09 vs. 0.84 ± 0.08 vs. 0.88 ± 0.09 vs. 0.91 ± 0.04, respectively; P < 0.0001).[29]

However, clinical studies investigating the impact of LVH on FFR have found no significant difference in values between those with and without LVH.[30] Further, in a substudy of the DANAMI-3 PRIMULTI, those with cardiac magnetic resonance defined LVH did not seem to interact with the correlation of diameter stenosis to FFR.[31] Furthermore, the presence of LVH did not seem to impact the clinical benefits of FFR-guided complete revascularization as compared with angiographic revascularization in this substudy. These clinical findings may be related to the fact that LVH is related to microvascular dysfunction and decreased coronary flow. With systole comes shortening and thickening accompanied by elevated cardiac muscle strain. This in addition to high intraventricular pressures is responsible for systolic flow impairment that can be seen in LVH.[16] Extravascular compression (in both systole and diastole) of the microvascular circulation in theory could elevate FFR.

The hemodynamic effects of elevated LVEDP and increased central venous pressure in the setting of diastolic dysfunction associated with LVH are also thought to complicate the reliability of FFR. Leonardi and colleagues[32] compared FFR preuse and postuse of nitroprusside (meant to reduce afterload) to evaluate the effects of increased LVEDP on FFR values in 528 cardiac cycles. The study showed that in multivariate analysis LVEDP was positively associated with FFR, increasing by 0.008 for every 1 mm Hg increase in LVEDP (p < 0.001), with a stronger correlation of 0.01 for every 1 mm Hg increase in LVEDP for those lesions with an FFR less than 0.80 (p < 0.001). These findings suggest in the setting of increased LVEDP (LVH, AS, and decompensated HF), evaluating moderate severity lesions with FFR could underestimate the hemodynamic significance. Central venous pressure had been included in the experimental validation of myocardial FFR [(Pd-right atrial pressure)/(Pa-right atrial pressure)],[33] the predecessor of the clinically used FFR. Central venous pressure was excluded in the commonly used (and clinical trial proved) FFR calculation as it was thought to be negligible. Toth and colleagues[34] largely proved this negligibility when comparing myocardial FFR to clinically used FFR in 1,676 stenoses. The median difference, although statistically significant, was an FFR difference of 0.01 when comparing myocardial FFR to FFR across a wide range of right atrial pressures. Nonetheless, there were larger differences between myocardial FFR to FFR as the right atrial pressure approached 12 mm Hg (median difference 0.02, IQR 0.01 to 0.03). These findings suggest that those with markedly elevated central venous pressures may have ischemic reclassification. However, in this study, a central venous pressure greater than 10 mm Hg had limited clinical impact as only 9% of those classified with an FFR greater than 0.80 were reclassified with a myocardial FFR of less than 0.80.

The degree of the myocardium, microvascular dysfunction, and hemodynamic effects associated with LVH plays a complex role in obtaining the simple hyperemic Pd/Pa calculation for FFR. It is possible that in patients with LVH, the FFR-decreasing effects that a myocardial territory a stenosed vessel may be balanced out by the FFR-increasing effects that occur with increased LVED and microvascular resistance. Ultimately, FFR seems to be reliable and useful when evaluating intermediate coronary lesions in those with LVH.

Older age

Increasing age leads to increased microvascular dysfunction and increased flow velocity, which in turn leads to reduced coronary filling. In nonhyperemic states, these findings would affect the evaluation of Pd/Pa. However, even with hyperemia, studies have suggested that in those with increased age with intermediate stenosis similar to their younger counterparts, FFR values were higher.[35] Lin and colleagues showed that in 178 left anterior descending evaluations with FFR that elderly patients (aged >70 years) had a smaller difference in the resting Pd/Pa and FFR (ΔFFR) compared with a younger age group (0.13 ± 0.05 vs. 0.15 ± 0.05, P = 0.014) and age was independently associated with FFR and ΔFFR in multivariate analysis. It is hypothesized that elderly patients have a reduced hyperemic response to adenosine. This, in turn, could lead to underestimation of lesion severity, although myocardial resistance should still be minimal in the presence of microvascular disease. Whether the difference in FFR values in older adults translates to clinical differences is unclear. A substudy of the FAME trial showed that although FFR is less likely to be abnormal in older adults for any given stenosis, FFR-guided PCI was equally beneficial compared with angiography-guided PCI for those aged more than 65 years as compared with those aged less than 65 years. These findings have spurred the FIRE trial which has been enrolling those aged more than 75 years to evaluate the difference in clinical outcomes between FFR guidance complete revascularization versus culprit only revascularization in those presenting with ST or non-ST elevation MI as has been done in prior trials in a younger population.[36,37]

SUMMARY

With the dramatic increase of FFR use in the cath laboratory coupled with the more recent emergence of NHPRs, accurate interpretation of these hemodynamic indices has become paramount. As additional evidence supporting the use of NHPRs emerges, more clinicians are using these indices in addition to FFR or in-lieu of FFR when relative or absolute contra-indications exist to induce hyperemia. However, both FFR and NHPRs have limitations that operators need to be cognizant of. Particular clinical and procedural scenarios may call for use of one over the other. For example, FFR seems to have more accuracy and reproducibility in those with AF undergoing evaluation of an intermediate lesion, whereas the future may show iFR to be superior to FFR when evaluating which lesion in series has a higher ischemic burden. Importantly, the outcome data for use of FFR or NHPRs in patients with special clinical scenarios are limited, let alone using one over the other in these scenarios. Ultimately, the goal moving forward in patients undergoing physiologically guided revascularization is accuracy, reliability, and translation to improvement in clinical outcomes. Understanding pitfalls, limitations, and strengths for FFR and NHPRs will help guide us to that goal.

CLINICS CARE POINTS

- Post-transcatheter aortic valve replacement (TAVR) for aortic stenosis, there seems to be an average decrease in fractional flow reserve (FFR) values for coronary lesions; however, this change is rarely clinically relevant and the decision to defer revascularization based on pre-TAVR seems to be safe.

- When comparing pre-TAVR versus post-TAVR, nonhyperemic pressure ratio (NHPR) for coronary lesions has significant variability, suggesting that FFR may be a more reliable alternative.

- FFR evaluation remains reproducible and reliable in patients with atrial fibrillation (AF), whereas the reproducibility of NHPR like instantaneous wave-free ratio (iFR) in patients with AF is far less.

- FFR evaluation seems to be a reliable marker of hemodynamic significance in patients with left ventricular hypertrophy and a coronary lesion, despite the concern of coronary territories providing large myocardial territories.

- Evaluation of left main coronary artery disease during FFR and NHPR is best evaluated with the pressure wire down a branch vessel with minimal-to-no disease.

- Serial coronary lesions affect the accurate evaluation of FFR for each individual lesion.

- iFR pullback may provide a more reliable modality to evaluate the hemodynamic significance of individual coronary lesions in series as compared with FFR, especially when comparing focal versus diffusely diseased lesions in series. However, whether intervening on these lesions based on iFR change leads to improved clinical outcomes is unknown.

DISCLOSURE

Dr D.M. Tehrani reports no disclosures. Dr A.H. Seto has received research grants from Philips and Acist, consulting fees from Medtronic and Medicure, and is a speaker for Terumo, General Electric, and Janssen

REFERENCES

1. Tonino PA, Bruyne BD, Pijls NH, et al. Fractional flow reserve versus angiography for guiding percutaneous coronary intervention. N Engl J Med 2009; 360(3):213–24.

2. Smith CR, Leon MB, Mack MJ, et al. Transcatheter versus surgical aortic-valve replacement in high-risk patients. N Engl J Med 2011;364(23):2187–98.
3. Leon MB, Smith CR, Mack MJ, et al. Transcatheter versus surgical aortic-valve replacement in intermediate-risk patients. N Engl J Med 2016; 374(17):1609–20.
4. Mack MJ, Leon MB, Thourani VH, et al. Transcatheter versus surgical aortic-valve replacement in low-risk patients. N Engl J Med 2019;380(18): 1695–705.
5. Kotronias RA, Kwok CS, George S, et al. Transcatheter aortic valve implantation with or without percutaneous coronary artery revascularization strategy: a systematic review and meta-analysis. J Am Heart Assoc 2017;6(6):e005960.
6. Pesarini G, Scarsini R, Zivelonghi C, et al. Functional assessment of coronary artery disease in patients undergoing transcatheter aortic valve implantation: Influence of pressure overload on the evaluation of lesion severity. Circ Cardiovasc Interv 2016;9(11): e004088.
7. Scarsini R, Pesarini G, Zivelonghi C, et al. Physiologic evaluation of coronary lesions using instantaneous wave-free ratio (iFR) in patients with severe aortic stenosis undergoing transcatheter aortic valve implantation. Eurointervetion 2018;13(13):1512–9.
8. Camuglia AC, Syed J, Garg P, et al. Invasively assessed coronary flow dynamics improved following relief of aortic stenosis with transcatheter aortic valve implantation. J Am Coll Cardiol 2014;63(17):1808–9.
9. Wiegerinck EM, van de Hoef TP, Rolandi MC, et al. Impact of aortic valve stenosis on coronary hemodynamics and instantaneous effect of transcatheter aortic valve implantation. Circ Cardiovasc Interv 2015;8(8):e002443.
10. Sabbah M, Joshi FR, Minkkinen M, et al. Long-term changes in Invasive Physiological Pressure Indices of stenosis severity following transcatheter aortic valve implantation. Circ Cardiovasc Interv 2022; 15(1):e011331.
11. Lunardi M, Scarsini R, Venturi G, et al. Physiological vesrus angiographic guidance for myocardial revascularization in patients undergoing transcatheter aortic valve implantation. J Am Heart Assoc 2019; 8(22):e012618.
12. Range FT, Schafers M, Acil T, et al. Impaired myocardial perfusion and perfusion reserve associated with increased coronary resistance in persistent atrial fibrillation. Eur Heart J 2007;28(18): 2223–30.
13. Kochiadakis GE, Skalidis EI, Kalebubas MD, et al. Effect of acute atrial fibrillation on phasic coronary blood flow pattern and flow reserve in humans. Eur Heart J 2002;23(9):734–41.
14. Berry C, Veer MV, Witt N, et al. VERIFY (VERification of instantaneous wave-free ratio and fractional flow reserve for the assessment of coronary artery stenois severity in everyday practice): a multicenter study in consecutive patients. J Am Coll Cardiol 2013;61(13):1421–7.
15. Bentea GP, Berdaoui B, Samyn S, et al. Reliability of fractional flow reserve and instantaneous wave-free ratio in assessing intermediate coronary stenosis in patients with atrial fibrillation. Am J Cardiol 2022; 162:105–10.
16. De Bruyne B, Bartunek J, Sys SU, et al. Simultaneous coronary pressure and flow velocity measurements in humans. Feasibility, reproducibility, and hemodynamic dependence of coronary flow, velocity reserve, hyperemic flow versus pressure slope index, and fractional flow reserve. Circulation 1996; 94(8):1842–9.
17. Hamilos M, Muller O, Cuisset T, et al. Long-term clinical outcome after fractional flow reserve-guided treatment in patients with angiographically equivocal left main coronary artery stenosis. Circulation 2009;120(15):1505–12.
18. Oviedo C, Maehara A, Mintz GS, et al. Intravascular ultrasound classification of plaque distribution in left main coronary artery bifurcations: where is the plaque really located? Circ Cardiovasc Interv 2010; 3(2):105–12.
19. De Bruyne B, Pijls NH, Heyndrickx GR, et al. Pressure-derived fractional flow reserve to assess serial epicardial stenoses: theoretical basis and animal validation. Circulation 2000;101(15):1840–7.
20. Pijls NH, de Bruyne B, Bech GJ, et al. Coronary pressure measurement to assess the hemodynamic significance of serial stenoses within one coronary artery: validation in humans. Circulation 2000; 02(19):2371–7.
21. Yong AS, Daniels D, de Bruyne B, et al. Fractional flow reserve assessment of left main stenosis in tpihe presence of downstream coronary stenoses. Circ Cardiovasc Interv 2013;6(2):161–5.
22. Fearon WF, Yong AS, Lenders G, et al. The impact of downstream coronary stenosis on fractional flow reserve assessment of intermediate left main coronary artery disease: human validation. JACC Cardiovasc Interv 2015;8(3):398–403.
23. Concordance between FFR and iFR for the assessment of intermediate lesions in the left main coronary artery. A prospective validation of a default value for iFR (iLITRO). 2022. Available at: https://clinicaltrials.gov/ct2/show/NCT03767621. Accessed February 21, 2022.
24. Davies JE, Sen S, Dehbi HM, et al. Use of the Instantaneous wave-free ratio or fractional flow reserve in PCI. N Engl J Med 2017;376(19):1824–34.
25. Gotberg M, Christiansen EH, Gudmundsdottir IJ, et al. Instantaneous wave-free ratio versus fractional flow reserve to guide PCI. N Engl J Med 2017; 376(19):1813–23.

26. Kikuta Y, Cook CM, Sharp AS, et al. Pre-angioplasty instantaneous wave-free ratio pullback predicts hemodynamic outcome in humans with coronary artery disease: Primary results of the international multicenter iFR GRADIENT registry. JACC Cardiovasc Interv 2018;11(8):757–67.

27. Jeremias A, Davies JE, Maehara A, et al. Blinded physiological assessment of residual ischemia after successful angiographic percutaneous coronary intervention: The DEFINE PCI study. JACC Cardiovasc Interv 2019;12(20):1991–2001.

28. Distal evaluation of functional performance with intravascular sensors to assess the narrowing effect: guided physiologic stenting (DEFINE GPS). 2022. Available at: https://clinicaltrials.gov/ct2/show/NCT04451044. Accessed February 21, 2022.

29. Leone AM, De Caterina AR, Basile E, et al. Influence of the amount of myocardium subtended by a stenosis on fractional flow reserve. Circ Cardiovasc Interv 2013;6(1):29–36.

30. Chhatriwalla AK, Ragosta M, Powers ER, et al. High left ventricular mass index does not limit the utility of fractional flow reserve for the physiologic assessment of lesion severity. J Invasive Cardiol 2006;18(11):544–9.

31. Sabbah M, Nepper-Christensen L, Lonborg J, et al. Fractional flow reserve-guided PCI in patients with and without left ventricular hypertrophy: a DANAMI-3-PRIMULTI substudy. Eurointervention 2020;16(7):584–90.

32. Leonardi RA, Townsend JC, Patel CA, et al. Left ventricular end-diastolic pressure affects measurement of fractional flow reserve. Cardiovasc Revasc Med 2013;14(4):218–22.

33. Pijls NH, van Son JA, Kirkeeide RL, et al. Experimental basis of determining maximum coronary, myocardial, and collateral blood flow by pressure measurements for assessing functional stenosis severity before and after percutaneous transluminal coronary angioplasty. Circulation 1993;87:1354–67.

34. Toth GG, de Bruyne B, Rusinaru D, et al. Impact of right atrial pressure on fractional flow reserve measurements: comparison of fractional flow reserve and myocardial fractional flow reserve in 1,600 coronary stenoses. JACC Cardiovasc Interv 2016;9(5):453–9.

35. Jin X, Lim HS, Tahk SJ, et al. Impact of age on the functional significance of intermediate epicardial artery disease. Circ J 2016;80(7):1583–9.

36. Biscaglia S, Guiducci V, Santarelli A, et al. Physiology-guided revascularization versus optimal medical therapy of nonculprit lesions in elderly patients with myocardial infarction: rationale and design of the FIRE trial. Am Heart J 2020;229:100–9.

37. Smits PC, Abdel-Wahab M, Neumann FJ, et al. Fractional flow reserve-guided multivessel angioplasty in myocardial infarction. N Engl J Med 2017;376(13):1234–44.

What About All the Recent "Negative" FFR Trials?

Nils P. Johnson, MD, MS

KEYWORDS

- Fractional flow reserve • Randomized controlled trial • Percutaneous coronary intervention
- Coronary artery bypass grafting

KEY POINTS

- Study design for diagnostic strategies must focus on discordant decisions.
- Composite endpoints for percutaneous coronary intervention (PCI) should discard mortality and focus on vessel-level outcomes for spontaneous myocardial infarction.
- Initial PCI must be included when calculating the total amount of target vessel revascularization.
- Ultrahigh rates of fractional flow reserve <=0.8 do not change treatment decisions from an angiographic-based strategy.
- Although PCI is a reasonable option for patients with severe multivessel disease, coronary artery bypass grafting remains better.

INTRODUCTION

Since its introduction in 1993,[1] fractional flow reserve (FFR) has gained a class IA recommendation from European guidelines[2] in 2010 and from American guidelines[3] in 2020. Nevertheless, the year 2021 saw the presentation or publication of several randomized trials widely considered "negative" for FFR.

In May, the FLOWER-MI trial was published suggesting no benefit from FFR-guided treatment over an angiographic-based strategy for nonculprit lesions noted at the time of acute ST-segment elevation myocardial infarction (STEMI).[4] Then, in September, the RIPCORD-2 trial was presented and interpreted as having no advantage for systematic FFR at the time of invasive diagnostic angiography.[5] In November, 2 studies were published: the FUTURE trial claimed no advantage to an FFR-guided strategy over angiographic decisions for multivessel disease[6] and the FAME 3 trial did not meet its noninferiority endpoint comparing FFR-guided percutaneous coronary intervention (PCI) against traditional angiographic-selection for coronary artery bypass grafting (CABG).[7]

Has FFR exceeded its "expiration date" after nearly 30 years on the cath laboratory shelf? This review critically examines each of these 4 randomized clinical trials (RCTs) to draw insights not only about FFR but also about study design and interpretation. Our conclusion mirrors the title of an excellent editorial from 15 years ago: "not all randomized trials are equal."[8]

FLOWER-MI: Fractional Flow Reserve for ST-Segment Elevation Myocardial Infarction Nonculprit Vessels

Overview

The immediate goal for a patient presenting with acute STEMI remains reperfusion of the culprit vessel. Even in cases successfully treated with fibrinolytic therapy, guidelines recommend invasive coronary catheterization within 3 to 24 hours.[3] Because almost all patients with STEMI ultimately undergo angiography, physicians routinely uncover nonculprit atherosclerotic disease outside of the infarct-related artery. Optimal treatment of these bystander lesions has changed during the past decade with a series of RCT-comparing

This article originally appeared in *Interventional Cardiology Clinics*, Volume 12 Issue 1, January 2023.
Division of Cardiology, Department of Medicine, Weatherhead PET Center, McGovern Medical School at UTHealth and Memorial Hermann Hospital, 6431 Fannin Street, Room MSB 4.256, Houston, TX 77030, USA
E-mail address: Nils.Johnson@uth.tmc.edu

Cardiol Clin 42 (2024) 31–39
https://doi.org/10.1016/j.ccl.2023.07.009

strategies: expectant management pending symptoms (wait and see), routine noninvasive evaluation, intracoronary physiology, or angiographic severity.

The FLOWER-MI trial randomized patients with STEMI and a lesion in a nonculprit artery to either an FFR-guided strategy or PCI. It enrolled 1171 subjects during a 2-year period from about 40 centers in France, and reported 1-year clinical follow-up. Nonculprit lesions had to be in a sizable vessel of at least 2.0 mm diameter with a visual severity of 50% or more diameter stenosis.

Endpoint

What endpoint is appropriate for these nonculprit vessels? FLOWER-MI used a composite of all-cause mortality, myocardial infarction (MI), and unplanned hospitalization leading to urgent revascularization. However, we must critically consider each component individually.

PCI instead of medical therapy (the only treatment difference between the 2 strategies in FLOWER-MI) has never been shown to reduce all-cause mortality. A patient-level pooled analysis of 2400 subjects from 3 RCT comparing FFR-guided PCI against medical therapy found no difference in all-cause death after a median follow-up of 2.9 years: hazard ratio 1.03 (95% confidence interval [CI] 0.69–1.54, $P = .89$).[9] Similarly the COMPLETE trial randomized 4041 subjects with STEMI and nonculprit vessels to either expectant management or PCI but found no difference in death from any cause after a median follow-up of 3.0 years: hazard ratio 0.91 (95%CI 0.69–1.20).[10] Consequently, incorporating death into a composite endpoint adds an equal number of events to both groups, thereby biasing the hazard ratio toward unity. FLOWER-MI observed a total of 19 deaths with similar distribution between treatment strategies: hazard ratio 0.89 (95%CI 0.36–2.20).

Coronary physiology evaluates a specific vessel, and PCI treats a portion of that vessel. There is no mechanistic basis for physiology to cause events in separate vessels. For example, an FFR of 0.86 in a nonculprit right coronary artery enrolled in FLOWER-MI cannot produce an infarct or revascularization in the left anterior descending artery. Therefore, endpoints of MI or revascularization should focus on the target vessel (TVMI or TVR), not off-target distributions.

Myocardial infarctions arise by different mechanisms that can largely be grouped into spontaneous or periprocedural. Although beyond the scope of this review, the definition and utility of periprocedural MI remains uncertain. Importantly, the recent ISCHEMIA trial demonstrated that neither procedural MI by their definition nor type 4a or 5 MI by the universal definition increased all-cause mortality, unlike MI due to plaque rupture, stent thrombosis, or severe in-stent restenosis (so-called type 1, 4b, and 4c mechanisms).[11]

The above discussion clarifies that spontaneous TVMI provides a relevant endpoint, unlike non-TVMI and periprocedural events. Previous studies have demonstrated that PCI instead of medical therapy reduces relevant infarcts, albeit without explicit data on TVMI. The patient-level pooled analysis of 2400 subjects from 3 RCT comparing FFR-guided PCI against medical therapy found a hazard ratio of 0.62 (95%CI 0.46–0.85, $P = .003$) after the initial 7 days (to exclude periprocedural events).[9] Similarly, COMPLETE trial demonstrated a hazard ratio for MI of 0.68 (95%CI 0.53–0.86) favoring PCI.[10] Conversely, FLOWER-MI found no increased hazard from an FFR-guided strategy with hazard ratio 1.77 (95%CI 0.82–3.84), indicating that PCI of high-FFR lesions does not attenuate their progression to infarction.

Finally, revascularization must not only focus on the target vessel but also include the initial procedures when comparing a strategy of more versus less PCI.[12,13] Initially for the nonculprit artery in FLOWER-MI a total of 591 stents were placed by an FFR-guided strategy while 865 stents were placed using an angiography-based strategy. During 1 year of follow-up, another 8 subjects in the FFR arm underwent urgent TVR compared with 3 in the other group. Assuming 1 additional stent per late TVR, the total number of stents placed is (591 + 8)/980 for FFR versus (865 + 3)/891 for angiography, equal to 0.6 stents/vessel compared with 1.0 stents/vessel — approximately 40% relative reduction. Focusing on the small number of non-TVR (7 vs 8 subjects) or late TVR (8 vs 3 vessels) distracts from a basic and obvious message: an angiographic-guided strategy in FLOWER-MI led to higher rates of total TVR.

Potentially PCI of the nonculprit vessel with FFR>0.8 might improve symptoms, even if it does not reduce TVMI. However, FLOWER-MI showed no differences here either, with similar average number of antianginal medications (mean 1.0 in each group, hazard ratio 1.01, 95% CI 0.90–1.14), quality of life survey (scores 0.86 vs 0.87), and class II or greater angina (63% vs 68% of subjects).

Design

Regardless of randomization, vessels with FFR≤0.8 received PCI in both arms of the FLOWER-MI trial. Only vessels with FFR>0.8 received PCI in the angiography-guided group, whereas comparable vessels received medical therapy after FFR assessment. Consequently, any changes in clinical outcome between the 2 groups must have arisen from the vessels with FFR>0.8 because only their treatment differed. Vessels with FFR≤0.8 contributed an equal number of events in both groups, biasing the hazard ratio toward unity. This mechanism and its consequence for the design of RCT for diagnostic tests (here FFR and angiography) has been articulated for more than 20 years[14] but remains underappreciated.

What would a more effective design have been for FLOWER-MI? Measure FFR for all vessels and either randomize only if FFR>0.8 or keep the FFR blinded as in CompareAcute.[15] Notably FLOWER-MI found that only 56% of nonculprit vessels had an FFR≤0.8, indicating that the effective sample size (discordant treatment) was less than half of the randomized population. **Table 1** summarizes the rate of FFR≤0.8 in nonculprit vessels uncovered at the time of STEMI.[4,15–17] Together the literature shows that FLOWER-MI was not an outlier but rather just more than 40% of all angiographically significant vessels have an intact FFR. This large minority must remain the subject of investigation, unmixed with the 60% of vessels with reduced FFR that would be suitable for PCI either way.

Logistics
Although the FLOWER-MI protocol "encouraged [FFR assessment] to be done during the index procedure but if necessary can be performed during another procedure as soon as possible during the index hospital admission, usually within 5 days" (quote from the protocol), ultimately 97% of FFR evaluations were staged. By comparison, the CompareAcute RCT in a similar population performed FFR-guided treatment (not just its measurement) of the nonculprit vessel in 83% of acute STEMI procedures.[15] Because FLOWER-MI found that only 56% of nonculprit vessels had an FFR≤0.8, it implies that almost half of all staged

FFR assessments resulted in essentially a diagnostic angiogram, with its attendant cost, delay, and small risk associated with repeat vascular access and coronary instrumentation.

Relatedly, we would expect that the procedure duration and amount of contrast used to assess and treat the nonculprit vessel would have been lower, because 44% of such cases had an FFR>0.8 and received medical therapy. However, the median procedure duration (35 vs 30 minutes) and contrast (110 mL for both groups) for the nonculprit vessel did not differ.

What unexpectedly differed between the arms was the number of culprit vessels, namely 980 in the FFR-guided group compared with 891 in the angiographic-guided arm—10% higher despite a comparable number of subjects (586 vs 577). Likely this difference arose as vessels were selected after randomization, not before, and could have been avoided by asking operators to identify target vessels first as done in prior FFR trials.[18] Operators appeared more willing to bring patients back for FFR assessment than angiographic-based PCI. Potentially this higher number of lesions in the FFR group may have contributed to equalizing the procedure duration and contrast use mentioned earlier.

Finally, 154 of the 980 FFR values were missing, almost 16%. Although data quality is never perfect in any RCT, the fact that a central parameter such as FFR could be missing from nearly 1 in 5 lesions seems surprisingly large given that these vessels received FFR-guided therapy.

Summary of FLOWER-MI
From an improper endpoint (not focusing on spontaneous TVMI) to design issues (not focusing on the 40% of FFR vs angiographic discordances) to several logistical limitations, FLOWER-MI did not live up to its expectations. Despite these numerous flaws, the trial showed us that an FFR- instead of an angiographic-guided strategy reduced the number of stents in the nonculprit vessel, with no penalty on death, TVMI, or symptoms. In that sense, FLOWER-MI provides the same message as FAME,[18] namely an FFR>0.8 does not benefit from PCI.

Practically at least 80% of nonculprit vessels noted at the time of STEMI can undergo immediate FFR assessment.[15] As summarized in **Table 1**, approximately 60% will have low FFR and need consideration for revascularization, either at that time or during a staged procedure depending on clinical circumstances. No meaningful evidence exists that PCI of a vessel with an FFR>0.8— even a nonculprit noted at the time of STEMI— brings any clinical advantage.

Table 1
Abnormal FFR frequency among nonculprit vessels noted at the time of ST-segment elevation myocardial infarction

Trial	Vessels	FFR≤0.8
PRIMULTI[16]	314	217 (69%)
CompareAcute[15]	867	433 (50%)
FLOWER-MI[4]	826	460 (56%)
FULL-REVASC[17]	742	446 (60%)
Pooled	2749	1556 (57%)

Abbreviation: FFR, fractional flow reserve.

RIPCORD-2: Systematic Versus Selective Fractional Flow Reserve

Overview

Diagnostic tests can be used as part of 3 general pathways.[19] First, the new test can replace an existing test, usually by being more accurate, cheaper, faster, and/or less invasive. Second, the test can serve as triage to another diagnostic test, usually whereby a negative test excludes patients from further evaluation. Third, the test can add information to the preceding clinical pathway and serve as a final link with treatment.

From its beginning, FFR has operated along this final "add-on" pathway. Seminal FFR outcomes trials have generally enrolled patients with symptoms despite medical therapy, often with preceding equivocal or abnormal noninvasive testing, and a significant angiographic lesion in a sizable vessel on invasive catheterization. Only then was FFR added to make a final decision: "... *investigator first indicated which stenoses were thought to require stenting on the basis of the clinical and angiographic data*" (emphasis added to original quote).[20] Thus FFR augments, not replaces, clinical judgment—what might be called "*selective*" FFR.

In contrast, the RIPCORD-2 trial mandated "*systematic*" FFR for all vessels of approximately 2.25 mm diameter or larger with any stenosis greater than 30% diameter reduction by visual assessment.[21] It randomized 1100 subjects enrolled from almost 20 centers in the United Kingdom.[5] Operators could select among treatment plans of medical therapy, PCI, or CABG.

Endpoint

Coprimary endpoints included both total hospital costs and quality of life. A key secondary endpoint was composite all-cause mortality, MI, unplanned revascularization, and stroke at 1 year. The motivation for prioritizing both economics and clinical outcomes was that "given that there is a financial burden associated with FFR measurement compared with angiography alone, as well as the small procedural risk involved, such a profound change in routine clinical practice would require evidence not just of clinical benefit but also of cost effectiveness."[21]

Design

Several prior trials have examined patient-level treatment decisions before and after measuring FFR.[22–26] Each study had the same general concept: operators incorporated clinical and angiographic data and selected one of medical therapy, PCI, or CABG; then FFR was measured and the plan could change. The decisions can be viewed in a 3-by-3 grid, as in **Fig. 1**. Unchanged decisions fall along the diagonal, whereas changed decisions appear above or below.

From 5245 patients pooled from 5 studies,[22–26] including the pilot RIPCORD trial[26] that informed the design of RIPCORD-2, operators kept the same patient-level decision in 63% of cases. In 23% of cases the decision was "downgraded," namely changed from a more aggressive treatment such as PCI to a less invasive treatment such as medical therapy. However, in 14% of cases the decision was "upgraded," that is, changed from less invasive to more invasive treatment such as medical therapy's becoming CABG.

It is important to contrast "downgrading" versus "upgrading" based on FFR assessment. Foundational trials such as FAME[18] only allowed operators to downgrade therapy based on FFR. For example, a lesion thought to require PCI based on the totality of clinical and angiographic data was selected for inclusion. Then, if FFR was negative, medical therapy was substituted for PCI—a "downgrade" to less invasive treatment. In no previous randomized trial was the operator allowed to measure FFR in a vessel thought most suitable for medical therapy after review of all clinical and angiographic information and then, based on FFR, to select a more invasive treatment such as PCI (an "upgrade").

Therefore, the untested component of RIPCORD-2 was neither keeping the same therapy after FFR assessment (as could have been anticipated in roughly 60% of cases) nor using FFR to downgrade from PCI to medical therapy (as could have been anticipated in roughly 25% of cases) as already validated in an existing RCT.[18] Instead, the novel hypothesis was using FFR to escalate invasive treatment largely in vessels deemed suitable for medical therapy, which applies to approximately 15% of patients. As designed, we cannot separate these 3 groups: the 60% where FFR did not make a difference, the 25% where FFR de-escalated invasive treatment, and the 15% where FFR led to more invasive therapy. An alternative design would have focused completely on this unproven and unstudied question by only including patients selected for medical therapy, and either performing an FFR then randomizing if abnormal or first measuring a blinded FFR in everyone and then unblinding half of cases.

The composite treatment decisions in RIPCORD-2 indicate a modest swing from PCI to both medical therapy and CABG through the systematic use of FFR. Although the percentage of subjects treated with PCI dropped from 61% with angiography alone to 56% after an FFR assessment, this 5% split into a 2% increase in

	after FFR					with FFR		
	medical	PCI	CABG			medical	PCI	CABG
medical	1429	**638**	**70**		medical	same	?	?
before FFR PCI	1072	1746	**42**	*without* FFR PCI	FAME	same	?
CABG	65	62	121		CABG	?	?	same

same 63%
"downgrade" 23%
"upgrade" 14%
**NEVER TESTED IN RCT

Fig. 1. Changes in treatment after FFR. A total of 5 trials with 5245 patients[22–26] tabulated treatment decisions before and after measuring FFR. These 3 × 3 tables present the choices of medical therapy, PCI, or CABG (some studies allowed for a decision to obtain additional testing). In more than 60% of cases, treatment did not change. The most common change in treatment was to switch from PCI to medical therapy—what might be called a "downgrade" from more invasive to less invasive treatment, as seen in just more than 20% of cases. However, measuring FFR also led to some decision for more invasive treatment, such as switching to PCI instead of medical therapy—what might be called an "upgrade" and was seen in approximately 15% of cases. Most of the time treatment does not change, so neither will clinical outcomes. Already switching from angiographic-based PCI to FFR-guided medical therapy has been validated as safe and beneficial in the FAME trial.[18] CABG, coronary artery bypass grafting; FFR, fractional flow reserve; PCI, percutaneous coronary intervention; RCT, randomized controlled trial. **, adds emphasis.

medical therapy but also a 3% increase in CABG. Could some of these additional CABG referrals have arisen from borderline or "gray zone" FFR values in the LAD from diffuse disease and/or higher flow due to its larger mass of supplied myocardium?[27] Without further details regarding the FFR distributions among vessels and across treatment decisions, we can only speculate. However, the net shift was too small to influence total hospital cost ($P = .137$), quality of life metrics ($P = .88$), or clinical outcomes ($P = .64$ for hierarchical composite major adverse cardiac events).

Summary of RIPCORD-2

As with any test, the value of FFR depends on the pretest probability. A key lesson from RIPCORD-2 is that *systematic* FFR should not replace *selective* FFR. Always performing a test adds costs, complexity, and confusion compared with using it after a thoughtful integration of all available information. Clinical judgment still matters—wires are no substitute for being a doctor.

FUTURE: Systematic Fractional Flow Reserve for Multivessel Disease

Overview

In many ways, the FUTURE trial[6] mimicked RIPCORD-2 by studying *systematic* FFR, albeit this time in a population with mandatory multivessel disease. A total of 941 subjects from more than 30 French centers were enrolled with at least 50% diameter stenosis visually in either the left main or in 2 to 3 sizable vessels 2.5 mm diameter or larger. As in RIPCORD-2, subjects were randomized to a treatment decision based on integration of clinical and angiographic data, or to a treatment decision altered by systematic FFR. Operators could select among treatment plans of medical therapy, PCI, or CABG.

Endpoint

The primary composite endpoint of all-cause mortality, MI, stroke, or unplanned revascularization after 1 year shares all the same fundamental limitations as discussed earlier for FLOWER-MI and RIPCORD-2. This endpoint did not differ significantly between the 2 arms of the trial: hazard ratio 0.97 (95%CI 0.69–1.36, $P = .85$). Notably recruitment was halted early by an independent monitoring board due to a suggestion of adverse outcomes not born out by the full analysis—a false-positive emphasizing the hazards of monitoring trial "safety," no matter how well intentioned.

Design

As in RIPCORD-2,[5] the FUTURE trial[6] only permitted composite decisions in each group, with both "upgrading" and "downgrading" possible. Due to this design, we cannot understand which decisions would have differed with versus without FFR information. Alternative designs, such as the pilot RIPCORD study,[26] would have obtained blinded FFR values or only randomized "upgrade" discordances. **Fig. 1** again emphasizes that FUTURE incorporated an undersized trial analogous to FAME[18] but mixed together and also underpowered.

Logistics

The net impact of systematic FFR assessment in FUTURE was to shift 8% of decisions from PCI to medical therapy, with no change in net 12% CABG. This magnitude is smaller than anticipated by trials such as FAME that shifted 37% of patients from PCI to medical therapy.[18] A key explanation for the blunted impact arises from the large number of subjects not treated consistently with the protocol: "Despite finding FFR>0.80, 127 (11.5%) lesions were managed by PCI and stenting; likewise, 38 (16.9%) bypass grafts were performed."[6]

Furthermore in the 12% of subjects treated by CABG, no FFR impact was seen in terms of procedural complexity (2.9 total grafts in each group, P = .81). This finding differs greatly from RCT in which FFR before CABG reduced total grafts: 2.5 versus 2.9, P < .001.[28] As with the 11.5% protocol violations for FFR-guided PCI treatment, this result emphasizes that FFR was also ignored when planning CABG.

Summary of FUTURE

FUTURE mixed treatment decisions (60% of which would have been the same with or without FFR), contained an underpowered trial analogous to FAME,[18] ignored negative FFR results (greater than 10% PCI and greater than 15% CABG despite an FFR>0.8), and included nonmodifiable events in a composite endpoint (all-cause death). What can we learn from such a trial apart from how not to do it?

FAME 3: Fractional Flow Reserve-Guided Percutaneous Coronary Intervention Versus Traditional Coronary Artery Bypass Grafting

Overview

The past several years have seen the publication of patient-level pooled analyses from several RCT comparing CABG to PCI for left main and/or multivessel disease.[29–31] Although published during the course of FAME 3, these massive analyses have provided several relevant results. First, PCI increases all-cause mortality compared with CABG in 11,528 subjects: hazard ratio 1.20 (95% CI 1.06–1.37, P = .0038).[29] Notably, the additional risk of PCI over CABG accrues after the first year (hazard ratio 1.39, 95%CI 1.17–1.62, P < .0001) but not during the first year (hazard ratio 0.97, 95%CI 0.80–1.19, P = .80) and is driven by patients with diabetes (hazard ratio 1.44, 95%CI 1.20–1.74, P = .0001) and multivessel disease (hazard ratio 1.28, 95% CI 1.09–1.49, P = .0019). Second, stroke occurs less often after PCI than CABG but only during the first 30 days (hazard ratio 0.33, 95%CI 0.20–0.53, P < .001) and not during the next 59 months (hazard ratio 1.05, 95%CI 0.80–1.38, P = .72).[30] Interestingly, the additional stroke risk is driven by exactly the same patients who gain additional mortality benefit from CABG: diabetes and multivessel disease. Third, PCI increases the risk of spontaneous MI (hazard ratio 2.35, 95%CI 1.71–3.23, P < .0001) and repeat revascularization (hazard ratio 1.78, 95%CI 1.51–2.10, P < .0001), albeit in an analysis of patients with left main disease.[31]

Therefore, although PCI for left main or severe multivessel disease is a reasonable therapy with less stroke during the first month, CABG reduces mortality, spontaneous MI, and repeat revascularization in patients suitable for either procedure. During the period in which these new, pooled syntheses from CABG versus PCI trials were appearing, the FAME 3 trial in almost 50 global centers enrolled 1500 patients with severe multivessel disease (but not left main) in whom either CABG or PCI was a reasonable technical option.[32] Subjects were randomized to traditional angiographic-guided CABG or FFR-guided PCI. As summarized in **Table 2**, the characteristics of the FAME 3 population largely matched prior CABG versus PCI trials, albeit smaller in size (1500 vs 11,518 subjects), less diabetes (29% vs 38%), and no left main disease.

Endpoint

Because it took more than 11,000 patients and 5 years of follow-up to reach definitive insights into the specific benefits of CABG over PCI,[29] the use of a composite endpoint for the 1500 subjects in FAME 3 followed for just 1 year[7] reflects the difficult reality of doing these types of studies. Even with this more modest size, all-cause mortality, MI, stroke, and repeat revascularization did not meet the prespecified threshold for noninferiority of PCI compared with CABG: hazard ratio 1.5 (95%CI 1.1–2.2, P = .35 for noninferiority). Each

Table 2
Comparison of FAME 3 to a massive pooled analysis of coronary artery bypass grafting versus percutaneous coronary intervention trials

	FAME 3[7]	Pooled[29]
Sample size	1500	11,518
Age (y)	65	64
male	82%	76%
Diabetes	29%	38%
EF<50%	18%	16%
Recent ACS	39%	34%
Left main	0%	39%
SYNTAX		
Average	26	26
Score>32	18%	21%
CABG/PCI		
# Stent	3.7	3.1
LIMA	97%	96%
Off pump	24%	28%

Abbreviations: ACS, acute coronary syndrome; CABG, coronary artery bypass grafting; EF, ejection fraction; LIMA, left internal mammary artery; PCI, percutaneous coronary intervention; SYNTAX, anatomic scoring system for coronary artery disease.

component of the endpoint, although individually underpowered and therefore not strictly significant, matched the expected direction seen in pooled analyses: more death after PCI (hazard ratio 1.7), higher rates of MI (hazard ratio 1.5), more frequent repeat revascularization (hazard ratio 1.5), and similar stroke (hazard ratio 0.9). Eventually FAME 3 will be followed for a total of 4 years if funding permits,[32] allowing more events to occur among the components of the composite endpoint.

Design

Unlike the diagnostic strategy trials discussed earlier such as FLOWER-MI,[4] RIPCORD-2,[5] and FUTURE,[6] the FAME 3 trial[7] cannot focus only on "discordances" between FFR and angiography because the treatments differ as well (PCI or CABG). The percentage of vessels with high FFR can be estimated from the FFR-guided arm that encountered 21% chronic total occlusions (whose FFR has been historically deemed positive as in the FAME trial[18]) plus only 24% of stenotic vessels with an FFR>0.8 among 82% of vessels that underwent physiologic measurement.[7] Therefore, 21% + (1−0.24) × 82% equals 83% of vessels with an FFR≤0.8, and a mean value of 0.70 similar to 0.71 in FAME[18] and 0.68 in FAME 2.[20]

What is the consequence of this extremely high rate of FFR≤0.8 and severe average value near 0.7? If the FFR≤0.8 rate had been 100%, then FAME 3 would have been a typical PCI versus CABG trial. If the FFR≤0.8 rate had been 0%, then FAME 3 would have compared CABG against medical therapy (one cell in the 3 × 3 grid depicted by **Fig. 1**). Although FFR details have not yet been published by vessel, we can assume that the mandate to have a mammary graft to the left anterior descending (LAD) artery in FAME 3 pushed the FFR≤0.8 rate in this vessel close to 100%. Therefore a composite rate of 83%—and likely even higher in the LAD—indicates that FAME 3 was essentially a typical PCI versus CABG trial. Physiology made almost no difference because so few vessels had a negative FFR>0.8.

Logistics

A subgroup analysis of FAME 3 suggested potential heterogeneity of treatment benefit stratified by the anatomic SYNTAX score. Namely, subjects with less anatomic complexity indicated by a SYNTAX score <22 had a lower composite event rate with PCI versus CABG (5.5% vs 8.6%) compared with intermediate 23 to 32 (13.7% vs 6.1%) or high >33 (12.1% vs 6.6%) complexity. This heterogeneity has been sought in much larger series of more than 11,000 subjects[29] without finding a

significant interaction with all-cause mortality for all patients (interaction $P = .21$) or just those with multivessel disease ($P = .32$) as enrolled in FAME 3. Given the smaller sample size and shorter duration of follow-up in FAME 3, and its discordance with larger pooled results with 5-year of outcomes, we should be cautious regarding this subgroup finding.

Summary of FAME 3

Did FFR "fail" in the FAME 3 trial? No, it simply confirmed that severe multivessel disease benefits from CABG more than PCI, as seen in more than 11,000 patients from other RCTs.[29] If a test is almost always abnormal (such as FFR in FAME 3), then you do not really need it!

SUMMARY

What can we learn from 4 recent RCT of FFR published or presented in 2021? First, study design for diagnostic strategies must focus on discordant decisions.[14] Second, composite endpoints for PCI should discard mortality and focus on vessel-level outcomes for spontaneous MI. Third, initial PCI must be included when calculating the total amount of TVR. Fourth, ultrahigh rates of FFR≤0.8 do not change treatment decisions from an angiographic-based strategy. Finally, although PCI is a reasonable option for patients with severe multivessel disease, CABG remains better.

CLINICS CARE POINTS

- Study design for diagnostic strategies must focus on discordant decisions.
- Composite endpoints for PCI should discard mortality and focus on vessel-level outcomes for spontaneous MI.
- Initial PCI must be included when calculating the total amount of TVR.
- Ultrahigh rates of FFR (0.8) do not change treatment decisions from an angiographic-based strategy.
- Although PCI is a reasonable option for patients with severe multivessel disease, CABG remains better.

DISCLOSURE

N.P. Johnson received internal funding from the Weatherhead PET Center for Preventing and

Reversing Atherosclerosis; received significant institutional research support from St. Jude Medical (CONTRAST, NCT02184117), Philips Volcano Corporation (DEFINE-FLOW, NCT02328820), and CoreAalst (PPG Registry, NCT04789317) for studies using intracoronary pressure and flow sensors; has an institutional licensing agreement with Boston Scientific for the smart-minimum FFR algorithm commercialized under 510(k) K191008; and has pending patents on diagnostic methods for quantifying aortic stenosis and TAVI physiology, and also algorithms to correct pressure tracings from fluid-filled catheters.

REFERENCES

1. Pijls NH, van Son JA, Kirkeeide RL, et al. Experimental basis of determining maximum coronary, myocardial, and collateral blood flow by pressure measurements for assessing functional stenosis severity before and after percutaneous transluminal coronary angioplasty. Circulation 1993;87:1354–67.

2. Wijns W, Kolh P, Danchin N, et al. Guidelines on myocardial revascularization. Eur Heart J 2010;31: 2501–55.

3. Lawton JS, Tamis-Holland JE, Bangalore S, et al. 2021 ACC/AHA/SCAI Guideline for Coronary Artery Revascularization: A Report of the American College of Cardiology/American Heart Association Joint Committee on Clinical Practice Guidelines. J Am Coll Cardiol 2022;79:e21–129.

4. Puymirat E, Cayla G, Simon T, et al. Multivessel PCI Guided by FFR or Angiography for Myocardial Infarction. N Engl J Med 2021;385:297–308.

5. Stables RH, Mullen LJ, Elguindy M, et al. Routine Pressure Wire Assessment Versus Conventional Angiography in the Management of Patients With Coronary Artery Disease: The RIPCORD 2 Trial. Circulation 2022;46:687–98.

6. Rioufol G, Dérimay F, Roubille F, et al. Fractional Flow Reserve to Guide Treatment of Patients With Multivessel Coronary Artery Disease. J Am Coll Cardiol 2021;78:1875–85.

7. Fearon WF, Zimmermann FM, De Bruyne B, et al. Fractional Flow Reserve-Guided PCI as Compared with Coronary Bypass Surgery. N Engl J Med 2022;386:128–37.

8. Gould KL. Not all randomized trials are equal. J Am Coll Cardiol 2007;50:2013–5.

9. Zimmermann FM, Omerovic E, Fournier S, et al. Fractional flow reserve-guided percutaneous coronary intervention vs. medical therapy for patients with stable coronary lesions: meta-analysis of individual patient data. Eur Heart J 2019;40:180–6.

10. Mehta SR, Wood DA, Storey RF, et al. Complete Revascularization with Multivessel PCI for Myocardial Infarction. N Engl J Med 2019;381:1411–21.

11. Chaitman BR, Alexander KP, Cyr DD, et al. Myocardial Infarction in the ISCHEMIA Trial: Impact of Different Definitions on Incidence, Prognosis, and Treatment Comparisons. Circulation 2021;143: 790–804.

12. Goodney PP, Woloshin S, Schwartz LM. Fractional flow reserve-guided PCI in stable coronary disease. N Engl J Med 2012;367:2355.

13. Johnson NP, Collison D. Is Target Vessel Failure a Failure? JACC Cardiovasc Interv 2022;15:1044–6.

14. Bossuyt PM, Lijmer JG, Mol BW. Randomised comparisons of medical tests: sometimes invalid, not always efficient. Lancet 2000;356:1844–7.

15. Smits PC, Abdel-Wahab M, Neumann FJ, et al. Fractional Flow Reserve-Guided Multivessel Angioplasty in Myocardial Infarction. N Engl J Med 2017;376: 1234–44.

16. Engstrøm T, Kelbæk H, Helqvist S, et al. Complete revascularisation versus treatment of the culprit lesion only in patients with ST-segment elevation myocardial infarction and multivessel disease (DANAMI-3—PRIMULTI): an open-label, randomised controlled trial. Lancet 2015;386:665–71.

17. Böhm F, Mogensen B, Östlund O, et al. The Full Revasc (Ffr-gUidance for compLete non-cuLprit REVASCularization) Registry-based randomized clinical trial. Am Heart J 2021;241:92–100.

18. Tonino PA, De Bruyne B, Pijls NH, et al. Fractional flow reserve versus angiography for guiding percutaneous coronary intervention. N Engl J Med 2009; 360:213–24.

19. Van den Bruel A, Cleemput I, Aertgeerts B, et al. The evaluation of diagnostic tests: evidence on technical and diagnostic accuracy, impact on patient outcome and cost-effectiveness is needed. J Clin Epidemiol 2007;60:1116–22.

20. De Bruyne B, Pijls NH, Kalesan B, et al. Fractional flow reserve-guided PCI versus medical therapy in stable coronary disease. N Engl J Med 2012;367: 991–1001.

21. Elguindy M, Stables R, Nicholas Z, et al. Design and Rationale of the RIPCORD 2 Trial (Does Routine Pressure Wire Assessment Influence Management Strategy at Coronary Angiography for Diagnosis of Chest Pain?): A Randomized Controlled Trial to Compare Routine Pressure Wire Assessment With Conventional Angiography in the Management of Patients With Coronary Artery Disease. Circ Cardiovasc Qual Outcomes 2018;11:e004191.

22. Nakamura M, Yamagishi M, Ueno T, et al. Modification of treatment strategy after FFR measurement: CVIT-DEFER registry. Cardiovasc Interv Ther 2015; 30:12–21.

23. Layland J, Oldroyd KG, Curzen N, et al. Fractional flow reserve vs. angiography in guiding management to optimize outcomes in non-ST-segment elevation myocardial infarction: the British Heart

Foundation FAMOUS-NSTEMI randomized trial. Eur Heart J 2015;36:100–11.

24. Baptista SB, Raposo L, Santos L, et al. Impact of Routine Fractional Flow Reserve Evaluation During Coronary Angiography on Management Strategy and Clinical Outcome: One-Year Results of the POST-IT. Circ Cardiovasc Interv 2016;9:e003288.

25. Van Belle E, Rioufol G, Pouillot C, et al. Outcome impact of coronary revascularization strategy reclassification with fractional flow reserve at time of diagnostic angiography: insights from a large French multicenter fractional flow reserve registry. Circulation 2014;129:173–85.

26. Curzen N, Rana O, Nicholas Z, et al. Does routine pressure wire assessment influence management strategy at coronary angiography for diagnosis of chest pain?: the RIPCORD study. Circ Cardiovasc Interv 2014;7:248–55.

27. Collet C, Johnson NP, Mizukami T, et al. Fractional Flow Reserve After Percutaneous Coronary Intervention: A Pooled, Individual-Patient Analysis and Expert Opinion. Under journal review.

28. Toth GG, Collet C, Langhoff Thuesen A, et al. Influence of fractional flow reserve on grafts patency: Systematic review and patient-level meta-analysis. Catheter Cardiovasc Interv 2022;99:730–5.

29. Head SJ, Milojevic M, Daemen J, et al. Mortality after coronary artery bypass grafting versus percutaneous coronary intervention with stenting for coronary artery disease: a pooled analysis of individual patient data. Lancet 2018;391:939–48.

30. Head SJ, Milojevic M, Daemen J, et al. Stroke Rates Following Surgical Versus Percutaneous Coronary Revascularization. J Am Coll Cardiol 2018;72:386–98.

31. Sabatine MS, Bergmark BA, Murphy SA, et al. Percutaneous coronary intervention with drug-eluting stents versus coronary artery bypass grafting in left main coronary artery disease: an individual patient data meta-analysis. Lancet 2021;398:2247–57.

32. Zimmermann FM, De Bruyne B, Pijls NH, et al. Rationale and design of the Fractional Flow Reserve versus Angiography for Multivessel Evaluation (FAME) 3 Trial: a comparison of fractional flow reserve-guided percutaneous coronary intervention and coronary artery bypass graft surgery in patients with multivessel coronary artery disease. Am Heart J 2015;170:619–26.e2.

Using Physiology Pullback for Percutaneous Coronary Intervention Guidance
Is this the Future?

Sukhjinder Singh Nijjer, BSc, MB ChB, FRCP, PhD

KEYWORDS

• PCI optimization • Pressure wire pullback • Physiology pullback • iFR • FFR • PPG

KEY POINTS

- Coronary physiology identifies ischemia at a vessel, but most coronary intervention is performed using the angiogram alone, leaving 20% to 30% of vessels with residual ischemia.
- Physiology pullback can identify lesion level ischemia to better target coronary intervention.
- Fractional flow reserve (FFR) pullback will identify the lesion with the greatest gradient; once intervention has been performed, FFR pullback should be repeated to assess residual disease.
- Instantaneous wave-free ratio (iFR) pullback is a strong predictor of post-percutaneous coronary intervention physiology and strategies should aim to achieve an iFR greater than 0.95 as it is associated with reduced clinical events.
- Co-registration between physiology and angiography enables faster interrogation of the data to determine interventional strategies.

NATURE OF THE PROBLEM

It is well established that coronary angiography has limits on identifying physiologically significant stenoses.[1] Coronary physiology, as measured using an intracoronary pressure wire, can readily identify vessel-level ischemia.[2,3] However, once measured, operators frequently rely upon angiographic appearance alone to select lesions for percutaneous coronary intervention (PCI). More refined operators may optimize coronary intervention by supplementing with intracoronary imaging to ensure the deployed stent is well expanded and well apposed. In this manner, Modern PCI approaches combining pressure wire and imaging together improved outcomes in the SYNTAX-II study compared with a historical cohort.[4,5] However, approximately 20% to 30% of vessels undergoing coronary intervention remain ischemic despite stenting.[6–8] Furthermore, around 20% to 30% of patients have residual angina post-procedure.[9] This may be because physiologically important stenoses have been underappreciated. Further intervention could improve outcomes in this setting. In others, residual ischemia results from diffuse atherosclerotic disease meaning an optimal result is unlikely. Therefore, there remains a clinical need to better identify stenoses for coronary intervention as well as identify those patients most likely to have residual ischemia to intensify medical therapy or consider surgical revascularization.

Physiologic pullback, the use of pressure wire data accumulated by slowly withdrawing the sensor through the coronary vessel, offers a potential solution. Physiologic pullback, performed *before* coronary intervention can help identify physiologically important lesions throughout the

This article originally appeared in *Interventional Cardiology Clinics*, Volume 12 Issue 1, January 2023.
Department of Cardiology, Imperial College London, Hammersmith Hospital, Du Cane Road, London, W12 0HS, United Kingdom
E-mail address: s.nijjer@imperial.ac.uk
Twitter: @SukhNijjer (S.S.N.)

Cardiol Clin 42 (2024) 41–53
https://doi.org/10.1016/j.ccl.2023.07.008

vessel.[10–14] Knowledge before intervention can guide treatment decisions. With the use of non-hyperemic pressure ratios such as instantaneous wave-free ratio (iFR) it is possible to credibly predict the physiologic outcome for a given stenting strategy.[15,16] This means operators can see, before placing any stents, the potential outcome of any given approach. Those patients likely to remain ischemic can be identified and treatment decisions can be altered accordingly. Alternatively, if a good outcome is predicted and not achieved, it readily identifies those patients in which further intervention is required—potentially reducing future angina.

Physiologic pullback is readily available in all cases in where a pressure wire is used. It can be performed under both resting or hyperemic conditions (**Fig. 1**). Used alone, the operator can scrutinize the pressure trace to identify focal and diffuse disease and determine treatment decisions. When combined with automated co-registration with angiographic appearances, resting ratios such as iFR, can provide a clear prediction of the post-PCI physiologic values for a given PCI strategy. Studies have demonstrated that the prediction is within acceptable clinical tolerances. Ongoing randomized studies are assessing the merits of this guided approach versus a more traditional approach. Incremental innovations such as this, will subtly improve coronary intervention to be more targeted and to reduce residual ischemia which may then improve patient outcomes.

PHYSIOLOGIC MEASUREMENT

Invasive coronary physiology remains the established gold-standard for assessing ischemia in patients who have not had definitive ischemia testing performed before coronary angiography. It has a Level 1A recommendation by both the European Society of Cardiology and American College of Cardiology/American Heart Association guidelines for coronary revascularization.[17,18]

FRACTIONAL FLOW RESERVE

Fractional flow reserve (FFR), measured as a pressure ratio of distal coronary pressure to proximal aortic pressure during hyperemia, is an established parameter that correlates well with non-invasive markers of ischemia.[3] A value of ≤ 0.80 is typically considered significant. FFR has been shown to improve outcomes when patients with multi-vessel disease selected for PCI have coronary intervention guided by the FFR value compared with angiographic guidance alone.[19] Patients in whom the FFR is nonsignificant can

often be managed medically with a low rate of major adverse events.[20–22] Contrary to this, those with significant ischemia on FFR who are medically managed are more likely to have revascularization in the short-term and more significant adverse events in the longer-term.

INSTANTANEOUS WAVE-FREE RATIO

iFR is a resting pressure ratio that measures distal coronary pressure during diastole without the use of exogenous hyperemic agents.[23] It identifies ischemia as least as well as FFR and a value of ≤ 0.89 is considered significant.[24] In two large randomized controlled studies, DEFINE-FLAIR and iFR-SwedeHeart, has been shown to be non-inferior to FFR in the management of coronary disease.[25,26] Outcome data are available to 5 years and show clear safety without a concerning increase in mortality or myocardial infarction (**Fig. 2**).[27]

SETTING UP FOR PHYSIOLOGIC ASSESSMENT

Performing physiologic assessment is a simple and easy to perform procedure. However, there are many steps in which the values measured can be artificially affected. Care and attention are essential for reliable measurements that can alter clinical decisions.

Operators are recommended to use 6Fr guiding catheters. Although modern smaller catheters can be used, there can be pressure damping impacting on the aortic pressure trace. Should a complication occur, a 6Fr system permits more rapid treatment. Weight-adjusted heparin and liberal use of intracoronary nitrates is essential. Nitrates do not induce long-lived hyperemia and reduce the impact of epicardial vasospasm such that the measured pressure gradients reflect only the epicardial stenoses proximal to the pressure sensor.

The pressure wire system should be activated and calibrated to atmospheric pressure at the level of the heart prior insertion into the patient. The pressure sensor should be calibrated against the central aortic pressure trace at the ostium of the vessel or in the aorta itself. Damping from the guiding catheter must be avoided and contrast should be expunged before making readings. In the case of iFR, multiple readings can be performed; each will represent an average of five heartbeats. In the case of FFR, hyperemia should be induced in a consistent manner between patients. A fixed dose infusion is recommended for consistency and to match the reported protocols in the pivotal trials. In laboratories using adenosine, 140 mcg/

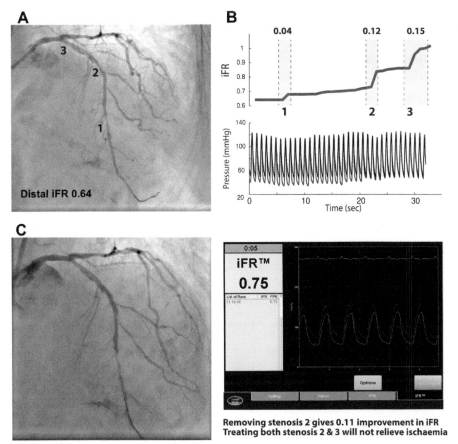

Fig. 1. Multiple lesions within this vessel contribute to ischemia. The angiogram (*A*) shows a left anterior descending artery with at least 3 discrete angiographic stenoses and diffuse atherosclerosis. Pressure wire assessment at rest demonstrates an iFR of 0.64 confirming significant ischemia but taken alone, it does not suggest which lesion should have intervention. (*B*) iFR pullback demonstrates there are 3 discrete pressure gradients correlating with angiographic disease. (*C*) Stenting stenosis 2 generates 0.11 unit gain (0.12 was predicted but assumes perfect resolution of gradients) meaning the vessel iFR is 0.75. Treatment of lesion 2 and 3, the most angiographically significant stenoses, would generate an iFR around 0.80—which remains ischemic. Lesion 3, although angiographically moderate is causing significant pressure loss and warrants further assessment. Therefore, interrogation pullback information can alter revascularization techniques and strategy before it is undertaken.

kg/min is typical. Central infusions are ideal but require additional large bore venous access. Peripheral infusions take longer to induce hyperemia and a prolonged infusion may be required. The traces should be inspected and recorded to observe for clarity and quality of the pressure trace.

PERFORMING PULLBACK PHYSIOLOGY

Physiologic pullback can be performed in every pressure wire case but provides the greatest utility in those vessels which are significant (iFR ≤0.89, FFR <0.80) and it can suggest an interventional strategy. In nonischemic vessels, a pullback trace can help confirm that a stenosis of interest is only contributing minimally to the pressure loss in the vessel. Regardless of whether a formal pullback is performed, it is recommended that after completing a pressure wire assessment, that the sensor is withdrawn to the ostium to ensure that pressure calibration has been maintained. A pressure ratio of 1.0 is expected at the ostium.

When performing physiologic pullback, the angiographic view should lay out the coronary vessel with the least amount of foreshortening. Constant radioscopic fluoroscopy should be maintained to enable co-localization of pressure gradients with the angiographic location of the sensor. The pressure wire should be withdrawn slowly, at a rate of 1-2 mm per second. This means a typical left anterior descending (LAD) vessel would take

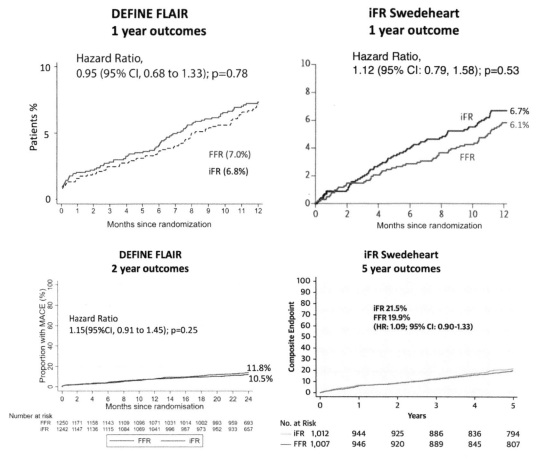

Fig. 2. iFR outcome data at 1, 2 and 5 years. iFR has been compared with FFR in 2 major randomized controlled studies, DEFINE FLAIR[25] and IFR-SwedeHeart.[26] There is no significant difference in major adverse clinical events (MACE) a composite of death, non-fatal myocardial infarction or unplanned revascularization. Image has been adapted from published studies.[25-27]

30 to 40 s to complete. In patients undergoing FFR, intravenous infusion of adenosine is recommended as intracoronary injections cannot produce sufficiently long hyperemia. Longer acting agents such as Regadenoson have been used but have not gained significant traction in the catheter lab due to a variable duration of hyperemia.

RECOGNIZING COMMON ERRORS DURING PULLBACK PHYSIOLOGY

It is common for the rate of pullback to vary and, when crossing through very tight stenoses, there may be a jumping of the sensor that can cause artifact on the pressure trace. It is also common for operators to rush the last stage of the pullback as they reach the guiding catheter (**Fig. 3**). Caution is needed as a rapid withdrawal can cause the pressure sensor to strike the guiding catheter leading to artifact. In systems with integrated

artificial intelligence, such artifacts may be automatically corrected. In older systems, the operator will need to interpret the data taking account of the artifact or repeat the pullback.

When performing a physiologic pullback, the physiologic parameter is computed in multiple locations throughout the vessel. For resting indices, such as iFR, the value at a given location will represent the iFR value of the epicardial coronary lesions proximal to the sensor with only a modest impact on the value imposed by the distal disease.[15,16,28,29] The offset between predicted and observed values for a chosen intervention are small (**Fig. 4**). Caution is needed when residual disease is close to the diagnostic threshold for ischemia, that is around 0.89 as small variations can have a larger impact on classification.[30]

For hyperemic indices, such as FFR, the raw FFR value measured during pullback is only a crude estimate of the significance of the proximal

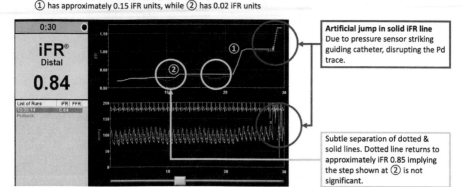

Pullback trace shows two apparent physiological lesions:
① has approximately 0.15 iFR units, while ② has 0.02 iFR units

Artificial jump in solid iFR line
Due to pressure sensor striking guiding catheter, disrupting the Pd trace.

Subtle separation of dotted & solid lines. Dotted line returns to approximately iFR 0.85 implying the step shown at ② is not significant.

Fig. 3. iFR Pullback with artifact from guiding catheter. A typical iFR pullback screen is shown. The distal IFR is 0.84 with two discrete steps on the iFR pullback trace (marked 1 and 2). A solid iFR line is shown reflecting the highest iFR value measured during the pullback process. A more subtle dotted line shows the live iFR value at the given location. When the dotted iFR line returns a lower value, it suggests the step on the solid line is artificial. The red circles denote artifact generated by the pressure sensor striking the guiding catheter or other electrical noise. The iFR trace exceeds 1.10 at this location. As the sensor had reached an iFR of 1.0 at the ostium, then the artifact can be disregarded.

disease.[10,11] This is because more distal coronary disease alters the hyperemic response of individual lesions such that is not readily calculable. Studies have suggested that the raw FFR value will under-estimate the true FFR by 40%.[31] There are formulae available to correct for the difficulties imposed by hyperemia but they are not practical as they require balloon occlusion of a stenosis to compute wedge pressure. Alternative equations have been suggested and may have utility.

UNIQUE ISSUES FOR INSTANTANEOUS WAVE-FREE RATIO PULLBACK

When performing an iFR pullback, a dedicated mode activates beat to beat iFR measurements. As this removes averaging, the distally measured value during pullback can be at variance from the formally measured iFR value that is averaged over five beats. If there is a large deviation between these values at the beginning of the pullback, it is recommended to start the process again.

When starting the pullback, a solid animated line is displaying on the console. It is recommended that a few seconds are allowed to elapse to generate a consistent line without fluctuation. This will improve the accuracy of predictions of post-PCI iFR values. The wire should be withdrawn slowly as he slower the pullback, the more heart beats and iFR readings are computed, increasing the fidelity as more iFR values are computed at a given location (**Fig. 5**). Once the pressure sensor has reached the guiding catheter

and the value of 1.0 is recorded, the pullback can be stopped and analyzed. In those with co-registration available, an angiogram should be performed without moving the image intensifier or panning to trigger automated co-registration.

During pullback, if there is ventricular ectopy or pulse irregularity, the algorithms may express caution on the associated iFR value. The pullback trace may mark areas of caution but the recording may still be valid (**Fig. 6**). If there is concern, the pullback should be repeated.

The iFR pullback systems have evolved over time. In the majority of installed systems, the operator will observe two lines being plotted—a solid and dotted line. The dotted line represents the raw iFR value. The solid line represents the highest iFR measured so far. Typically, both lines should overlie each other without significant variation and newer systems choose only to present the solid iFR line. However, if during pullback, there is an artifact due to ventricular ectopy or a whipping artifact from the pressure sensor striking a calcified coronary lesion, the solid line can jump closer to unity, whereas the true iFR represented by the dotted line may still be much lower (**Fig. 7**). In this situation, it can appear as if there is a step-up on the pressure trace and represent a focal lesion. Further pullback data will continue to produce a solid line from that point—even if it was erroneous. Vigilance is required to correct for this. In pullback traces where there has been large separation of the solid and dotted lines, the operator should consider repeating the pullback trace for reliable computation of a post PCI result.

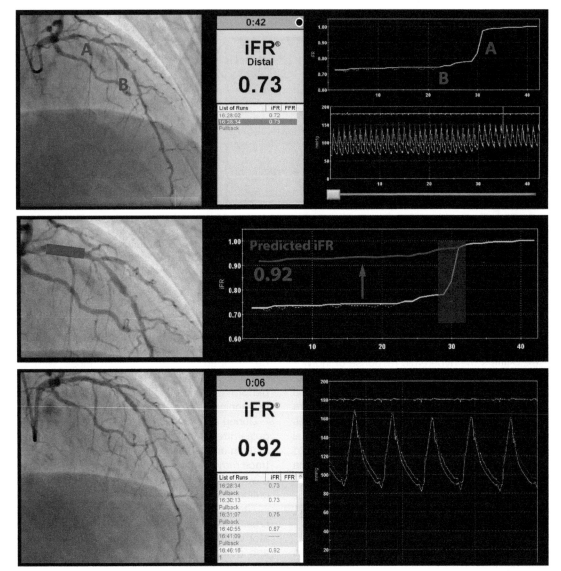

Fig. 4. iFR Pullback with prediction of post PCI result. A significantly diseased LAD vessel is shown with a combination of focal disease (marked A & B) and diffuse disease. The distal iFR is 0.73 confirming ischemia. The pullback trace shows that lesion B contributes minimally to the total vessel ischemia. Removing lesion A would not alter the pressure loss imposed by B or by the distal diffuse disease. The pressure trace therefore moves upward assuming perfect resolution of the pressure loss caused by lesion A. The predicted iFR of 0.92 is achieved intervention. This is in the non-ischemic zone although DEFINE-PCI has shown an association of lower clinical events with a post-PCI iFR ≥0.95.

CO-REGISTRATION OF ANGIOGRAPHY AND PHYSIOLOGIC DATA

Although operators can readily perform pressure wire pullback, interpreting the data can be challenging. One may not recall where a given pressure gradient corresponds to specific locations on the angiogram. Co-registration of the physiologic data with the coronary angiogram allows intuitive interpretation of both sets of data together (**Fig. 8**).

iFR co-registration is a mature technology that is readily available in many cardiac catheter laboratories world-wide. By activating co-registration at the time of wire pullback, the additional information is available without additional steps. The operator should avoid movement of the image intensifier or panning during the wire pullback. The angiographic field of view should show the entirety of the coronary vessel as well as the guiding catheter and avoid significant overlapping vessels. The presence of another intracoronary wire does

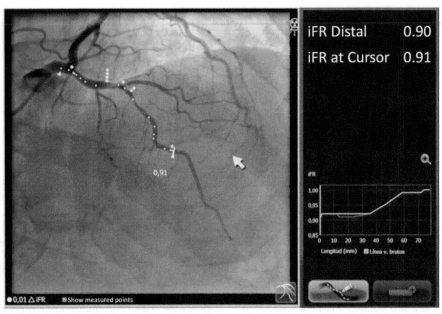

Fig. 5. iFR Pullback data depends on the speed of pullback. As iFR is measured beat to beat, the slower the pullback, the greater the fidelity. This can be visualized on co-registered pullbacks. The console can show measured points as white dots' on the angiogram. Areas of pressure loss or gradients will be between the white dots. In the shown example, there is a paucity of white dots in the lesion of interest. This is likely because the sensor was moved too quickly within the lesion. This means the co-registered pressure loss is labeled more proximal than the angiographically evident lesion. A repeat pullback would be recommended if there is doubt.

not preclude co-registration and it is also possible to co-register onto prior angiographic views or even views without contrast in cases of zero-contrast PCI.

The added value of co-registration is readily evident to operators in real-time cases. The operator can easily visualize where the greatest pressure loss occurs within the vessel and relate this to angiographic appearance. Virtual PCI can be performed to remove a given stenosis or stenoses and the system will compute an estimated post-PCI iFR, under the assumption that any performed PCI is perfect (with no residual pressure loss in the stented segment). The length of the required stenting is highly accurate. The system computes the length by tracking changes in radio-opaque marker as it moves through vessel tortuosity meaning that foreshortening is corrected.

In some cases, operators may be concerned about the loss of wire position during pullback measurement. This is particular evident in high grade stenoses that are challenging to re-wire. The pullback trace can be performed alongside a work-horse buddy wire. Provided TIMI III flow is maintained within the vessel, the presence of an additional wire does not have significant impact on the measured physiology. Caution is needed in highly tortuous vessels as the combination of dual wires may have a kinking effect on the vessel.

INTERROGATING INSTANTANEOUS WAVE-FREE RATIO PULLBACK AND PREDICTING POST-PERCUTANEOUS CORONARY INTERVENTION INSTANTANEOUS WAVE-FREE RATIO VALUES

The iFR pullback traces computes a beat-to-beat iFR value in the vessel. At every location, the measured iFR represents the physiologic significance of the stenoses proximal to the stenosis—with minimal impact of the distal disease. Removing a given stenosis has modest impact on the resting physiologic values of distal stenoses.[15,16,29] Therefore, in most circumstances it is possible to predict the post-PCI iFR value with good accuracy. In vessels with highly significant iFR values—for example, ≤0.50, the change in resting flow conditions after PCI is sufficient for the prediction to be clinically inaccurate. It should be noted that the accuracy of the post-PCI iFR value will depend on where the pressure sensor is placed before and after PCI. Care should be taken to ensure that before and after PCI values are measured at the same location.

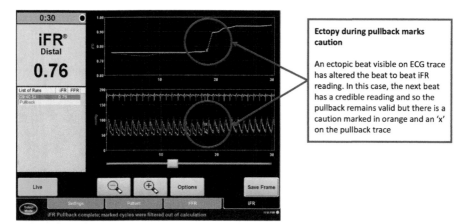

Ectopy during pullback marks caution

An ectopic beat visible on ECG trace has altered the beat to beat iFR reading. In this case, the next beat has a credible reading and so the pullback remains valid but there is a caution marked in orange and an 'x' on the pullback trace

Fig. 6. Ectopy marking caution. This figure demonstrates an iFR pullback where ventricular ectopy has marked caution. During pressure wire pullback, if there is ventricular ectopy or pulse irregularity, the algorithms may express caution on the associated iFR value with an X. In this case, the area of caution impacts the most significant area of pressure loss. Operators should review the raw pressure trace. The next heart beat is normal with a valid IFR reading and so the over observed step is likely to be valid.

The accuracy of predicted iFR values with those that are observed after real world PCI is has been shown in two non-randomized studies in which lesions were carefully selected.[15,16] More work is required to understand the real world application and how technology tolerates all-comer stenoses. The predicted post-PCI iFR value can represent a target for operators to achieve. When operators have not achieved what was predicted before PCI, this may be because there is residual pressure loss within the stented segment or important residual disease. A repeat pullback should be performed when intervention has not achieved the expected non-ischemic iFR value to identify the residual pressure loss. Adequate intracoronary nitrates and flushing of the catheter before repeat measurements is essential. In cases where intervention is performed on the pressure wire, one should consider electrical drift on the wire as this becomes more likely the longer the wire remains in situ.

USING INSTANTANEOUS WAVE-FREE RATIO TO IDENTIFY RESIDUAL ISCHEMIA AFTER PERCUTANEOUS CORONARY INTERVENTION

DEFINE PCI studied residual ischemia after routine angiographically guided PCI. 467 patients across the United States, with confirmed

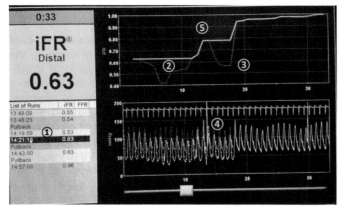

① - Large variance between initial iFR (0.53-0.54) with starting pullback value (0.63)
② & ③ - large separation of dotted & solid lines; both return to an average of 0.55, consistent with the true distal IFR value
④ & ⑤ - sensor striking severe stenosis causes an artefact that incorrectly moves solid iFR line upwards to 0.77, creating appearance of a step. However, no true physiological step at this location

Fig. 7. Artifact causing apparent stenosis on pullback trace. This pullback trace demonstrates several issues. There is a large variation between the resting iFR before pullback and the value measured during pullback. This implies a high grade stenosis and some beat to beat variation in the resting iFR value (marked 1). Moving the wire back reveals the raw iFR value is around 0.55 consistent with the raw iFR value (marked 2 and 3). There is artifact on the pressure trace, (marked 4), possibly from the pressure sensor striking the lesion. This causes the solid iFR line (which indicates the highest value measured within the vessel) to jump to 0.77 creating the appearance of two physiologic lesions within the vessel. When repeated, the artifact was removed.

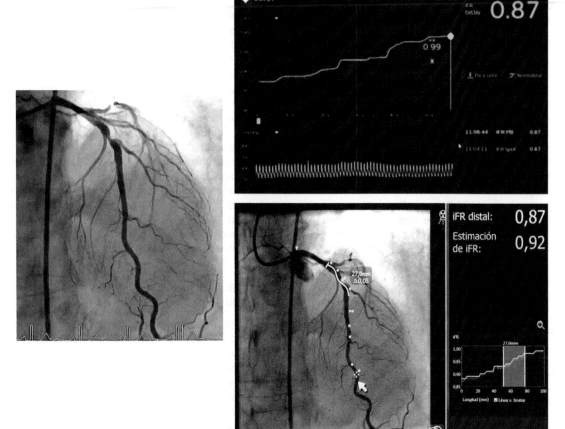

Fig. 8. Co-registration helps interpretation of pressure traces. In this left anterior descending vessel, a focal stenosis is evident in the proximal to mid-segment. iFR assessment confirms ischemia (iFR 0.87) but the pullback trace as the appearance of predominantly diffuse disease with no clear focal step. Co-registration reveals that although there is diffuse pressure loss, the vessel can be brought into the non-ischemic zone by placing a 27 mm stent in angiographically evident lesion.

ischemia on a pre-PCI iFR assessment, proceeded to PCI by angiographic appearance only.[32] After the PCI was considered complete, iFR and iFR-pullback were performed but operators were blinded to the results. were blinded to the result. As seen in other studies, 24% of patients remained ischemic with the post-PCI iFR ≤0.89. Analysis of the pullback traces showed that over 80% of these ischemic vessels were due to focal disease, defined as ≥0.03 iFR units lost across ≤15 mm. The implication of focal disease is that further intervention to these areas of focal loss with a further stent. Approximately 60% of the ischemic vessels had pressure loss outside of the already stented segment with 38% having residual pressure loss within the stent.[32] This latter point is likely explained by the modest levels of post-dilatation (only 58%).

The 1-year clinical outcome assessment of the study demonstrated that those patients with an iFR ≥0.95 post-PCI was associated with higher event free survival with 0% cardiac death or spontaneous MI and 1.8% rate of MACE vessel revascularization.[33] Those patients with iFR less than 0.95 post-PCI had a higher rate of MACE at 5.7% ($P = .04$). There was a suggestion that patients with worse angina had less symptoms when post-PCI iFR greater than 0.95.[33]

Although a useful mechanistic study, DEFINE PCI cannot provide clear evidence that a pre-PCI pullback approach would lead to improved outcomes. Furthermore, it cannot answer the question whether clinical decisions based on the post-PCI pullback would have altered outcome. A further randomized study, DEFINE-GPS is required to answer this question.

ONGOING RESEARCH IN INSTANTANEOUS WAVE-FREE RATIO PULLBACK AND CO-REGISTRATION

The DEFINE GPS study is a randomized controlled study that is currently recruiting patients across over 100 international centers.[34] It seeks to randomize approximately 3000 patients with confirmed ischemia to PCI by either standard angiographic means or to PCI guided by iFR pullback measurement. iFR co-registration will be used and those in the physiology arm will target an iFR $\geq$0.95 post-PCI or iFR greater than 0.90 in the presence of diffuse disease. The primary endpoint will assess MACE or hospitalization for unstable angina at 2 years. Secondary endpoints will assess quality of life and cost-effectiveness. This study will establish whether a pre-PCI physiology pullback adds value over and above standard angiographic PCI and is much anticipated in the field.

UNIQUE ISSUE FOR FRACTIONAL FLOW RESERVE PULLBACK

FFR uses exogenous hyperemia to maximize the pressure gradient measured across the whole cardiac cycle. As FFR relies upon maximal hyperemia to be valid, the pressure sensor should be distal within the vessel to compute a value that is valid for the whole vessel. When FFR is measured between two coronary stenoses, the presence of a distal stenosis reduces the extent of hyperemia experienced by the more proximal stenosis. Similarly, the flow presented to the distal stenosis is not maximal in the presence of a significant proximal stenosis. This 'interaction' or 'cross-talk' between stenoses means the FFR measured at a given place is not a true reflection of the significance of the lesions proximal to the sensor. Removing a stenosis will also increase hyperemic flow and alter the pressure-flow relationship within the vessel. Although there is a change in resting flow after PCI, the magnitude of the change is much smaller compared with the change in hyperemic flow. This means predicting FFR values after removing a given stenosis is less clearly computed.

When using FFR pullback, the locations causing the largest pressure gradient should be targeted for intervention first. Once intervention has be done, the FFR and FFR-pullback should be repeated to identify the next area with most pressure loss. In many cases, a lesion that previously appeared nonsignificant with an apparent FFR greater than 0.80, will now have an FFR $\leq$0.80.

PULLBACK PRESSURE GRADIENTS

A further attempt to understand the nature of coronary disease has been lead to the development of pullback pressure gradient (PPG).[35] This is computed by withdrawing a pressure wire at 1 mm/s using a motorized pullback device during maximal hyperemia. The pressure gradients measured across the whole vessel can then be assessed to identify the largest pressure gradient over a length of 20 mm. This pressure gradient can then be indexed by the pressure gradient measured across the whole vessel. The PPG index describes the extent of coronary disease in the vessel as a continuous metric. PPG index values close to 1 suggest focal disease, whereas values closer to 0 suggest diffuse disease.

Pullback pressure gradient index is calculated using the formulae given below:

$$PPG\ index = \{MaxPPG_{20mm}/\Delta FFR_{vessel}+(1-\text{length with functional disease(mm)/total vessel length (mm)})/2.$$

Early work using this approach shows the angiographically defined disease is frequently reclassified. In a cohort of 100 vessels, 30% of angiographically defined Focal disease was physiologically diffuse. It is likely PPG will be a useful research tool in numerically describing the atherosclerotic process.

It should be acknowledged, however, that PPG does not offer a solution to revascularization decisions for tandem disease. Although the pressure gradient can be mapped over the motorized pullback much like the iFR-pullback work, as hyperemia triggers crosstalk between stenoses, the gradients do not predict the post-PCI physiology.

USING POST-PERCUTANEOUS CORONARY INTERVENTION FRACTIONAL FLOW RESERVE VALUES TO OPTIMIZE PERCUTANEOUS CORONARY INTERVENTION

The value of a physiology pullback guided approach to intervention remains under-tested with few randomized studies. One study, TARGET-FFR, added a complex algorithm to guide further intervention *after* PCI was performed.[36] In this study, PCI was performed in the usual manner based on angiographic appearances and a post-PCI FFR measurement was made. Patients were randomized to one of two groups. In the control group, the post-PCI FFR value was not disclosed to the operator. In those allocated the physiologic arm, the results were disclosed and a strict protocol followed. If the recorded FFR was not $\geq$0.90, then further PCI was performed according to a pullback and pre-determined criteria. Those with residual pressure gradient within the stented segment had high pressure non-compliant balloon dilatation. Those with pressure loss of ≥ 0.05 within a <20 mm length of vessel had further stent placed. After each step, a repeat hyperemic pressure pullback was performed.

After PCI, 29% of vessels were still frankly ischemic with FFR less than 0.80 and 32% had FFR 0.81 to 0.89.[36] In the 131 patients randomized to the physiologic optimization protocol, only 40 patients (31% of the cohort) had the PCI optimization protocol followed. The operator declining in 15% cases and diffuse disease being found in 33%.[36] In the 29 patients with valid paired FFR values before and after optimized PCI, a small but statistically significant increase in FFR was noted from 0.76 ± 0.08 to 0.82 ± 0.06 ($P < .001$). Those lesions which had a further stent placed had higher gains in FFR than those having further post-dilatation to the already placed stent. 10% more patients were noted to be in the optimal FFR$\geq$0.90 range and 11% less patients in the FFR less than 0.80 range compared with controls. However, despite these small gains, procedure time was dramatically increased as was total contrast and radiation dose. Given the challenges posed by the protocol and the modest gain it remains to be seen if this approach could be introduced in more routine clinical work.

SUMMARY

As coronary disease becomes increasingly complex, there is a clear need for innovations that drive improved clinical outcomes. There remains the need to better selecting treatment strategies that will alleviate ischemia and reduce patient symptoms. The use of pressure wire pullback may support this and improve patient care. Although readily available and practically easy to perform, to date, the data to support physiology pullback has been limited. Studies have established that FFR pullback is a poor predictor of post-PCI FFR values and has a cumbersome multi-stepped approach to use the data. iFR pullback is quick to perform and has reassuring findings regarding prediction of post-PCI outcomes but only in small studies and it requires major randomized controlled data. Systems that co-register angiographic and intravascular imaging data with physiology represent a true paradigm shift in how we treat coronary stenoses and likely represents the future of PCI.

CLINICS CARE POINTS

- Careful preparation of pressure wires and a fixed protocol with appropriate normalisation of pressures and intracoronary nitrates should be used in every case.
- When analysing pressure wire pullback, look for artefact and pressure drift as this may alter clinical decision making
- Very severe coronary stenoses can cause cross-talk between lesions at both rest and hyperaemia which can limit accuracy of post-PCI prediction
- PCI strategy should ensure plaque is covered and avoid landing stents within significant disease as this impacts on the durability of the result.

DISCLOSURE

Dr S.S. Nijjer has received honoraria for speaking for Philips and has an ongoing Consulting agreement.

REFERENCES

1. Toth G, Hamilos M, Pyxaras S, et al. Evolving concepts of angiogram: fractional flow reserve discordances in 4000 coronary stenoses. Eur Heart J 2014;35(40):2831–8. https://doi.org/10.1093/eurheartj/ehu094.
2. Pijls NHJ, Gelder BV, Voort PV der, et al. Fractional Flow Reserve A Useful Index to Evaluate the Influence of an Epicardial Coronary Stenosis on Myocardial Blood Flow. Circulation 1995;92(11):3183–93. https://doi.org/10.1161/01.CIR.92.11.3183.
3. Pijls NH, De Bruyne B, Peels K, et al. Measurement of fractional flow reserve to assess the functional severity of coronary-artery stenoses. N Engl J Med 1996;334(26):1703–8. https://doi.org/10.1056/NEJM199606273342604.
4. Escaned J, Collet C, Ryan N, et al. Clinical outcomes of state-of-the-art percutaneous coronary revascularization in patients with de novo three vessel disease: 1-year results of the SYNTAX II study. Eur Heart J 2017;38(42):3124–34. https://doi.org/10.1093/eurheartj/ehx512.
5. Banning AP, Serruys P, De Maria GL, et al. Five-year outcomes after state-of-the-art percutaneous coronary revascularization in patients with de novo three-vessel disease: final results of the SYNTAX II study. Eur Heart J 2022;43(13):1307–16. https://doi.org/10.1093/eurheartj/ehab703.

6. Lee JM, Hwang D, Choi KH, et al. Prognostic Implications of Relative Increase and Final Fractional Flow Reserve in Patients With Stent Implantation. JACC: Cardiovasc Interventions 2018;11(20):2099–109. https://doi.org/10.1016/j.jcin.2018.07.031.

7. Agarwal SK, Kasula S, Hacioglu Y, et al. Utilizing Post-Intervention Fractional Flow Reserve to Optimize Acute Results and the Relationship to Long-Term Outcomes. JACC: Cardiovasc Interventions 2016;9(10):1022–31. https://doi.org/10.1016/j.jcin.2016.01.046.

8. Pijls NHJ. Coronary Pressure Measurement After Stenting Predicts Adverse Events at Follow-Up: A Multicenter Registry. Circulation 2002;105(25):2950–4. https://doi.org/10.1161/01.CIR.0000020547.92091.76.

9. Boden WE, O'Rourke RA, Teo KK, et al. Optimal medical therapy with or without PCI for stable coronary disease. N Engl J Med 2007;356(15):1503–16. https://doi.org/10.1056/NEJMoa070829.

10. Pijls NHJ, Bruyne BD, Bech GJW, et al. Coronary Pressure Measurement to Assess the Hemodynamic Significance of Serial Stenoses Within One Coronary Artery Validation in Humans. Circulation 2000;102(19):2371–7. https://doi.org/10.1161/01.CIR.102.19.2371.

11. De Bruyne B, Pijls NHJ, Heyndrickx GR, et al. Pressure-Derived Fractional Flow Reserve to Assess Serial Epicardial Stenoses Theoretical Basis and Animal Validation. Circulation 2000;101(15):1840–7. https://doi.org/10.1161/01.CIR.101.15.1840.

12. Kim HL, Koo BK, Nam CW, et al. Clinical and Physiological Outcomes of Fractional Flow Reserve-Guided Percutaneous Coronary Intervention in Patients With Serial Stenoses Within One Coronary Artery. JACC: Cardiovasc Interventions. 2012;5(10):1013–8. https://doi.org/10.1016/j.jcin.2012.06.017.

13. Park SJ, Ahn JM, Pijls NHJ, et al. Validation of Functional State of Coronary Tandem Lesions Using Computational Flow Dynamics. Am J Cardiol 2012;110(11):1578–84. https://doi.org/10.1016/j.amjcard.2012.07.023.

14. Nam CW, Koo BK. Fractional Flow Reserve Assessment of Serial Lesions. 2014. Available at: http://www.radcliffecardiology.com/articles/fractional-flow-reserve-assessment-serial-lesions. Accessed May 13, 2014.

15. Nijjer SS, Sen S, Petraco R, et al. Pre-Angioplasty Instantaneous Wave-Free Ratio Pullback Provides Virtual Intervention and Predicts Hemodynamic Outcome for Serial Lesions and Diffuse Coronary Artery Disease. JACC: Cardiovasc Interventions. 2014;7(12):1386–96. https://doi.org/10.1016/j.jcin.2014.06.015.

16. Kikuta Y, Cook CM, Sharp ASP, et al. Pre-Angioplasty Instantaneous Wave-Free Ratio Pullback Predicts Hemodynamic Outcome In Humans With Coronary Artery Disease: Primary Results of the International Multicenter iFR GRADIENT Registry. JACC: Cardiovasc Interventions 2018;11(8):757–67. https://doi.org/10.1016/j.jcin.2018.03.005.

17. Knuuti J, Wijns W, Saraste A, et al. 2019 ESC Guidelines for the diagnosis and management of chronic coronary syndromes. Eur Heart J 2019;100(k504):106. https://doi.org/10.1093/eurheartj/ehz425.

18. Lawton JS, Tamis-Holland JE, Bangalore S, et al. 2021 ACC/AHA/SCAI Guideline for Coronary Artery Revascularization: A Report of the American College of Cardiology/American Heart Association Joint Committee on Clinical Practice Guidelines. Circulation 2022;145(3):e18–114. https://doi.org/10.1161/CIR.0000000000001038.

19. Tonino PAL, De Bruyne B, Pijls NHJ, et al. Fractional Flow Reserve versus Angiography for Guiding Percutaneous Coronary Intervention. New Engl J Med 2009;360(3):213–24. https://doi.org/10.1056/NEJMoa0807611.

20. Bech GJ, De Bruyne B, Bonnier HJ, et al. Long-term follow-up after deferral of percutaneous transluminal coronary angioplasty of intermediate stenosis on the basis of coronary pressure measurement. J Am Coll Cardiol 1998;31(4):841–7.

21. Pijls NHJ, van Schaardenburgh P, Manoharan G, et al. Percutaneous coronary intervention of functionally nonsignificant stenosis: 5-year follow-up of the DEFER Study. J Am Coll Cardiol 2007;49(21):2105–11. https://doi.org/10.1016/j.jacc.2007.01.087.

22. Zimmermann FM, Ferrara A, Johnson NP, et al. Deferral vs. performance of percutaneous coronary intervention of functionally non-significant coronary stenosis: 15-year follow-up of the DEFER trial. Eur Heart J 2015;36(45):3182–8. https://doi.org/10.1093/eurheartj/ehv452.

23. Sen S, Escaned J, Malik IS, et al. Development and validation of a new adenosine-independent index of stenosis severity from coronary wave-intensity analysis: results of the ADVISE (ADenosine Vasodilator Independent Stenosis Evaluation) study. J Am Coll Cardiol 2012;59(15):1392–402. https://doi.org/10.1016/j.jacc.2011.11.003.

24. Gotberg M, Cook CM, Sen S, et al. The Evolving Future of Instantaneous Wave-Free Ratio and Fractional Flow Reserve. J Am Coll Cardiol 2017;70(11):1379–402. https://doi.org/10.1016/j.jacc.2017.07.770.

25. Davies JE, Sen S, Dehbi HM, et al. Use of the Instantaneous Wave-free Ratio or Fractional Flow Reserve in PCI. New Engl J Med 2017;376(19):1824–34. https://doi.org/10.1056/NEJMoa1700445.

26. Gotberg M, Christiansen EH, Gudmundsdottir IJ, et al. Instantaneous Wave-free Ratio versus Fractional Flow Reserve to Guide PCI. New Engl J Med

2017;376(19):1813–23. https://doi.org/10.1056/NEJMoa1616540.

27. Götberg M, Berntorp K, Rylance R, et al. 5-Year Outcomes of PCI Guided by Measurement of Instantaneous Wave-Free Ratio Versus Fractional Flow Reserve. J Am Coll Cardiol 2022;79(10):965–74. https://doi.org/10.1016/j.jacc.2021.12.030.

28. Nijjer SS, de Waard GA, Sen S, et al. Coronary pressure and flow relationships in humans: phasic analysis of normal and pathological vessels and the implications for stenosis assessment: a report from the Iberian-Dutch-English (IDEAL) collaborators. Eur Heart J 2016;37(26):2069–80. https://doi.org/10.1093/eurheartj/ehv626.

29. Nijjer SS, Petraco R, van de Hoef TP, et al. Change in Coronary Blood Flow After Percutaneous Coronary Intervention in Relation to Baseline Lesion Physiology Results of the JUSTIFY-PCI Study. Circ Cardiovasc Interv 2015;8(6):e001715. https://doi.org/10.1161/CIRCINTERVENTIONS.114.001715.

30. Modi BN, De Silva K, Rajani R, et al. Physiology-Guided Management of Serial Coronary Artery Disease: A Review. JAMA Cardiol 2018;3(5):432–8. https://doi.org/10.1001/jamacardio.2018.0236.

31. Modi BN, Sankaran S, Kim HJ, et al. Predicting the Physiological Effect of Revascularization in Serially Diseased Coronary Arteries. Circ Cardiovasc Interventions 2019;12(2):e007577. https://doi.org/10.1161/CIRCINTERVENTIONS.118.007577.

32. Jeremias A, Davies JE, Maehara A, et al. Blinded Physiological Assessment of Residual Ischemia After Successful Angiographic Percutaneous Coronary Intervention. DEFINE PCI Study 2019;12(20):1991–2001. https://doi.org/10.1016/j.jcin.2019.05.054.

33. Patel MR, Jeremias A, Maehara A, et al. 1-Year Outcomes of Blinded Physiological Assessment of Residual Ischemia After Successful PCI: DEFINE PCI Trial. JACC: Cardiovasc Interventions 2022;15(1):52–61. https://doi.org/10.1016/j.jcin.2021.09.042.

34. Philips Clinical, Medical Affairs Global. *Distal Evaluation of Functional Performance With Intravascular Sensors to Assess the Narrowing Effect: Guided Physiologic Stenting.* clinicaltrials.gov. 2022. Available at: https://clinicaltrials.gov/ct2/show/NCT04451044. Accessed April 14, 2022.

35. Collet C, Sonck J, Vandeloo B, et al. Measurement of Hyperemic Pullback Pressure Gradients to Characterize Patterns of Coronary Atherosclerosis. J Am Coll Cardiol 2019;74(14):1772–84. https://doi.org/10.1016/j.jacc.2019.07.072.

36. Collison D, Didagelos M, Aetesam-ur-Rahman M, et al. Post-stenting fractional flow reserve vs coronary angiography for optimization of percutaneous coronary intervention (TARGET-FFR). European Heart Journal 2021;42(45):4656–68. https://doi.org/10.1093/eurheartj/ehab449.

Physiologic Assessment After Percutaneous Coronary Interventions and Functionally Optimized Revascularization

Doosup Shin, MD[a,1], Seung Hun Lee, MD, PhD[b,1], David Hong, MD[c],
Ki Hong Choi, MD[c], Joo Myung Lee, MD, MPH, PhD[c,*]

KEYWORDS

- Percutaneous coronary intervention • Fractional flow reserve • Non-hyperemic pressure ratios
- Instantaneous wave-free ratio

KEY POINTS

- Post-PCI physiologic indexes have important prognostic values.
- Post-PCI physiologic assessment enables functional optimization of PCI.
- Physiology-guided pre-PCI planning and post-PCI optimization will improve outcomes.

INTRODUCTION

The primary goal of percutaneous coronary intervention (PCI) in patients with coronary artery disease (CAD) is to resolve myocardial ischemia, providing symptom relief and improved prognosis. As angiographic assessment of CAD has limited predictability for the presence of ischemia due to the dissociation of anatomic and functional measures of coronary stenosis severity,[1] coronary physiologic assessment has been used to define ischemia-causing stenoses, and physiology-guided PCI has been well validated in multiple randomized clinical trials.[2–5] Therefore, recent guidelines for revascularization recommended using fractional flow reserve (FFR) or non-hyperemic pressure ratios (NHPRs), such as instantaneous wave-free ratio (iFR), to assess the hemodynamic relevance of intermediate-grade stenosis.[6,7]

However, physiology-guided PCI does not guarantee functionally optimized PCI. Multiple studies have shown that a substantial proportion of patients who underwent angiographically successful PCI had evidence of residual ischemia manifested by suboptimal post-PCI FFR[8–10] or iFR values,[11] which were associated with worse clinical outcomes.[8–10,12–18] Therefore, post-PCI physiologic assessment would not only provide crucial information on the effect of revascularization but also allow us to identify the presence of residual disease causing myocardial ischemia that cannot be determined by angiogram, thereby providing a potential opportunity to achieve functionally optimized revascularization. In this comprehensive review, we discuss the importance of post-PCI physiologic assessment and its potential role to improve PCI patient outcomes and prognosis.

This article originally appeared in *Interventional Cardiology Clinics*, Volume 12 Issue 1, January 2023.
^a Division of Cardiology, Duke University Medical Center, 2301 Erwin Rd, Durham, NC 27710, USA;
^b Department of Internal Medicine and Cardiovascular Center, Chonnam National University Hospital, 42, Jebong-ro, Dong-gu, Gwangju 61469, Republic of Korea; ^c Division of Cardiology, Department of Internal Medicine, Heart Vascular Stroke Institute, Samsung Medical Center, Sungkyunkwan University School of Medicine, 81 Irwon-ro, Gangnam-gu, Seoul 06351, Republic of Korea
¹ Contributed equally to this work.
* Corresponding author.
E-mail addresses: drone80@hanmail.net; joomyung.lee@samsung.com

Prognostic Implications of Post-Percutaneous Coronary Intervention Physiologic Indexes

Table 1 summarizes previous studies on post-PCI physiologic indexes and their prognostic implications.[12–17,19–33] Regardless of stent type used, low post-PCI FFR values have consistently been associated with worse clinical outcomes. In a patient-level meta-analysis, post-PCI FFR showed an inverse relationship with subsequent events (hazard ratio [HR]: 0.86, 95% confidence interval [CI]: 0.80 to 0.93; $P < .001$).[8] One of the limitations is that the optimal cut-off values for the post-PCI FFR varied among the studies, although they were slightly lower among the studies using second-generation drug-eluting stent (DES) (0.84–0.90) compared with earlier reports with bare-metal stent or mainly first-generation DES. The heterogeneity of the optimal cut-off values of post-PCI FFR stems from the fact that the values were set to predict subsequent clinical events that would be affected by study population, event rates, and the definition of clinical events of each study, whereas the optimal cut-off value of pre-PCI FFR was determined to identify the presence of ischemia using non-invasive stress tests.[34] Also, the optimal cut-off value of post-PCI FFR could be lower in the left anterior descending (LAD) artery than non-LAD,[17] because the LAD generally supplies a larger subtended myocardium, which is one of the key determinants of hyperemic coronary flow and consequently FFR.[35] Nevertheless, it is apparent that suboptimal post-PCI FFR values have consistently been shown as an independent predictor for worse clinical outcomes.

Recent studies have also reported the prognostic implications of post-PCI NHPRs. In the study by Hakeem and colleagues,[36] patients with suboptimal post-PCI resting distal-to-aortic pressure ratio (Pd/Pa) ($\leq$ 0.96) had a significantly higher risk of major adverse cardiovascular events compared with patients having optimal post-PCI resting Pd/Pa greater than 0.96 (24% vs 15%; $P = .0006$).[36] Similarly, a multicenter study from the PERSPECTIVE-PCI (Prognostic Perspective of Invasive Hyperemic and Non-Hyperemic Physiologic Indices Measured After Percutaneous Coronary Intervention) registry showed a significant difference in target vessel failure (TVF) according to ischemic cut-off values for Pd/Pa ($\leq$ 0.92 vs > 0.92; 6.2% vs 2.5%; $P = .029$).[37] In DEFINE-PCI (Physiologic Assessment of Coronary Stenosis Following PCI) study where angiographically successful PCI was achieved, post-PCI iFR $\geq$ 0.95 was associated with a significant reduction in the composite of cardiac death, spontaneous

myocardial infarction, or clinically driven target vessel revascularization compared with post-PCI iFR less than 0.95 (1.8% vs 5.7%; $P = .04$).[18]

When interpreting post-PCI physiologic indexes, it is important to understand they can be affected by transient changes in boundary conditions, such as driving pressure, microcirculatory resistance, or coronary flow.[38] Studies reported that procedure-related transient microcirculatory dysfunction can influence myocardial perfusion imaging and post-PCI FFR values.[39,40] Therefore, caution needs to be used when assessing post-PCI FFR values or FFR gains in the presence of severe underlying microvascular disease or transient microvascular dysfunction during PCI manifested as no-reflow or slow-flow.[38] Similarly, post-PCI NHPRs can also be influenced by transient changes in boundary conditions such as increased heart rate, elevated sympathetic tone, or post-occlusion reactive hyperemia.[38] A recent study by Shin and colleagues[37] showed discordance between post-PCI FFR and resting Pd/Pa values which could, in part, be explained by an increased resting coronary flow in post-PCI phase due to reactive hyperemia, resulting in falsely low resting Pd/Pa values. Therefore, it would be important to ensure sufficient recovery time before measuring the NHPRs, and rechecking with post-PCI FFR if uncertainty remains.

Prognostic Implications of Post-Percutaneous Coronary Intervention Physiologic Gain

A few studies showed that not only the absolute value of post-PCI physiologic indexes but also the degree of their changes after PCI affected outcomes and prognosis. Compared with post-PCI FFR which reflects the presence of residual disease in the entire target vessel after PCI, increase in FFR values after PCI (or FFR gain) reflects the degree of net physiologic benefits from the revascularization procedure itself. FFR gain can be calculated as an absolute increase of FFR values (ΔFFR: post-PCI FFR – pre-PCI FFR) or a relative increase of FFR values (percent FFR increase: [post-PCI FFR – pre-PCI FFR]/pre-PCI FFR $\times$ 100).[15,16,41] In the combined cohort of FAME and FAME 2 trials, higher ΔFFR after PCI was associated with improvement of quality of life and anginal symptoms, as well as reduced risk of vessel-oriented clinical events.[16,41] In a study by Lee and colleagues,[15] patients with low percent FFR increase ($\leq$ 15%) showed a significantly higher risk of TVF than those with a high percent FFR increase. Furthermore, a percent FFR increase was independently associated with TVF risk, and adding a percent FFR increase to

Table 1
Clinical studies evaluating prognostic impact of post-percutaneous coronary intervention fractional flow reserve or non-hyperemic pressure ratios

Study	Inclusion	Device	Follow-up, Months	Post-PCI Index	Results	Comment
Clinical studies evaluating prognostic impact of post-PCI fractional flow reserve						
Bech et al,[19] 1999	60 SIHD with SVD	Balloon angioplasty	24	FFR<0.90	MACE rates between post-PCI FFR<0.90 vs ≥0.90 were 41% vs 12% ($P = .012$).	Post-PCI FFR after successful balloon angioplasty with residual %DS<50% on visual assessment. Post-PCI FFR≥0.90 was achieved in 48% of patients.
Pijls et al,[20] 2002	750 SIHD or ACS	BMS	6	FFR<0.90	MACE rates were 4.9% in post-PCI FFR>0.95, 6.2% in FFR 0.90%–0.95%, 20.3% in FFR<0.90, and 29.5% in FFR<0.80.	Post-PCI FFR after successful stent implantation with residual %DS<10% on visual assessment. Post-PCI FFR>0.95 was achieved in 36% and >0.90 in 68% of patients.
Dupouy et al,[21] 2005	100 SIHD with SVD	BMS	6	FFR ≤ 0.95	Post-PCI FFR >0.95 at 6 mo showed lower angina frequency than ≤ 0.95 (19% vs 52%).	To achieve post-PCI FFR>0.95, higher inflation pressure was needed. Only 52% patients with residual %DS<20% had FFR>0.95.
Klauss et al,[22] 2005	119 SIHD	BMS	6	FFR<0.95	Post-PCI FFR<0.95 was independent predictor of MACE (OR 6.22, 95% CI 1.79–1.62, $P = .004$).	Post-PCI FFR after residual %DS<10% on visual assessment. Post-PCI FFR≥0.95 was achieved in 55% of patients.

(continued on next page)

Table 1
(continued)

Study	Inclusion	Device	Follow-up, Months	Post-PCI Index	Results	Comment
Jensen et al,[23] 2007	98 SIHD with SVD	BMS	9	NR	Patients with step-up in FFR between distal vessel and distal stent edge showed higher binary restenosis (44.0% vs 8.1%, $P < .001$).	Post-PCI FFR was measured after residual %DS 0% on visual assessment. The prognostic impact of residual diffuse atherosclerotic disease after PCI was evaluated by FFR step-up amount in the distal segment of vessel.
Nam et al,[26] 2011	80 SIHD or ACS (non-culprit)	First-generation DES	12	FFR $\leq$ 0.90	MACE rates between post-PCI FFR $\leq$ 0.90 vs >0.90 were 12.5% vs 2.5% ($P < .01$). Target vessel location (LAD vs non-LAD) was independent predictor of post-PCI FFR.	Post-PCI FFR was measured after residual %DS <20% on visual assessment. Post-PCI FFR>0.90 was achieved in 50% of patients.
Leesar et al,[25] 2011	66 SIHD with SVD	BMS (43%) or First-generation DES (57%)	24	FFR<0.96	MACE rates between post-PCI FFR<0.96 vs $\geq$0.96 were 28% vs 6% ($P = .02$). After stenting, FFR step-up across the stent was measured in patients with post-PCI FFR<0.96.	If there was trans-stent FFR gradient, further adjunctive balloon was performed using non-compliant balloon. The additional procedure increased the proportion of patients with post-PCI FFR $\geq$0.96 from 48% to 53%.

Source	Population	DES Type	Follow-up (mo)	FFR Cutoff	Results	Comments
Ishii et al,[24] 2011	33 SIHD	First-generation DES	8	NR	Patients with 8-mo angiographic restenosis had lower post-PCI FFR (0.81 ± 0.12 vs 0.92 ± 0.06, $P = .029$). Trans-stent FFR gradient was higher in the restenosis group. Distal segment FFR step-up was not associated with restenosis in stented segment.	Adjunctive high-pressure balloon inflation was performed until angiographic residual stenosis <25%. IVUS-guided DES implantation. Prognostic impact of trans-stent FFR gradient was evaluated.
Ito et al,[27] 2014	97 SIHD or ACS (non-culprit)	Second-generation DES	Median 17.8	FFR ≤ 0.90	MACE rate was significantly higher in patients with post-PCI FFR ≤ 0.90 vs >0.90 were 17% vs 2% ($P = .02$).	Post-PCI FFR was measured after residual %DS <30% on QCA. IVUS-guided DES implantation. Mainly second-generation DES was used (96.9%).
Doh et al,[28] 2015	107 SIHD or ACS (non-culprit)	First- (60.5%) or second- (39.5%) generation DES	36	FFR<0.89	TVF rates between post-PCI FFR<0.89 vs ≥0.89 were 11% vs 39% ($P = .03$). Cut-off of IVUS minimum stent area for post-PCI FFR≥0.89 was 5.4 mm².	Post-PCI FFR was measured after residual %DS <10% on visual assessment. IVUS-guided DES implantation. Post-PCI FFR≥0.89 was achieved in 83% of patients.

(continued on next page)

Table 1
(*continued*)

Study	Inclusion	Device	Follow-up, Months	Post-PCI Index	Results	Comment
Reith et al,[29] 2015	66 SIHD	DES	20	FFR ≤ 0.905	MACE rates between post-PCI FFR ≤ 0.905 vs >0.905 were 35.9% vs 5.3% (P = .01). Cut-off of OCT percent area stenosis after PCI for MACE was ≤ 16.85%.	Post-PCI FFR was measured after residual %DS <10% on visual assessment. OCT-guided DES implantation. Post-PCI FFR>0.905 was achieved in 61% of patients. DES type was not specified.
Agarwal et al,[12]	574 SIHD or ACS	BMS (21%) or DES (79%)	31	FFR ≤ 0.86	MACE rates between post-PCI FFR ≤ 0.86 vs >0.86 were 23% vs 17% (P = .02). Subsequent procedure based on post-PCI FFR increased final-PCI FFR from 0.78 ± 0.07– 0.87 ± 0.05 (42% post dilatation, 33% additional stenting, 18% both dilatation and stenting, 9% IVUS or OCT).	Post-PCI FFR>0.86 was achieved in 68% of patients. FFR<0.86 had incremental prognostic value over clinical and angiographic variables for MACE prediction. DES type was not specified. The authors showed that additional interventions targeting a higher post-PCI FFR would improve patient outcome.

Study	Population	Stent type	FFR cutoff	Results	Comments
Kasula et al,[30] 2016	390 SIHD and 189 ACS (NSTEMI or UA)	BMS (26%) or DES (74%) in ACS patients	FFR ≤ 0.91 for ACS	Patients with final FFR values > 0.91 had significantly less adverse events than those with final FFR ≤ 0.91 after ACS (19% vs 30%; $P = .03$). Patients with ACS who achieved final FFR of >0.91 had similar outcomes compared with patients with SIHD (19% vs 16%; $P = .51$).	This study appears to use a similar database of the study by Agarwal et al. 2016(12), but focused on ACS population. The authors showed prognostic value of post-PCI FFR in patients with ACS. This study measured FFR in presumed culprit vessel of NSTEMI or UA patients. DES type was not specified.
Piroth et al,[14]	639 SIHD or ACS	First- or second-generation DES	FFR<0.92	VOCE rates between post-PCI FFR<0.92 vs ≥0.92 were 8.7% vs 4.2% (HR 2.14, 95% CI 1.19–3.84, $P = .011$). However, positive likelihood ratio of post-PCI FFR for predicting VOCE was limited (<1.4).	Post-hoc analysis from FAME (69.2% of FFR-guided arm) and FAME 2 (64.2% of FFR-guided PCI plus medical treatment arm) trials.
Li et al,[13] 2017	1476 SIHD or UA	Second-generation DES	FFR ≤ 0.88	TVF rates between post-PCI FFR<0.88 vs ≥0.88 were 12.3% vs 6.1% ($P = .002$), driven by differences in cardiac death (1.9% vs 0.6%, $P = .018$) and target vessel revascularization	Post-PCI FFR was measured after residual %DS <10% on visual assessment. Post-PCI FFR>0.88 was achieved in 67.6% of patients. Post-PCI FFR was measured 10 mm distal to the lesion

(continued on next page)

Table 1
(continued)

Study	Inclusion	Device	Follow-up, Months	Post-PCI Index	Results	Comment
					(11.8% vs 5.2%, P = .001). Post-PCI FFR<0.88 was independent predictor of TVF at 3 y.	or stent edge, not at the distal segment of the vessel.
Nishi et al,[41] 2018	716 SIHD	First- or second-generation DES	12	Tertile value of Δ FFR	There was significant association between ΔFFR (post-PCI FFR – pre-PCI FFR) and quality of life (EQ-5D index) at 1 mo and 1 yr after PCI (P for trend = 0.047 and 0.009 for 1 mo and 1 yr analysis, respectively).	Post-hoc analysis of patient-level pooled data of FAME and FAME 2 trials, similar to the study by Piroth et al.[14] or Fournier et al.[16] The larger FFR gain from PCI (higher ΔFFR), the greater improvement of quality of life after PCI.
Lee JM et al,[15] 2018	621 SIHD or ACS (non-culprit)	Second-generation DES	24	FFR<0.84	TVF rates between post-PCI FFR<0.84 vs ≥0.84 were 9.1% vs 2.6%, HR 3.37, 95% CI 1.41–8.03, P = .006. Percent FFR increase also had prognostic impact (≤ 15% vs >15%, 9.2% vs 3.0%, HR 3.61, 95% CI 1.54–8.46, P = .003). Percent FFR increase had incremental prognostic value in	Post-PCI FFR was measured after residual %DS <20% on visual assessment. Post-PCI FFR≥0.84 was achieved in 66.0% of patients. Percent FFR increase>15% was achieved in 69.2% of patients. Among the post-PCI FFR≥0.84 group, there were no significant

					addition to clinical risk factors and post-PCI FFR for TVF prediction.	differences in clinical outcomes according to percent FFR increase
Hwang et al,[17] 2019	835 SIHD or ACS (non-culprit)	Second-generation DES	24	FFR ≤ 0.84	TVF rates were significantly different between FFR ≤ 0.84 vs >0.84 in all vessels (8.3% vs 3.1%, $P < .001$). LAD (≤ 0.82) and non-LAD (≤ 0.88) showed different best cut-off value for predicting TVF.	Post-PCI FFR was measured after residual %DS <20% on visual assessment.
von Bommel et al,[33] 2019	637 SIHD or ACS	Second-generation DES	1	FFR ≤ 0.90	Post-PCI FFR>0.90 was achieved in 50% of lesions. No significant difference in MACE between post-PCI FFR ≤ 0.90 vs >0.90 at 1 mo (2.0% vs 1.5%, $P = .636$).	Post-PCI FFR was measured using microcatheter system (Navvus RXi, ACIST Medical System) at 20 mm distal from distal edge of the stent. Irrespective of post-PCI FFR, no further treatment was allowed.
Azzalini et al,[31] 2019	65 SIHD or unstable angina	Second-generation DES	12	FFR<0.90	MACE rates between post-PCI FFR<0.90 vs ≥0.90 were 31.6% vs 9.1% ($P = .047$). Residual distal lesion was the most common reason of post-PCI FFR<0.90 (42%), followed by residual uncovered	Post-PCI FFR was measured using microcatheter system (Navvus RXi, ACIST Medical System). Operators decided further treatment after post-PCI FFR and then final post-PCI FFR was measured.

(continued on next page)

Table 1
(continued)

Study	Inclusion	Device	Follow-up, Months	Post-PCI Index	Results	Comment
					proximal (14%) and distal plaques (2%), stent under-expansion (2%), and edge dissections (2%). No plausible reason was identified in 37%.	Post-PCI FFR≥0.90 was achieved in 33.8% of patients.
Hoshino et al,[32] 2019	201 SIHD with de novo LAD lesions	Second-generation DES	Median 24	FFR<0.86	VOCE was significantly higher if post-PCI FFR <0.86 (log-rank $P = .002$) but not MACE (log-rank $P = .084$). D-index (difference of post-PCI FFR between distal vessel and distal stent edge divided by the length between the 2 points) was significantly lower in vessels with clinical events. The optimal D-index cutoff value for VOCE was 0.017/ cm and was a significant predictor for VOCE.	Only LAD lesions were included. Study included patients who underwent IVUS-guided second-generation DES implantation in LAD. The prognostic impact of residual diffuse atherosclerotic disease after successful IVUS-guided PCI was evaluated by the D-index.

| Fournier et al,[16] 2019 | 639 SIHD | First- or second-generation DES | 24 | Δ FFR ≤ 0.24 | The ΔFFR (post-PCI FFR – pre-PCI FFR) was significantly associated with improvement of angina class and the risk of VOCE at 2 y. The risk of VOCE was significantly higher in the lowest tertile (ΔFFR ≤ 0.18) than the highest tertile (ΔFFR >0.31) (HR 2.01, 95% CI 1.03–3.92, $P = .04$). ΔFFR ≤ 0.24 was the most closely associated value with VOCE. | Post-hoc analysis of patient-level pooled data of FAME and FAME 2 trials, similar to the study by Piroth et al.[14] or Nishi et al.[41] The larger FFR gain from PCI (higher ΔFFR), the higher the symptomatic relief and the lower the event rate. |
| Yang et al,[50] 2020 | 135 SIHD or UA with LAD lesions | Second-generation DES | 72 | Trans-stent FFR gradient ≥0.04 | Trans-stent FFR gradient ≥0.04 was independent predictor of IVUS MSA<5.5 mm². Patients with trans-stent FFR gradient ≥0.04 showed significantly higher risk of MACE than those with trans-stent FFR gradient <0.04 (30.4% vs 6.6%, $P = .031$). | Only LAD lesions were included. Study included patients who underwent IVUS-guided second-generation DES implantation in LAD. Prognostic impact of trans-stent FFR gradient was evaluated. |

(continued on next page)

Table 1
(continued)

Clinical studies evaluating prognostic impact of post-PCI non-hyperemic pressure ratios

Study	Inclusion	Device	Follow-up, Months	Post-PCI Index	Results	Comment
Hakeem et al,[36] 2019	574 SIHD or ACS	Second-generation DES	30	FFR ≤ 0.86 Resting Pd/Pa ≤ 0.96	MACE rates between post-PCI FFR ≤ 0.86 vs >0.86 were 23% vs 17% (P = .02). MACE rates between post-PCI resting Pd/Pa ≤ 0.96 vs >0.96 were 24% vs 15% (P = .0006). Patients with resting Pd/Pa ≤ 0.96 and FFR ≤ 0.86 had the highest event rate (25%).	Post-PCI resting Pd/Pa had incremental prognostic value in addition to clinical/angiographic variables and post-PCI FFR for MACE prediction.
Jeremias et al,[11] 2019 and Patel et al,[18] 2022	500 SIHD or ACS	Second-generation DES	12	iFR ≤ 0.89 for detection of ischemia iFR <0.95 for clinical outcomes	24.0% of patients showed post-PCI iFR ≤ 0.89 after operator judged angiographically successful PCI. Among these patients, iFR pullback showed 81.6% had untreated focal stenosis (38.4% within stent, 31.5% in proximal, 30.1% in distal segment) and 18.4% had diffuse disease.	Post-PCI iFR was measured after operator judged the procedure was completed. Post-PCI iFR pullback recording classified the patterns into focal (iFR gradient ≥0.03 within ≤ 15 mm length) or diffuse disease (iFR gradient ≥0.03 over >15 mm length). Optimal cut-off value of post-PCI iFR was <0.95 (AUC 0.74,

Study	Patients	Stent	Follow-up	Threshold	Results
					Patients with post-PCI iFR<0.95 showed significantly higher risk of cardiac death or spontaneous MI (3.2% vs 0.0%, log rank P = .02) or higher risk of cardiac death, spontaneous MI, or clinically driven TVR (5.7% vs 1.8%, log rank P = .04) than those with post-PCI iFR≥0.95.	95% CI 0.61–0.88) for 1-y cardiac death or spontaneous MI.
Shin et al.[37] 2020	588 SIHD or ACS (non-culprit)	Second-generation DES	24	FFR ≤ 0.80 Resting Pd/Pa ≤ 0.92	After angiographically successful PCI, 18.5% had post-PCI FFR ≤ 0.80 and 36.9% showed post-PCI Pd/Pa ≤ 0.92. In post-PCI Pd/Pa>0.92 group, 93.8% of patients showed concordant results with post-PCI FFR>0.80. Conversely, in post-PCI Pd/Pa ≤ 0.92 group, 60.4% of patients showed post-PCI FFR >0.80.	Post-PCI resting Pd/Pa and FFR was measured after residual %DS <20% on visual assessment. Among patients with abnormal post-PCI Pd/Pa ≤ 0.92, only patients with positive post-PCI FFR ≤ 0.80 showed significantly higher risk of TVF than did those with post-PCI Pd/Pa>0.92.

(continued on next page)

Table 1
(continued)

Study	Inclusion	Device	Follow-up, Months	Post-PCI Index	Results	Comment
					Post-PCI FFR ≤ 0.80 showed significantly higher risk of TVF (10.3% vs 2.5%, $P < .001$) than >0.80. Post-PCI resting Pd/Pa ≤ 0.92 showed significantly higher risk of TVF (6.2% vs 2.5%, $P = .029$) than >0.92. Post-PCI iFR and dPR showed same results with resting Pd/Pa.	

Abbreviations: ACS, acute coronary syndrome; AUC, area under curve; BMS, bare metal stent; CI, confidence interval; DES, drug-eluting stent; EQ-5D, European Quality of Life five dimension; FFR, fractional flow reserve; HR, hazard ratio; iFR, instantaneous wave-free ratio; IVUS, intravascular ultrasound; LAD, left anterior descending artery; MACE, major adverse cardiac events; NR, not reported; NSTEMI, non-ST-segment elevation myocardial infarction; OCT, optical coherence tomography; %DS, percent diameter stenosis; PCI, percutaneous coronary intervention; QCA, quantitative coronary angiography; resting Pd/Pa, resting distal coronary pressure/aortic pressure; SIHD, stable ischemic heart disease; SVD, single vessel disease; TVF, target vessel failure; UA, unstable angina; VOCE, vessel-oriented composite events.

the prediction model with post-PCI FFR significantly increased the discriminant and reclassification ability for TVF.[15] More recently, the TARGET-FFR trial (The Trial of Angiography vs pressure-Ratio-Guided Enhancement Techniques—Fractional Flow Reserve) showed that percent FFR increase had a modest but significant correlation with angina score, and a larger percent FFR increase was associated with a reduced burden of patient-reported angina.[42] These results support the importance of degree of physiologic gain from PCI on the improvement of symptoms and prognosis.

Post-PCI physiologic indexes and physiologic gains after PCI are determined by underlying disease patterns in the target vessels and relative physiologic contribution of focal stenosis and diffuse atherosclerotic disease before and after PCI (Fig. 1).[38] After successful PCI, physiologic gain (eg, ΔFFR or percent FFR increase) is expected to be high in patients with severe focal stenosis (see Fig. 1A). Although post-PCI physiologic index can still be low if residual diffuse disease is in the non-stented segment, these patients reasonably benefit from PCI as determined by high physiologic gain and show modest outcomes despite suboptimal post-PCI physiologic index (see Fig. 1B). Conversely, both post-PCI physiologic index and physiologic gain can be low in patients with higher relative contribution of diffuse atherosclerotic disease than focal stenosis, and these patients are least likely to benefit from PCI and more likely to have worse outcomes (see Fig. 1C). Therefore, consideration of physiologic gains, in addition to post-PCI physiologic indexes, allow us to understand the nature of disease and physiologic appropriateness of PCI results, which would be important for functionally optimized revascularization and better stratification of high-risk patients.[15,38]

Post-Percutaneous Coronary Intervention Physiologic Assessment and Functionally Optimized Percutaneous Coronary Intervention

To achieve functionally optimized PCI, it is important to evaluate the correctable causes of suboptimal post-PCI physiologic results. Suboptimal post-PCI physiologic results could be due to suboptimal stent deployment and/or presence of residual focal or diffuse disease in the non-stented segments in the target vessel. However, post-PCI FFR and NHPRs reflect hemodynamic compromise in the entire target vessel, so cannot differentiate the relative contribution of residual disease burden between the stented and non-stented segments.[38] Furthermore, post-PCI FFR and NHPRs cannot provide specific information on the cause(s) of suboptimal physiologic results. From this perspective, pressure-wire pullback and intravascular imaging can be useful to assess the distribution and location of the ischemia-causing residual disease and evaluate the underlying mechanisms of suboptimal stent placement. Fig. 2 shows case examples of suboptimal post-PCI physiologic results and physiology-guided optimization using pressure-wire pullback and intravascular imaging.

In FFR-SEARCH (Fractional Flow Reserve—Stent Evaluated at Rotterdam Cardiology Hospital) study with 100 vessels with post-PCI FFR ≤ 0.85,[43] intravascular ultrasound (IVUS) identified stent underexpansion in 74%, significant residual focal lesion in proximal or distal segment in 29% and 30%, respectively, stent malapposition in 23%, vascular spasm in 9%, lumen compromising intramural hematoma in 3%, and residual diffuse atherosclerotic disease in 8%.[43] In a study by Wolfrum and colleagues,[44] 61.9% of patients with suboptimal post-PCI FFR less than 0.90 were found to have suboptimal stent results in optical coherence tomography (OCT), which included stent underexpansion (46%), incomplete lesion coverage (39%), stent malapposition (54%, whereby all cases of malapposition were accompanied by stent underexpansion and/or incomplete lesion coverage), stent distal edge dissection (15%), and tissue protrusion (8%).[44] Importantly, OCT-guided stent optimization significantly increased post-PCI FFR values from 0.80 ± 0.02 to 0.88 ± 0.01 ($P = .008$).[44] In a larger study by Agarwal and colleagues[12] with 664 lesions from 574 patients, 21% of lesions were found to have ischemic post-PCI FFR ≤ 0.80 after angiographically successful PCI. For these lesions with ischemic post-PCI FFR, functional optimization was attempted via adjunctive post-dilatation in 42%, additional stenting in 33%, and both in 18%. These additional procedures significantly increased post-PCI FFR values from 0.78 ± 0.08 to 0.87 ± 0.06 and decreased the proportion of lesions with ischemic FFR from 21% to 9%.[12] In lesions with persistently ischemic post-PCI FFR despite functional optimization, FFR pullback tracings revealed a significant pressure gradient distal to the stented segment, suggesting presence of diffuse disease in the distal non-stented segment.[12]

The concept of post-PCI functional optimization was prospectively evaluated in a study by Uretsky and colleagues,[45] which included 250 vessels in 226 consecutive patients. In this study, 36.5% of revascularized vessels showed immediate post-

A Severe Focal Stenosis

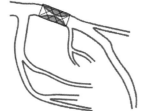

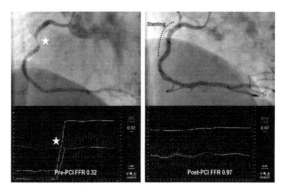

- Severe focal stenosis
  → High physiologic gain after PCI

- Minimal residual disease burden
  → High post-PCI physiologic index

- Favorable outcome

B Severe Focal Stenosis on Moderate Diffuse Disease

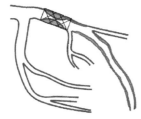

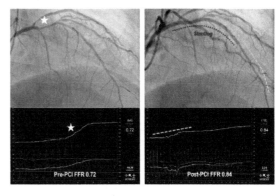

- Severe focal stenosis
  → High physiologic gain after PCI

- Moderate residual disease burden
  → Low post-PCI physiologic index

- Modest outcome

C Moderate Focal Stenosis on Predominant Diffuse Disease

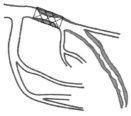

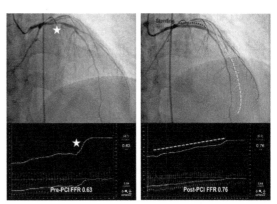

- Moderate focal stenosis
  → Low physiologic gain after PCI

- High residual disease burden
  → Low post-PCI physiologic index

- Unfavorable outcome

Fig. 1. Different post-PCI physiologic results according to the disease patterns. Post-PCI physiologic results are determined by disease patterns according to the degree of focal stenosis and the presence of residual diffuse disease. Integrated interpretation of both post-PCI physiologic index and physiologic gain from PCI is important to understand the physiologic nature of target vessel disease, assess net benefits from PCI, and predict patient prognosis.

PCI FFR ≤ 0.80, and approximately one-third of these vessels (34.5%) were considered appropriate for further intervention based on pullback tracings.[45] Additional optimization procedures, including noncompliant balloon dilatation, implantation of another stent, or both, significantly increased post-PCI FFR values from 0.73 (interquartile range [IQR] 0.69 to 0.77) to 0.80 (IQR 0.77–0.85) ($P < .0001$).[45] The feasibility and efficacy of post-PCI FFR-guided functional optimization strategy has recently been evaluated by randomized controlled trial (TARGET-FFR).[42] In

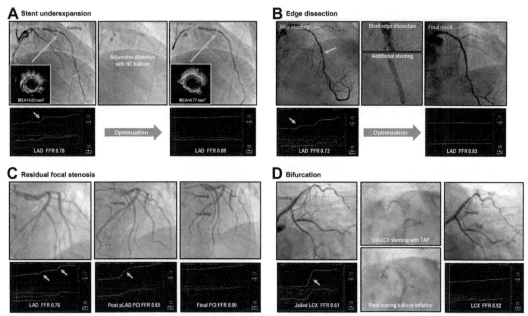

Fig. 2. Case examples of post-PCI physiology-guided procedural optimization. Illustrative case examples show optimization of PCI based on post-PCI physiologic assessment. (*A*) After stenting at the mid-LAD, immediate post-PCI FFR was 0.76 and pullback tracing showed a focal step-up within the stented segment. IVUS revealed stent underexpansion with MSA of 3.60 mm², which was optimized by adjunctive post-dilatation with an NC balloon. After procedural optimization, the final post-PCI FFR increased to 0.89. (*B*) After stenting at the mid-LAD, immediate post-PCI FFR was 0.72 and pullback tracing revealed a significant focal step-up at the distal edge of the stent. Careful examination of the angiogram revealed a distal edge dissection which was treated with additional stent implantation. This improved the final post-PCI FFR to 0.83. (*C*) Pre-PCI pullback showed tandem lesions with two distinct pressure step-ups at both proximal- and mid- LAD. After PCI for the proximal-LAD stenosis, post-PCI FFR was still suboptimal and pullback tracing showed significant pressure step-up across the mid-LAD stenosis. After additional stenting for the mid-LAD stenosis, final post-PCI FFR was much improved. (*D*) Provisional stenting from LM to LAD was performed for the LM bifurcation lesion. Post-PCI FFR for jailed LCX was 0.61 and pullback tracing showed a focal step-up at LCX ostium. After additional stenting for LM-LCX using TAP technique, the final post-PCI FFR was improved up to 0.92 without any focal step-up throughout LCX. *Abbreviations:* LCX, left circumflex artery; LM, left main stem; MSA, minimum stent area; NC, non-compliant; TAP, T and small protrusion.

this trial, patients were randomly assigned to either a physiology-guided incremental optimization strategy (PIOS) or a blinded coronary physiology assessment (control group) after angiographically guided PCI.[42] In PIOS group, operators reviewed the measurements if post-PCI FFR was less than 0.90 and planned additional intervention based on the FFR pullback tracing. If there was a hyperemic trans-stent gradient ≥0.05, post-dilation with a larger noncompliant balloon was performed in the stented segment. If there was a focal FFR step-up ≥.05 in a non-stented segment less than 20 mm, additional stents were deployed. These optimization procedures were repeated until post-PCI FFR became ≥0.90 or above criteria were no longer met. Although PIOS failed to increase the proportion of patients with post-PCI FFR greater than 0.90 by 20% (primary endpoint), it significantly reduced the proportion of patients

with post-PCI FFR ≤ 0.80 compared with the control group (18.6% vs 29.8%; *P* = .045).[42]

Results from this randomized clinical trial as well as observational and prospective studies suggest the feasibility and efficacy of functionally optimized PCI. One important question still unanswered is whether functionally optimized PCI can reduce TVF. One of the important findings from the DEFINE-PCI study, where blinded physiologic assessment was performed after angiographically successful PCI, was that 81.6% of cases with ischemic post-PCI iFR were attributable to angiographically inapparent focal lesions which could have been further optimized during the index procedure.[11,18] The ongoing large-scale, multicenter DEFINE-GPS trial (Distal Evaluation of Functional performance with Intravascular sensors to assess the Narrowing Effect: Guided Physiologic Stenting, NCT04451044), which is estimated to include up to 3200 participants, will investigate the clinical effectiveness of identification and treatment of angiographically inapparent residual ischemia using iFR co-registration platform.

Interpretation of Post-Percutaneous Coronary Intervention Pullback Tracings

As described above, the pressure-wire pullback is the key for post-PCI physiologic assessment and functionally optimized PCI, as it allows ocalization of functionally significant focal disease that causes residual ischemia after angiographically successful PCI. One of the practical questions when interpreting post-PCI pullback tracings is how to define the presence of residual focal disease that can be further optimized with additional procedures compared with residual diffuse disease. In the TARGET-FFR study, focal FFR increase ≥ 0.05 was considered to be significant for both stented and non-stented segments.[42] Regarding the non-stented segment, the length of disease responsible for the FFR increase ≥ 0.05 should be < 20 mm to be considered as focal disease.[42] In the DEFINE-PCI study, trans-stenotic iFR gradients of ≥ 0.03 were categorized as focal lesions when their length was ≤ 15 mm. When lesion length exceeded 15 mm, they were categorized as diffuse disease. Therefore, the degree of pressure gradient and the length of disease are key components to differentiate residual focal lesions from diffuse disease.

Recently, Lee and colleagues[46] suggested an objective method to analyze post-PCI FFR pullback tracing. In this study, the novel concept of instantaneous FFR changes across the target stenosis per unit time ($dFFR(t)/dt$) was applied to post-PCI pullback tracings, which can be easily and simultaneously calculated by software. The optimal cutoff value of $dFFR(t)/dt$ to define the presence of focal stenosis (major residual FFR gradient) was ≥ 0.035 per second, which corresponded with a trans-stenotic pressure gradient greater than 15 mm Hg.[46,47] Among 492 patients who underwent angiographically successful PCI, 33.9% were found to have a major residual FFR gradient defined by $dFFR(t)/dt$, and those patients had a significantly higher risk of TVF at 2 years than those without major residual FFR gradient (9.0% vs 2.2%; $P = .012$).[46] Interestingly, even in the subgroup of patients with the sufficient post-PCI physiologic result (post-PCI FFR ≥ 0.84 and percent FFR increase >15%), patients with major residual FFR gradient defined by $dFFR(t)/dt$ had a significantly higher risk of TVF compared with those without (10.4% vs 0.6%; $P = .019$),[46] which supported the unique value of $dFFR(t)/dt$. Despite

lack of standard method to define focal step-up in pullback tracings, all these studies provided objective criteria that can be used in daily practice, although $dFFR(t)/dt$ is not yet commercially available.

Proposed Algorithm for Post-Percutaneous Coronary Intervention Physiologic Assessment

As discussed above, numerous evidence exists supporting the prognostic values of post-PCI physiologic assessment and its role in functionally optimized PCI (**Fig. 3**). A proposed algorithm based on available evidence is shown in **Fig. 4**. Based on availability and operator preference, either FFR or NHPRs could be used as the initial evaluation tool to assess for presence of residual ischemia after successful PCI guided by angiography or intravascular imaging. As most patients with negative post-PCI NHPRs are likely to have negative post-PCI FFR as well, measuring NHPRs first could be beneficial, especially because it does not require hyperemia induction. In such cases, however, the operator should be aware of the possibility of the presence of post-occlusive reactive hyperemia that can lower NHPRs. Therefore, sufficient recovery time should be given before measuring the NHPRs, or confirmation with post-PCI FFR needs to be considered.

In cases of suboptimal post-PCI physiologic results, it is important to assess for presence of residual focal disease, in which case functional optimization with additional procedures could be beneficial. In this regard, pressure-wire pullback is required to discriminate focal step-up from diffuse gradual step-up. A significant focal step-up can be defined as increase of FFR ≥ 0.05 in less than 20 mm or increase of iFR ≥ 0.03 in ≤ 15 mm. The use of $dFFR(t)/dt$ could also be used with a cut-off value of ≥ 0.035 once it becomes commercially available. If significant focal step-up is identified in the stented and/or non-stented segments, intravascular imaging can help reveal the target of subsequent optimization procedures such as adjunctive post-dilatation with noncompliant or high-pressure balloon, additional stent implantation, or both. These additional optimization procedures can be repeated until sufficient physiologic results are obtained or focal step-up in pullback tracings is no longer present. If post-PCI FFR or NHPRs are suboptimal and there is only gradual step-up in pullback tracing, additional procedures may not provide significant benefit. In such cases, physiologic gain (absolute or relative increase in physiologic indexes) can be calculated for prognostication. If there is sufficient physiologic

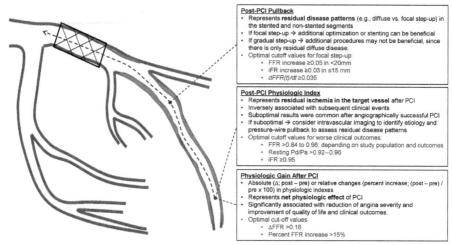

Post-PCI Pullback
- Represents **residual disease patterns** (e.g., diffuse vs. focal step-up) in the stented and non-stented segments
- If focal step-up → additional optimization or stenting can be beneficial
- If gradual step-up → additional procedures may not be beneficial, since there is only residual diffuse disease.
- Optimal cutoff values for focal step-up:
  - FFR increase ≥0.05 in <20mm
  - iFR increase ≥0.03 in ≤15 mm
  - *dFFR(t)/dt* ≥0.035

Post-PCI Physiologic Index
- Represents **residual ischemia in the target vessel** after PCI
- Inversely associated with subsequent clinical events
- Suboptimal results were common after angiographically successful PCI
- If suboptimal → consider intravascular imaging to identify etiology and pressure-wire pullback to assess residual disease patterns
- Optimal cutoff values for worse clinical outcomes:
  - FFR >0.84 to 0.96; depending on study population and outcomes
  - Resting Pd/Pa >0.92–0.96
  - iFR ≥0.95

Physiologic Gain After PCI
- Absolute (Δ; post – pre) or relative changes (percent increase; (post – pre) / pre × 100) in physiologic indexes
- Represents **net physiologic effect** of PCI
- Significantly associated with reduction of angina severity and improvement of quality of life and clinical outcomes.
- Optimal cut-off values
  - ΔFFR >0.18
  - Percent FFR increase >15%

Fig. 3. Summary of clinical implications of post-PCI physiologic assessment. Clinical implications of three important components of post-PCI physiologic assessment, including post-PCI physiologic index, physiologic gain, and pullback, are shown. ΔFFR is calculated as post-PCI FFR – pre-PCI FFR. Percent FFR increase is calculated as (post-PCI FFR – pre-PCI FFR)/pre-PCI FFR × 100. *Abbreviation: dFFR(t)/dt,* instantaneous FFR changes per unit time.

gain from PCI despite suboptimal post-PCI FFR or NHPRs, PCI can be considered to have been successful with improvement of symptoms. Aggressive medical treatment and risk factor modification would still be very important, as these patients have residual disease burden causing ischemia. If both post-PCI physiologic index and physiologic gain from PCI are suboptimal and there is no focal step-up in pullback tracing for further optimization, there would be minimal benefit from PCI and prognosis is expected to be poor.

Additional Consideration for Functionally Optimized Percutaneous Coronary Intervention

As discussed so far, post-PCI physiologic assessment plays a pivotal role in functionally optimized PCI. However, functionally optimized PCI needs to start at the beginning of the procedure before stent deployment, as studies have found that pre-PCI physiologic assessment allows prediction of post-PCI physiologic results.

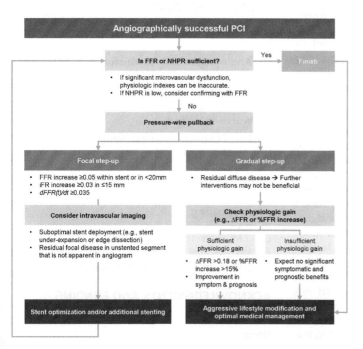

Fig. 4. Proposed flow diagram of post-PCI physiologic assessment. Proposed algorithm of post-PCI physiologic assessment based on available data is shown. ΔFFR is calculated as post-PCI FFR – pre-PCI FFR. %FFR increase is calculated as follows: (post-PCI FFR – pre-PCI FFR)/pre-PCI FFR × 100. *Abbreviation: dFFR(t)/dt,* instantaneous FFR changes per unit time.

Coronary flow is less affected under non-hyperemic conditions than hyperemic conditions, making a change in NHPRs after PCI more predictable than FFR.[48] This means that post-PCI value of NHPRs can be intuitively expected by adding step-up amount in pullback tracing into pre-PCI value.[38] Therefore, the degree of changes in NHPRs after treatment of individual lesions can be predicted in the pre-PCI phase, which allows procedural planning by selecting appropriate target lesions that need treatment to achieve optimal post-PCI physiologic results. A co-registration system incorporating both iFR pullback and angiographic images (SyncVision, Philips/Volcano, Amsterdam, The Netherlands) allows convenient procedural planning, and a clinical trial (DEFINE-GPS) is currently ongoing to clarify prognostic implications of iFR-based procedural planning and revascularization.

Pre-PCI physiologic characterization of disease patterns using pullback tracings of FFR or NHPRs can also help functionally optimized PCI. As PCI with stent implantation is a local treatment, discrimination of physiologic focal stenosis from diffuse disease would help select optimal targets for PCI. Visual assessment of the pullback tracing provides a rough idea of the presence of focal step-up, although this method is limited due to subjectivity and high inter-observer variability. For a more objective evaluation of disease patterns, Collet and colleagues[49] developed a pullback pressure gradient (PPG) index from the motorized FFR pullback. The PPG values approaching 1.0 represent predominantly focal disease, whereas values close to 0 represent predominantly diffuse disease.[49] Lee and colleagues[47] introduced an alternative method of quantifying local severity of disease by calculating instantaneous FFR gradient per unit time ($dFFR(t)/dt$) from the pre-PCI manual FFR pullback tracings. In this study, patients with major FFR gradients ($dFFR(t)/dt \geq 0.035/s$) were least likely to have suboptimal post-PCI physiologic results, supporting the role of characterization of disease patterns in predicting physiologic response to PCI.

Although concepts of the aforementioned methods and indexes have similarities and differences among each other, pre-PCI planning based on expected post-PCI physiologic results and disease patterns will increase achievement of functionally optimized PCI by[1] detecting the lesions that significantly contribute to myocardial ischemia but are not apparent on angiography and[2] reducing unnecessary stenting of lesions that would not result in sufficient physiologic gain and post-PCI physiologic results. Therefore, the concept of functionally optimized PCI should not be limited to the post-PCI phase, but really needs to be considered from the beginning of the procedure.

SUMMARY

Numerous evidence exists supporting the prognostic values of post-PCI physiologic assessment and its role in functionally optimized PCI. Post-PCI physiologic assessment would be particularly important, as a substantial proportion of patients who underwent angiographically successful PCI had evidence of residual ischemia manifested by suboptimal post-PCI FFR or NHPRs which were associated with worse clinical outcomes. Considering that the purpose of PCI is not just to alleviate angiographic stenosis but to resolve myocardial ischemia and improve prognosis, it is crucial to investigate the causes of suboptimal post-PCI physiologic results using pressure-wire pullback tracings and/or intravascular imaging. If there is a focal step-up in pullback tracings, additional optimization procedures will be required to achieve functionally optimized PCI. It is also important to note that functionally optimized PCI should be considered at the beginning of the procedure, as careful PCI planning using pre-PCI physiologic evaluation can increase the probability of functionally optimized PCI. Ongoing clinical trials will answer the remaining question regarding whether pre-PCI planning guided by pullback analysis and additional optimization procedures guided by post-PCI physiologic assessment will improve outcomes.[38]

CLINICS CARE POINTS

- Angiographically successful PCI does not necessarily result in functionally optimized PCI.
- Low post-PCI physiologic indexes predict worse outcomes.
- Post-PCI physiologic assessment enables optimization of PCI results and improves outcome.

DISCLOSURES

Dr J.M. Lee received a Research Grant from Abbott Vascular and Philips Volcano; has received consulting fees from RainMed and Zoll Medical.

ACKNOWLEDGMENTS AND FUNDING SOURCES

None

REFERENCES

1. Gould KL. Does coronary flow trump coronary anatomy? JACC Cardiovasc Imaging 2009;2:1009–23.
2. Tonino PA, De Bruyne B, Pijls NH, et al. Fractional flow reserve versus angiography for guiding percutaneous coronary intervention. N Engl J Med 2009; 360:213–24.
3. De Bruyne B, Pijls NH, Kalesan B, et al. Fractional flow reserve-guided PCI versus medical therapy in stable coronary disease. N Engl J Med 2012;367: 991–1001.
4. Davies JE, Sen S, Dehbi HM, et al. Use of the Instantaneous Wave-free Ratio or Fractional Flow Reserve in PCI. N Engl J Med 2017;376:1824–34.
5. Gotberg M, Christiansen EH, Gudmundsdottir IJ, et al. Instantaneous Wave-free Ratio versus Fractional Flow Reserve to Guide PCI. N Engl J Med 2017;376:1813–23.
6. Neumann FJ, Sousa-Uva M, Ahlsson A, et al. 2018 ESC/EACTS Guidelines on myocardial revascularization. Eur Heart J 2019;40:87–165.
7. de Waha S, Patel MR, Granger CB, et al. Relationship between microvascular obstruction and adverse events following primary percutaneous coronary intervention for ST-segment elevation myocardial infarction: an individual patient data pooled analysis from seven randomized trials. Eur Heart J 2017;38:3502–10.
8. Johnson NP, Toth GG, Lai D, et al. Prognostic value of fractional flow reserve: linking physiologic severity to clinical outcomes. J Am Coll Cardiol 2014;64: 1641–54.
9. Rimac G, Fearon WF, De Bruyne B, et al. Clinical value of post-percutaneous coronary intervention fractional flow reserve value: A systematic review and meta-analysis. Am Heart J 2017;183:1–9.
10. Wolfrum M, Fahrni G, de Maria GL, et al. Impact of impaired fractional flow reserve after coronary interventions on outcomes: a systematic review and meta-analysis. BMC Cardiovasc Disord 2016;16:177.
11. Jeremias A, Davies JE, Maehara A, et al. Blinded Physiological Assessment of Residual Ischemia After Successful Angiographic Percutaneous Coronary Intervention: The DEFINE PCI Study. JACC Cardiovasc Interv 2019;12:1991–2001.
12. Agarwal SK, Kasula S, Hacioglu Y, et al. Utilizing Post-Intervention Fractional Flow Reserve to Optimize Acute Results and the Relationship to Long-Term Outcomes. JACC Cardiovasc Interv 2016;9: 1022–31.
13. Li SJ, Ge Z, Kan J, et al. Cutoff Value and Long-Term Prediction of Clinical Events by FFR Measured Immediately After Implantation of a Drug-Eluting Stent in Patients With Coronary Artery Disease: 1- to 3-Year Results From the DKCRUSH VII Registry Study. JACC Cardiovasc Interv 2017;10:986–95.
14. Piroth Z, Toth GG, Tonino PAL, et al. Prognostic Value of Fractional Flow Reserve Measured Immediately After Drug-Eluting Stent Implantation. Circ Cardiovasc Interv 2017;10:e005233.
15. Lee JM, Hwang D, Choi KH, et al. Prognostic Implications of Relative Increase and Final Fractional Flow Reserve in Patients With Stent Implantation. JACC Cardiovasc Interv 2018;11:2099–109.
16. Fournier S, Ciccarelli G, Toth GG, et al. Association of Improvement in Fractional Flow Reserve With Outcomes, Including Symptomatic Relief, After Percutaneous Coronary Intervention. JAMA Cardiol 2019;4: 370–4.
17. Hwang D, Lee JM, Lee HJ, et al. Influence of target vessel on prognostic relevance of fractional flow reserve after coronary stenting. EuroIntervention 2019;15:457–64.
18. Patel MR, Jeremias A, Maehara A, et al. 1-Year Outcomes of Blinded Physiological Assessment of Residual Ischemia After Successful PCI: DEFINE PCI Trial. JACC Cardiovasc Interv 2022;15:52–61.
19. Bech GJ, Pijls NH, De Bruyne B, et al. Usefulness of fractional flow reserve to predict clinical outcome after balloon angioplasty. Circulation 1999;99:883–8.
20. Pijls NH, Klauss V, Siebert U, et al. Coronary pressure measurement after stenting predicts adverse events at follow-up: a multicenter registry. Circulation 2002;105:2950–4.
21. Dupouy P, Gilard M, Morelle JF, et al. Usefulness and clinical impact of a fractional flow reserve and angiographic targeted strategy for coronary artery stenting: FROST III, a multicenter prospective registry. EuroIntervention 2005;1:85–92.
22. Klauss V, Erdin P, Rieber J, et al. Fractional flow reserve for the prediction of cardiac events after coronary stent implantation: results of a multivariate analysis. Heart 2005;91:203–6.
23. Jensen LO, Thayssen P, Thuesen L, et al. Influence of a pressure gradient distal to implanted bare-metal stent on in-stent restenosis after percutaneous coronary intervention. Circulation 2007;116:2802–8.
24. Ishii H, Kataoka T, Kobayashi Y, et al. Utility of myocardial fractional flow reserve for prediction of restenosis following sirolimus-eluting stent implantation. Heart Vessels 2011;26:572–81.
25. Leesar MA, Satran A, Yalamanchili V, et al. The impact of fractional flow reserve measurement on clinical outcomes after transradial coronary stenting. EuroIntervention 2011;7:917–23.
26. Nam CW, Hur SH, Cho YK, et al. Relation of fractional flow reserve after drug-eluting stent implantation to one-year outcomes. Am J Cardiol 2011;107: 1763–7.
27. Ito T, Tani T, Fujita H, et al. Relationship between fractional flow reserve and residual plaque volume and clinical outcomes after optimal drug-eluting stent implantation: insight from intravascular

ultrasound volumetric analysis. Int J Cardiol 2014; 176:399–404.

28. Doh JH, Nam CW, Koo BK, et al. Clinical Relevance of Poststent Fractional Flow Reserve After Drug-Eluting Stent Implantation. J Invasive Cardiol 2015; 27:346–51.

29. Reith S, Battermann S, Hellmich M, et al. Correlation between OCT-derived intrastent dimensions and fractional flow reserve measurements after coronary stent implantation and impact on clinical outcome. J Invasive Cardiol 2015;27:222–8.

30. Kasula S, Agarwal SK, Hacioglu Y, et al. Clinical and prognostic value of poststenting fractional flow reserve in acute coronary syndromes. Heart 2016; 102:1988–94.

31. Azzalini L, Poletti E, Demir OM, et al. Impact of Post-Percutaneous Coronary Intervention Fractional Flow Reserve Measurement on Procedural Management and Clinical Outcomes: The REPEAT-FFR Study. J Invasive Cardiol 2019;31:229–34.

32. Hoshino M, Kanaji Y, Hamaya R, et al. Prognostic value of post-intervention fractional flow reserve after intravascular ultrasound-guided second-generation drug-eluting coronary stenting. EuroIntervention 2019;15:e779–87.

33. van Bommel RJ, Masdjedi K, Diletti R, et al. Routine Fractional Flow Reserve Measurement After Percutaneous Coronary Intervention. Circ Cardiovasc Interv 2019;12:e007428.

34. Pijls NH, De Bruyne B, Peels K, et al. Measurement of fractional flow reserve to assess the functional severity of coronary-artery stenoses. N Engl J Med 1996;334:1703–8.

35. Leone AM, De Caterina AR, Basile E, et al. Influence of the amount of myocardium subtended by a stenosis on fractional flow reserve. Circ Cardiovasc Interv 2013;6:29–36.

36. Hakeem A, Ghosh B, Shah K, et al. Incremental Prognostic Value of Post-Intervention Pd/Pa in Patients Undergoing Ischemia-Driven Percutaneous Coronary Intervention. JACC Cardiovasc Interv 2019;12:2002–14.

37. Shin D, Lee SH, Lee JM, et al. Prognostic Implications of Post-Intervention Resting Pd/Pa and Fractional Flow Reserve in Patients With Stent Implantation. JACC Cardiovasc Interv 2020;13: 1920–33.

38. Lee JM, Lee SH, Shin D, et al. Physiology-Based Revascularization. JACC: Asia 2021;1:14–36.

39. Murai T, Lee T, Yonetsu T, et al. Influence of micro-vascular resistance on fractional flow reserve after successful percutaneous coronary intervention. Catheter Cardiovasc Interv 2015;85:585–92.

40. Selvanayagam JB, Cheng AS, Jerosch-Herold M, et al. Effect of distal embolization on myocardial perfusion reserve after percutaneous coronary intervention: a quantitative magnetic resonance perfusion study. Circulation 2007;116:1458–64.

41. Nishi T, Piroth Z, De Bruyne B, et al. Fractional Flow Reserve and Quality-of-Life Improvement After Percutaneous Coronary Intervention in Patients With Stable Coronary Artery Disease. Circulation 2018;138:1797–804.

42. Collison D, Didagelos M, Aetesam-Ur-Rahman M, et al. Post-stenting fractional flow reserve vs coronary angiography for optimization of percutaneous coronary intervention (TARGET-FFR). Eur Heart J 2021;42:4656–68.

43. van Zandvoort LJC, Masdjedi K, Witberg K, et al. Explanation of Postprocedural Fractional Flow Reserve Below 0.85. Circ Cardiovasc Interv 2019; 12:e007030.

44. Wolfrum M, De Maria GL, Benenati S, et al. What are the causes of a suboptimal FFR after coronary stent deployment? Insights from a consecutive series using OCT imaging. EuroIntervention 2018;14: e1324–31.

45. Uretsky BF, Agarwal SK, Vallurupalli S, et al. Prospective Evaluation of the Strategy of Functionally Optimized Coronary Intervention. J Am Heart Assoc 2020;9:e015073.

46. Lee SH, Kim J, Lefieux A, et al. Clinical and Prognostic Impact From Objective Analysis of Post-Angioplasty Fractional Flow Reserve Pullback. JACC Cardiovasc Interv 2021;14:1888–900.

47. Lee SH, Shin D, Lee JM, et al. Automated Algorithm Using Pre-Intervention Fractional Flow Reserve Pullback Curve to Predict Post-Intervention Physiological Results. JACC Cardiovasc Interv 2020;13: 2670–84.

48. Nijjer SS, Petraco R, van de Hoef TP, et al. Change in coronary blood flow after percutaneous coronary intervention in relation to baseline lesion physiology: results of the JUSTIFY-PCI study. Circ Cardiovasc Interv 2015;8:e001715.

49. Collet C, Sonck J, Vandeloo B, et al. Measurement of Hyperemic Pullback Pressure Gradients to Characterize Patterns of Coronary Atherosclerosis. J Am Coll Cardiol 2019;74:1772–84.

50. Yang HM, Lim HS, Yoon MH, et al. Usefulness of the trans-stent fractional flow reserve gradient for predicting clinical outcomes. Catheter Cardiovasc Interv 2020;95:E123–9.

Physiology and Intravascular Imaging Coregistration—Best of all Worlds?

Tobin Joseph, MBBS, BSc[a,b], Michael Foley, MBBS, BSc[a,b,*],
Rasha Al-Lamee, MA, MBBS, PhD[a,b,c]

KEYWORDS

- Optical coherence tomography • Intravascular ultrasound • iFR • PCI • Coregistration

KEY POINTS

- Coregistration enables operators to incorporate data from invasive physiology or invasive imaging with coronary angiography to help deliver data-driven percutaneous coronary intervention (PCI) to patients.
- There is a limited but growing evidence base for the use of both hemodynamic instantaneous (iFR) coregistration or anatomic intravascular imaging coregistration.
- Both techniques of coregistration require angiography and a pullback sequence of either a pressure wire or an imaging catheter for data acquisition.
- Triregistration with coregistration of angiography, iFR, and intravascular imaging is also possible to further optimize lesion evaluation and PCI.
- Further research is required to validate the use of coregistration in clinical practice.

INTRODUCTION

Percutaneous coronary intervention (PCI) in modern practice is increasingly guided using coronary physiological indices.[1,2] This includes hyperemic pressure indices (ie, fractional flow reserve [FFR]) or nonhyperemic pressure indices (eg, instantaneous wave-free ratio [iFR]).[3] However, despite the evidence for physiology-based PCI, the utilization of these techniques is lagging behind. This might be, in part, due to the time-consuming nature of these methods and the additional consumption of resources.[2]

Alongside the development of pressure-based measurements, intravascular imaging is becoming increasingly commonplace. Techniques such as intravascular ultrasound (IVUS) and optical coherence tomography (OCT) can be used during PCI to assist plaque and vessel characterization, lesion preparation, stent sizing, positioning, and optimization to reduce the incidence of major adverse cardiovascular events.[4,5]

Coronary angiography, physiology, and intravascular imaging provide distinct, complementary data to target, guide, and optimize coronary artery intervention. The advent of coregistration has provided an even greater ability to deliver precision-PCI. The technology integrates data from coronary angiography with invasive

---

This article originally appeared in *Interventional Cardiology Clinics*, Volume 12 Issue 1, January 2023.

[a] National Heart and Lung Institute, Imperial College London, Du Cane Road, London, W120HS, UK; [b] Imperial College Healthcare NHS Trust, Du Cane Road, London, W120HS, UK; [c] Hammersmith Hospital, Du Cane Road, London W12 0HS, UK

* Corresponding author. National Heart and Lung Institute, Imperial College London, Du Cane Road, London, W120HS.

E-mail address: m.foley@imperial.ac.uk

Cardiol Clin 42 (2024) 77–87
https://doi.org/10.1016/j.ccl.2023.07.006

physiology or imaging or both. This provides various advantages mentioned above using each technique in isolation. This article will aim to review the use of iFR, IVUS, and OCT coregistration with coronary angiography to further guide intervention. We will also give practical advice on how to perform iFR and IVUS coregistration to ensure the best possible data acquisition for clinical decision-making.

INSTANTANEOUS WAVE-FREE RATIO COREGISTRATION

iFR allows instantaneous measurement of resting coronary pressure in the wave-free period.[6] Beyond the practical advantages offered of recording a single value across a stenosis without the need for induction of hyperemia, iFR also permits serial measurements to be made dynamically in a coronary artery with multiple or tandem stenoses, using a technology known as "iFR pullback" or "iFR scout." The alternative hyperemic FFR pullback is not only more practically challenging but can also be difficult to interpret given the interdependence of coronary stenoses during hyperemia.[7,8] iFR pullback allows operators to determine the individual contribution of a particular lesion to coronary pressure gradients without the issues of lesion "crosstalk" that is inevitable with FFR.[8,9]

A key advantage of iFR pullback over a single measurement taken in the distal coronary artery is the appreciation of residual diffuse or focal stenosis following angiographically successful PCI. When this was systematically investigated in the prospective, observational study Physiological Assessment of Coronary Stenosis following PCI study, as many as 1 in 4 patients had residual, post-PCI ischemia, with 81% of these patients having an unappreciated focal stenosis that was amenable to further PCI.[10] The 1-year outcomes

for this study were recently published.[11] It was found that achieving post-PCI iFR greater than 0.95 was associated with improved 1-year event-free survival. In this unblinded study, they also found that patients without residual ischemia post-PCI, measured by iFR, had a significantly lower symptom burden at 1 year when compared with those with residual ischemia.[11]

iFR pullback data has been demonstrated to modify the PCI strategy among contemporary interventional cardiologists. Beyond its ability to detect and localize post-PCI ischemia, iFR pullback can additionally modify, and potentially improve, the upfront PCI strategy in as many as a third of cases.[1]

The data from iFR pullback can be "coregistered" with coronary angiography to create a physiological map of a vessel. A pressure drop can then be visually depicted alongside the angiogram[8,12,13] (Fig. 1). This coregistration enables the modelling of stenting strategies and prediction of post-PCI outcome.[13]

Because iFR coregistration technology is relatively new, more data are awaited on its clinical use and how it might influence clinical outcomes. Matsuo and colleagues[12] investigated the use of the SyncVision system for iFR coregistration in a study of 70 lesions. They found that in 38% of stenoses, the classification of severity based on angiography alone changed when coregistered with iFR data. Higashioka and colleagues[8] investigated the reproducibility of iFR-coregistration in 51 coronary arteries from 39 patients where the coregistration was repeated twice. They demonstrated high reproducibility and the ability to precisely identify a target for PCI.

These early studies demonstrate the feasibility of iFR coregistration. Work is ongoing to further validate the technique. The theoretical and practical advantages of iFR coregistration enable

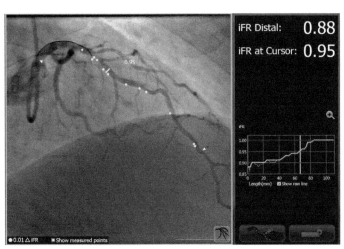

Fig. 1. iFR coregistered angiogram demonstrating diffuse LAD disease. Each yellow dot represents an increase in iFR of 0.01.

operators to quickly identify physiologically significant coronary artery disease (CAD) and determine suitability for PCI. Coregistration also allows for the prediction of post-PCI outcome, which enables operators to tailor their intervention strategy to the individual patient, using "virtual PCI" with accuracy and confidence that they can predict physiological outcomes using the software before stent insertion. A summary of these studies is shown in **Table 1**.

HOW TO USE INSTANTANEOUS WAVE-FREE RATIO COREGISTRATION

iFR coregistration is available as a component of the Volcano integrated physiology system (Philips Volcano, San Diego, USA).

Following standard arterial access, coronary angiography, and heparin administration, several steps are vital to good data acquisition:

1. A radiographic projection must be chosen in which the artery is fully visualized from guiding catheter proximally to the distal end of the artery, with minimal vessel overlap. This position should then be fixed until coregistration is complete.
2. The pressure wire must be flushed with saline, time must be allowed for the activation of the sensor and then the wire attached to the console.
3. The hemodynamic catheterization laboratory system and the pressure wire console must both be zeroed.
4. Intracoronary isosorbide dinitrate should be administered before instrumentation of the artery with the pressure wire.
5. The pressure wire is then advanced to the normalization position with the transition between the radio-opaque zone and the translucent zone just distal to the guiding catheter. Normalization between the proximal aortic pressure and distal pressure traces is then performed.
6. The pressure wire should be advanced into the distal coronary artery, at least 3 vessel diameters beyond the stenosis of interest.
7. iFR can now be recorded. With the SyncVision system activated, iFR pullback is performed. In iFR pullback mode, the wire should be slowly and steadily withdrawn under fluoroscopic guidance, until the pressure sensor is back in the normalization position.
8. A coronary angiogram image is then taken in the same projection.
9. The SyncVision system will then integrate the iFR pullback with the coronary angiogram, generating an iFR coregistration image (see **Figs. 1** and **2**).
10. The coregistration software will automatically select the pathway of the coronary artery. Occasionally, it is necessary to correct this path.
11. The coregistered images can then be used to determine the physiological distribution of disease, to plan PCI, and to predict post-PCI results.

Table 1
Summary of instantaneous wave-free ratio coregistration studies

Author (Year)	Study Population (Lesions/ Patients)	Study Design	Aim	Technology	Outcome
Matsuo et al,[12] 2021	70/70	Prospective cohort study	To evaluate utility and feasibility of physiological roadmaps coregistered with angiograms	SyncVision	Lesion morphology changes in 37% Post-iFR was significantly correlated with predicted post-iFR Post-iFR was lower than predicted with poor agreement
Higashioka et al,[8] 2020	51/39	Prospective cohort study	To assess the benefits of physiology-oriented PCI and assess reproducibility	SyncVision	iFR angio-coregistration is highly reproducible and can precisely identify a suitable target for PCI

Abbreviations: iFR, instantaneous wave-free ratio; PCI, percutaneous coronary intervention.

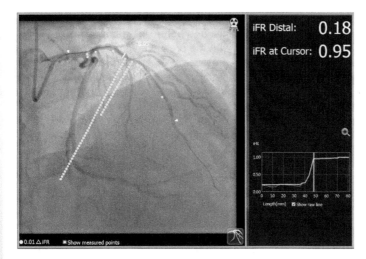

Fig. 2. iFR coregistered angiogram demonstrating focal pressure drop. Each yellow dot represents an increase in iFR of 0.01.

INSTANTANEOUS WAVE-FREE RATIO COREGISTRATION PITFALLS
Coronary Angiogram and Physiology Misalignment

The problem: The SyncVision system overlays the serially sampled iFR values with the coronary angiogram. To achieve this, the coronary angiogram must be from an identical projection as the iFR pullback conducted under continuous fluoroscopy. If the radiographic projection is altered between the pullback and the angiogram, then the physiological map will not be correctly overlayed on the coronary angiogram, leading to misleading results, or coregistration failure.

The solutions:

- Select a C arm position where the coronary artery of interest is well displayed with minimal overlap with other vessels.
- Perform an iFR pullback under continuous fluoroscopy.
- Do not move the C arm position, patient position, or magnification.
- Perform a coronary angiogram (alternatively, the "use last angiogram" function can be used, so long as it was taken in an identical projection).

Instantaneous wave-free ratio "jump" artifact

The problem: in order to correctly localize the lesion contributing to coronary artery pressure drop, the pressure wire must be withdrawn slowly and steadily. A rapid or staccato pullback of the pressure wire can lead to a "jump" across a region of physiological significance. If the withdrawal is faster than the iFR sampling frequency, then the physiological drop will be incorrectly mapped to a more proximal location.

The solutions are as follows:

- The pressure wire must be withdrawn slowly (<2 mm/s).
- If the pressure wire "jumps" across a stenosis, the wire should be readvanced and the iFR pullback repeated.
- If significant pressure drop seems to be associated with an area of coronary artery, proximal to an anatomically evident stenosis, jump artifact should be considered and the pullback data interpreted in this context.

Physiological Drift

The problem: as with a single iFR or FFR sample, the dynamic, coregistered iFR pullback is susceptible to physiological "drift" of the pressure sensor. Once the pullback and coregistration is complete, a physiological drift check should be completed. It is not uncommon to see physiological drift following iFR acquisition. This can lead to inaccurate iFR measurement, which can alter clinical decision-making.

The solutions are as follows:

- Flush the wire and allow to rest for around 20 seconds to allow the sensor to activate before instrumenting the coronary artery.
- If the pressure wire shows 0.02 units or greater of drift from normalization, the wire should be renormalized and readvanced.

Coronary pathway misidentification

The problem: in order to integrate coronary angiography with invasive physiology, the system must identify the true passage of the pressure wire through the coronary artery. In some cases, for example, overlapping or tortuous vessels, the system will incorrectly identify the coronary pathway.

The solutions are as follows:

- Choose a coronary projection before coregistration in which the coronary artery of interest can be seen with minimal overlap with other coronary vessels.
- Check the pathway identification at the end of coregistration acquisition and manually adjust the pathway if needed.

Intravascular ultrasound coregistration

IVUS can overcome some limitations of coronary angiography by enabling the cross-sectional imaging of potentially significant lesions seen on coronary angiography.[14,15] Frimerman and colleagues initially tested IVUS coregistration on phantoms simulating the coronary tree, before subsequently testing it in 42 arteries of 36 patients undergoing PCI for clinical reasons (using the SyncVision system). After statistical validation of the phantoms, their coregistration was successful in all cases and had an accuracy of 0.38 mm using a manual pullback method. They demonstrated ease of use, reliability, and ability to optimize stent landing zone and diameter as rated by the operators. The study demonstrated safety and feasibility of IVUS coregistration.

Prasad and colleagues[16] also conducted a small study into IVUS coregistration. They used an automated pullback method using a Siemens (Munich, Germany) system in 49 consecutive patients undergoing surveillance for cardiac allograft vasculopathy. The median interquartile range (IQR) coregistration distance mismatch measured at 108 bifurcations in 42 (85%) patients was 0.35 (0.00–1.16) mm. Seven patients were excluded. This study also demonstrated the feasibility of IVUS coregistration.

Houissa and colleagues[14] conducted another validation study for IVUS coregistration using a Siemens Axiom Artis (Munich, Germany). By the use of novel software, they were able to coregister IVUS and coronary angiography imaging from both phantom models and in vivo coronary arteries. The main characteristics of these studies are in **Table 2**.

A major advantage of coregistration of IVUS, which uses manual rather than automated pullback, is the ability to measure lesion length within the coronary artery, rather than simply cross-sectional imaging. There is less of an evidence base for the use of IVUS coregistration. There is a clear gap in the literature and further studies are warranted regarding the use of IVUS coregistration in PCI as well as head-to-head comparators with OCT.

HOW TO USE INTRAVASCULAR ULTRASOUND COREGISTRATION

IVUS coregistration is available as a component of the Philips SyncVision system. It is a simple procedure, and the following steps should be taken to ensure a good-quality IVUS coregistration acquisition, following standard techniques for arterial access and coronary angiography:

1. Acquire an appropriate roadmap image. The field of view should be maximized, with the collimator fully opened.
2. This roadmap should include the guiding catheter, and the entire length of the coronary artery of interest with the distal tip of the guidewire in view.
3. After acquisition, avoid changing the position of the C arm or the bed and do not alter the magnification.
4. Define the IVUS pathway on the SyncVision system—this should include the most proximal visible section of guiding catheter, the treatment area, and the distal guidewire tip.
5. Conduct an IVUS pullback. Set the fluoroscopy recording at 15 frames/s and press record on the IVUS console.
6. Withdraw the IVUS catheter at approximately 1 mm/s.
7. The SyncVision system will generate a coregistered IVUS pullback image. Cross-sectional coronary imaging can then be integrated with areas of angiographic importance to optimize PCI.

INTRAVASCULAR ULTRASOUND COREGISTRATION PITFALLS
Coronary Angiogram and Intravascular Ultrasound Misalignment

The problem: similar to iFR coregistration, the SyncVision system integrates the known location of the IVUS probe with a coronary artery roadmap. Movement of the C arm, bed or magnification alteration can lead to failed or incorrect coregistration.

The solution is as follows:

- Maintain the C arm and bed positions, and magnification settings, between roadmap acquisition and IVUS pullback.

Intravascular ultrasound "jump" artifact

The problem: similar to iFR coregistration, IVUS can miss key areas of anatomical interest by too rapid withdrawal or "jumping" back across a stenosis.

The solution is as follows:

Table 2
Summary of optical coherence tomographic studies

Author (Year)	Study Population (Lesions/Patients)	Study Design	Aim	Technology	Outcome
Houissa et al,[14] 2019	27/25	Initial phantom study with then prospective single-arm cohort study	To validate use of the system with phantoms and in the clinical setting	Siemens Axiom Artis	86% success rate of coregistration Differences between angiographic and IVUS landmarks were -0.22 ± 0.72 mm and 0.05 ± 1.01 mm, respectively. Interobserver variability was 0.23 ± 0.63 mm
Frimermanet al,[15] 2016	42/36	Initial phantom study with then prospective single-arm cohort study	To evaluate utility and feasibility of IVUS roadmaps coregistered with angiograms	SyncVision	They demonstrated ease of use, reliability, and ability to optimize stent landing zone and diameter—rated by the operators
Prasad et al,[16] 2016	108/49	Prospective single-arm cohort study	To determine the feasibility of automated coregistration of angiography and IVUS	Siemens	Demonstrated the feasibility of angio-IVUS coregistration which may be used as a clinical tool for localizing IVUS cross sections along an angiographic roadmap
Wang et al,[23] 2013	65	Initial phantom study with then prospective single-arm cohort study	To provide a computational framework for the coregistration of angiography with IVUS	Artis Zee, Siemens AG	The system is validated with a set of clinical cases and achieves good accuracy for coregistered of ECG-gated angiography and IVUS data

Abbreviations: ECG, electrocardiography.

- Slow, steady, withdrawal of the IVUS catheter at approximately 1 mm/s.

Coronary pathway misidentification

The problem: as with iFR, in order to integrate coronary angiography with IVUS, the system must identify the true passage of the pressure wire through the coronary artery. In some cases, for example, overlapping or tortuous vessels, the system will incorrectly identify the coronary pathway. The solutions are as follows:

- Choose a coronary projection before coregistration in which the coronary artery of interest can be seen with minimal overlap with other coronary vessels.
- Check the pathway identification at the end of coregistration acquisition and manually adjust the pathway if needed.

OPTICAL COHERENCE TOMOGRAPHY COREGISTRATION

Coronary angiography has been shown to underestimate lumen dimensions and boundaries of lipid core plaque, which has been associated with stent failure.[17] OCT can overcome this by providing detail regarding the vessel wall and nature of the disease including its composition. Coregistration allows data from OCT pullback to be paired with images obtained from angiography and allows operators to see an intracoronary cross section for a chosen point along a vessel. The concept of OCT coregistration was first reported in 2016; however, data on its impact on clinical outcomes are limited.[17] The largest studies are discussed below, with a summary in **Table 3**.

The real-time optical coherence tomography coregistration with angiography in percutaneous coronary intervention (OPTICO)-integration study demonstrated the concept of OCT coregistration to assist with PCI.[18] In 50 patients, PCI strategy was prospectively assessed with coronary angiography, OCT and OCT-coregistration. The use of coregistration significantly altered stent deployment strategy, sizing, and landing zone and demonstrated that with coregistration, PCI strategy often changes.

This study was further built on by the OPTICO-integration II trial.[19] This randomized study of 84 patients receiving either PCI guided by angiography-alone, conventional OCT or OCT coregistration, investigated longitudinal geographic mismatch, residual disease at stent edge. It demonstrated that OCT coregistration significantly reduced these outcomes when compared with both angiography-alone and conventional OCT. It

also demonstrated similar procedural and fluoroscopy times between the 3 cohorts.

Qin and colleagues[20] recently reported the use of a different coregistration system in a higher number of lesions (n = 1530). They found that mismatch between angiography-alone and OCT coregistration occurred in 4% of reference landmarks, and the mean time for coregistration was 20.7 seconds. This study, although not used in the PCI setting, further demonstrates the feasibility and accuracy of OCT coregistration and its potential in guiding PCI.

In a randomized trial of OCT-guided PCI versus OCT coregistered PCI in 200 de novo lesions, Koyama and colleagues[21] demonstrated that the use of OCT coregistered PCI did not significantly alter the rate of geographic miss. This was defined as angiographic $\geq$ type B dissection or diameter stenosis greater than 50% or OCT minimum lumen area less than 4.0 mm^2 with significant residual disease or dissection (dissection flap >60°) within 5 mm from the stent edge.

Clinical Cases

In this section, we will use real-world examples that demonstrate the value of coregistered data in clinical practice.

Case 1—Defining Physiologically Diffuse Coronary Disease

A 62-year-old man presented with stable angina and underwent coronary angiography. This revealed angiographically mild atheroma in the proximal left anterior descending (LAD) with moderate-to-severe stenosis in the mid-LAD. An iFR was performed in the distal vessel, showing significant flow limitation (iFR 0.88). The coregistered iFR pullback is shown below (see **Fig. 1**).

This data revealed that the pressure drop was distributed along the length of LAD demonstrating a diffuse pattern of disease. This data was used to inform the treatment strategy. Given that there was no focal pressure gradient that could be well treated with PCI, in this case, optimal medical therapy was selected as the best approach.

Case 2—Defining Physiologically Focal Coronary Disease

A 75-year-old man presented with severe stable angina. An angiogram was undertaken, revealing a severe stenosis in the proximal LAD with further angiographically moderate disease in the mid-LAD. An iFR was measured in the distal LAD confirming significant pressure gradient in this vessel (iFR 0.18). The coregistered iFR pullback is shown below (**Fig. 2**).

The coregistration image clarifies that the area of pressure drop is very focal. With this data, the

Table 3
Summary of optical coherence tomographic Coregistration studies

Author (Year)	Study Population (Lesions/Patients)	Study Design	Aim	Technology	Outcome
Schneider et al,[19] 2021	28/84	Randomized controlled trial (3 arms: coronary angiography, OCT-guided and OCT coregistration)	PCI strategy was prospectively assessed with coronary angiography, OCT, and OCT coregistration	OPTIS integrated system	The use of coregistration significantly altered stent deployment strategy, sizing, and landing zone and demonstrated that coregistration can be used successfully to augment PCI
Qin et al,[20] 2021	212/181	Post hoc validation of the coregistration approach from a retrospective, single center	To evaluate a novel approach for automatic coregistration of OCT and coronary angiography	AngioPlus Core and OctPlus, Pulse Medical Imaging Technology	The mismatch between OCT and coronary angiography occurred in 4% of reference landmarks, and the mean time for coregistration was 20.7 s
Koyama et al 2018	200/200	Randomized controlled trial (2 arms)	To evaluate whether automated coregistration of OCT with angiography reduces geographic miss during coronary stenting	OPTIS integrated system	The use of OCT coregistered PCI did not significantly alter rate of geographic miss
Leistner et al 2017	58/50	Prospective single-arm study	PCI strategy was prospectively assessed with coronary angiography, OCT, and OCT coregistration	OPTIS integrated system	The use of coregistration significantly altered stent deployment strategy, sizing, and landing zone and demonstrated that coregistration can be used successfully to augment PCI

iFR, instantaneous wave free ratio; IVUS, intravascular ultrasound; OCT, optical coherence tomography; PCI, percutaneous coronary intervention operators were able to plan a stenting strategy and select the correct stent length to relieve the focal stenosis in the LAD without extending to cover the long segment of moderate disease distally.

Case 3—Planning PCI with Coregistered IVUS with a Long Segment of Disease

A 79-year-old woman presented acutely with chest pain, shortness of breath, and inferior ST depression on her ECG. Her troponin was elevated, and she underwent urgent coronary angiography. This revealed a severe stenosis of the distal right coronary artery (RCA), involving the posterior descending artery bifurcation. She went on to have a pre-PCI coregistered IVUS assessment of her RCA (**Fig. 3**). This image demonstrated not only the vessel diameter and distal reference as with non-coregistered IVUS but also the length of the diseased segment. Because the IVUS data is mapped on the coronary angiogram, this can be used to aid both stent length selection and positioning.

Is There a Role for Intravascular Ultrasound/ Physiology Triregistration?

Coronary angiography, coronary physiology, and intracoronary imaging contribute distinct, complementary information that can be used to determine lesion significance, refine treatment options, and optimize PCI. In isolation, these technologies are useful; however, coregistration of iFR or intracoronary imaging with the coronary angiogram has the potential to improve our management of patients with CAD. We know that anatomical and physiological data are complementary but distinct. Angiography can overestimate and underestimate the severity of disease. Physiological data allows us to characterize the level of flow-limitation and determine the severity of disease. Although anatomic data from intravascular imaging allows us to

characterize the vessel, the plaque composition and plan our lesion preparation and PCI techniques. The relative advantages and disadvantages of these techniques are described in **Table 4**. All 3 modalities of angiography, invasive physiology and intravascular imaging provide important information that, when used in combination, can improve the way we select patients for PCI, determine which lesions need to be treated and make important decisions about how we perform PCI to improve clinical outcomes.

The Philips SyncVision system allows this integration. After completing an IVUS or iFR coregistration a second coregistration can be undertaken with the complementary technology, without moving C-arm position. The same angiogram should be used to coregister the second modality. This has been exemplified in a case report.[22]

Although triregistration of angiography, intravascular imaging, and coronary physiology data holds promise for improving PCI, there are no current data to support its use. Use of an additional technology has time and resource implications and whether this technique is of clinical benefit should be the subject of future clinical trials.

SUMMARY AND FURTHER DIRECTIONS

PCI has undergone numerous developments over the decades. Technological advances have enabled the synthesis of coregistration software—where we can overlay different data points to provide either a physiological roadmap or detailed anatomic roadmap to optimize PCI.

The technologies are quick and easy to use but further studies are required to evaluate their impact on clinical practice. Both iFR and IVUS coregistration are now regularly used in catheterization laboratories worldwide.

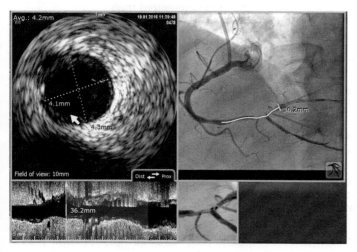

Fig. 3. IVUS coregistered angiogram demonstrating longitudinal and cross-sectional assessment of the RCA before stent deployment.

Table 4
Advantages and disadvantages of physiology and intravascular imaging coregistration

Coregistration Technique	Advantages	Disadvantages
iFR	A pressure drop can be visually depicted alongside the angiogram Allows for prediction of post-PCI outcome and enables tailoring of PCI approach Physiological data can be collected in single pullback	iFR coregistration technology s relatively new, more data is awaited on its clinical use and how it might influence clinical outcomes
IVUS	Provides detail regarding the vessel wall and nature of the disease including its composition No significant difference in fluoroscopy times versus OCT coregistration Images can be acquired in single pullback No need for blood clearance in vessel for image acquisition Theoretical reduced risk of dissection propagation (due to lack of blood displacement) Better placed to image left main, ostial lesions, chronic total occlusions	Smaller evidence-base for use of IVUS coregistration Requires some additional contrast injection for the coregistered images
OCT	Multiple RCTs investigating use of OCT coregistration Provides detail regarding the vessel wall and nature of the disease including its composition No significant difference in fluoroscopy times versus IVUS coregistration Images can be acquired in single pullback Better placed to image in-stent restenosis, calcium, thrombi, ruptured, and erosive plaques	Limited utility in patients with impaired renal function (contrast injection)

Triregistration, combining physiology, angiography, and intravascular imaging, has the ability to provide even more data for PCI optimization to further streamline our workflows but more data are needed to assess its clinical use.

CLINICS CARE POINTS

- iFR and IVUS coregistration are simple, practical, and quick adjuncts to conventional coronary angiography.
- iFR coregistration provides a physiological roadmap of a vessel, facilitating an optimized PCI strategy.
- IVUS coregistration has the ability to provide longitudinal anatomical data to support PCI decision-making and stent optimization.
- Performance of coregistration requires appropriate angiogram selection, consistency of fluoroscopic projection, and slow continuous pressure wire or catheter withdrawal.
- Continued clinical use of coregistration should be evidenced by improved clinical outcomes in randomized trials.

DISCLOSURE

Dr Michael Foley has received speaker's honoraria from Philips Volcano.

Dr Rasha Al-Lamee has received speaker's honoraria from Philips Volcano, Abbott Vascular, Medtronic, Janssen and Menarini Pharmaceuticals.

Dr Tobin Joseph does not have anything to disclose.

REFERENCES

1. Kikuta Y, Cook CM, Sharp ASP, et al. Pre-angioplasty instantaneous wave-free ratio pullback predicts

hemodynamic outcome in humans with coronary artery disease. JACC: Cardiovasc Interventions 2018;11(8): 757–67.

2. Demir OM, Rahman H, van de Hoef TP, et al. Invasive and non-invasive assessment of ischaemia in chronic coronary syndromes: translating pathophysiology to clinical practice. Eur Heart J 2022;43(2):105–17.

3. Davies JE, Sen S, Dehbi HM, et al. Use of the instantaneous wave-free ratio or fractional flow reserve in PCI. N Engl J Med 2017;376(19):1824–34.

4. Darmoch F, Alraies MC, Al-Khadra Y, et al. Intravascular ultrasound imaging–guided versus coronary angiography–guided percutaneous coronary intervention: a systematic review and meta-analysis. J Acad Hosp Adm 2020;9(5). https://doi.org/10.1161/JAHA.119.013678.

5. Ali ZA, Karimi Galougahi K, Maehara A, et al. Outcomes of optical coherence tomography compared with intravascular ultrasound and with angiography to guide coronary stent implantation: one-year results from the ILUMIEN III: OPTIMIZE PCI trial. EuroIntervention 2021;16(13):1085–91.

6. Sen S, Escaned J, Malik IS, et al. Development and validation of a new adenosine-independent index of stenosis severity from coronary wave–intensity analysis. J Am Coll Cardiol 2012;59(15):1392–402.

7. Nijjer SS, Sen S, Petraco R, et al. Pre-angioplasty instantaneous wave-free ratio pullback provides virtual intervention and predicts hemodynamic outcome for serial lesions and diffuse coronary artery disease. JACC: Cardiovasc Interventions. 2014;7(12):1386–96.

8. Higashioka D, Shiono Y, Kubo T, et al. The interstudy reproducibility of instantaneous wave-free ratio and angiography coregistration. J Cardiol 2020; 75(5):507–12.

9. Nijjer SS, Sen S, Petraco R, et al. The Instantaneous wave-Free Ratio (iFR) pullback: a novel innovation using baseline physiology to optimise coronary angioplasty in tandem lesions. Cardiovasc Revascularization Med 2015;16(3):167–71.

10. Jeremias A, Davies JE, Maehara A, et al. Blinded physiological assessment of residual ischemia after successful angiographic percutaneous coronary intervention. JACC: Cardiovasc Interventions 2019; 12(20):1991–2001.

11. Patel MR, Jeremias A, Maehara A, et al. 1-year outcomes of blinded physiological assessment of residual ischemia after successful PCI. JACC: Cardiovasc Interventions 2022;15(1):52–61.

12. Matsuo A, Kasahara T, Ariyoshi M, et al. Utility of angiography–physiology coregistration maps during percutaneous coronary intervention in clinical practice. Cardiovasc Interv Ther 2021;36(2):208–18.

13. Al-Lamee R, Rajkumar CA, Ganesananthan S, et al. Optimising physiological endpoints of percutaneous coronary intervention. EuroIntervention 2021;16(18): e1470–83.

14. Houissa K, Ryan N, Escaned J, et al. Validation of a novel system for Co-registration of coronary angiographic and intravascular ultrasound imaging. Cardiovasc Revascularization Med 2019;20(9):775–81.

15. Frimerman A, Abergel E, Blondheim D, et al. Novel method for real time Co-Registration of IVUS and coronary angiography. J Interv Cardiol 2016;29(2): 225–31.

16. Prasad M, Cassar A, Fetterly KA, et al. Co-registration of angiography and intravascular ultrasound images through image-based device tracking. Catheter Cardiovasc Interv 2016;88(7):1077–82.

17. van der Sijde JN, Guagliumi G, Sirbu V, et al. The OPTIS Integrated System: real-time, co-registration of angiography and optical coherence tomography. EuroIntervention 2016;12(7):855–60.

18. Leistner DM, Riedel M, Steinbeck L, et al. Real-time optical coherence tomography coregistration with angiography in percutaneous coronary intervention–impact on physician decision-making: the OPTICO-integration study. Catheter Cardiovasc Interv 2018; 92(1):30–7.

19. Schneider VS, Böhm F, Blum K, et al. Impact of real-time angiographic co-registered optical coherence tomography on percutaneous coronary intervention: the OPTICO-integration II trial. Clin Res Cardiol 2021;110(2):249–57.

20. Qin H, Li C, Li Y, et al. Automatic coregistration between coronary angiography and intravascular optical coherence tomography. JACC: Asia 2021;1(2): 274–8.

21. Koyama K, Fujino A, Maehara A, et al. A prospective, single-center, randomized study to assess whether automated coregistration of optical coherence tomography with angiography can reduce geographic miss. Catheter Cardiovasc Interv 2019;93(3):411–8.

22. Sacha J, Lipski P, Feusette P. Angiographic co-registration of instantaneous wave-free ratio and intravascular ultrasound improves functional assessment of borderline lesions in the coronary artery. pwki 2018;14(1):107–8.

23. Wang P, Ecabert O, Chen T, et al. Image-based Co-registration of angiography and intravascular ultrasound images. IEEE Trans Med Imaging 2013; 32(12):2238–49.

Intravascular Imaging-Derived Physiology—Basic Principles and Clinical Application

Annemieke C. Ziedses des Plantes, BSc[a], Alessandra Scoccia, MD[a],
Frank Gijsen, PhD[b], Gijs van Soest, PhD[b], Joost Daemen, MD, PhD[a],*

KEYWORDS

- Virtual FFR • IVUS-based FFR • OCT-based FFR • Percutaneous coronary intervention
- Functional lesion assessment • OFR

KEY POINTS

- Intravascular imaging-derived physiologic indices allow simultaneous morphologic and functional assessment with a single catheter.
- Recently developed intravascular imaging-derived physiologic indices have shown promising results.
- Validation in prospective outcome studies is required to demonstrate the clinical value of intravascular ultrasound-based and optical coherence tomography-based physiologic indices.

INTRODUCTION

The superiority of fractional flow reserve (FFR) as compared with coronary angiography (CAG)-guided percutaneous coronary intervention (PCI) has been established in several randomized trials.[1–5] However, the adoption of physiologic lesion assessment into clinical practice remains limited and has been linked to, among others, the need for a costly pressure wire and hyperemic agents with associated patient discomfort in case of FFR.[6,7] Recently, the estimation of coronary flow parameters based on 3D quantitative CAG through computational fluid dynamics (CFD) has gained interest and several imaging-derived physiologic indices have emerged with the intention to overcome the aforementioned limitations. The first clinical validation studies of angiography-derived physiologic indices show promising results, although classic limitations of angiography-based 3D reconstructions such as foreshortening and vessel overlap remain.[8–11]

High-resolution intravascular imaging techniques, such as intravascular ultrasound (IVUS) and optical coherence tomography (OCT), allow for accurate and comprehensive lesion assessment. Several randomized trials and meta-analyses have shown a reduction in major adverse cardiac events for both IVUS and OCT-guided PCI compared with angiography-guided PCI.[12–14] However, contemporary intravascular imaging systems preclude online physiologic lesion assessment. Combined use of FFR and intravascular imaging could be beneficial but requires 2 separate catheters. Recognizing that vessel caliber and geometry have a large influence on its functional characteristics, intravascular-imaging derived physiologic indices have been

This article originally appeared in *Interventional Cardiology Clinics*, Volume 12 Issue 1, January 2023.

[a] Department of Cardiology, Thoraxcenter, Erasmus University Medical Center, P.O. Box 2040, 3000 CA, Rotterdam, the Netherlands; [b] Department of Biomedical Engineering, Erasmus University Medical Center, P.O. Box 2040, 3000 CA, Rotterdam, the Netherlands
* Corresponding author. Department of Cardiology, Erasmus University Medical Center, room Rg-628, P.O. Box 2040, 3000 CA, Rotterdam, the Netherlands.
E-mail address: j.daemen@erasmusmc.nl

developed to provide a promising alternative allowing simultaneous morphologic and functional assessment. The present review aims to provide an overview of the currently available intravascular imaging-based physiologic indices, their diagnostic performance, and clinical application.

Intravascular Imaging-Derived Predictors of Fractional Flow Reserve

Several studies have investigated the ability of intravascular imaging techniques in predicting FFR. Both IVUS and OCT seem to be superior to CAG in determining lesion severity because they provide more accurate reference vessel dimensions and allow detailed assessment of lesion characteristics. IVUS-derived and OCT-derived minimal lumen areas (MLAs) have been proposed as a simple surrogate for physiologic assessment. However, the correlation and diagnostic performance of this index seems to be moderate. The corresponding optimal cutoff varied from 2.4 to 4.8 mm^2. Similarly, the AUC of OCT-derived MLA ranged from 0.74 to 0.91 for different cutoff values of MLA, whereas the corresponding optimal cutoff ranged between 1.59 and 2.88 mm^2. Moreover, in a head-to-head comparison between OCT and IVUS in predicting an FFR of 0.80 or less, both methods demonstrated a moderate diagnostic performance (AUC 0.70 for OCT vs 0.63 for IVUS, $P = .19$).[15] A systematic review by Chu and colleagues demonstrated that the correlation between IVUS-derived MLA and FFR ranged from weak to moderate (r 5 0.25–0.74), whereas the diagnostic performance of MLA, as expressed by the area under the curve (AUC), ranged from 0.76 to 0.87 in predicting an FFR of 0.75 or less and from 0.56 to 0.95 in predicting an FFR of 0.80 or less.[16]

From intravascular ultrasound/optical coherence tomography to Three-dimensional Geometric Models

In contrast to intravascular imaging-derived MLA, imaging-derived 3D morphologic assessment may provide a more accurate estimate of functional lesion significance. A crucial step in image-based FFR approaches is to create an accurate geometric model from the imaging data because the characteristics of blood flow in coronary arteries depend on 3D curvature, presence of bifurcations and lumen intruding plaques.[17] Due to the high quality and spatial resolution of intravascular imaging technologies such as IVUS and OCT, accurate lumen delineation and geometry reconstruction is possible. This geometric reconstruction can either contain only the main vessel

or include the ostia of side branches and adjust the reference diameter to consider the reference step-down phenomenon.[18] Li and colleagues generated a 3D reconstruction based on fusion of OCT and angiography, disregarding side branches, and a similar 3D reconstruction that included lumina of side branches derived from 3D angiography, and demonstrated that reconstruction of only the main vessel, disregarding flow loss through the side branches, may lead to underestimation of the CFD-based distal coronary pressure to aortic pressure (Pd/Pa) ratio and inaccurate regional shear stress calculations.[19] Because accurate coronary flow estimation is crucial for computation of pressure and velocity, a recent consensus statement on flow dynamics recommended that large side branches should be included in the 3D reconstruction.[17]

The motion of fluid, velocity, and pressure is described by the Navier-Stokes equations. The most common way to solve these equations is through CFD. In the context of computational FFR, this methodology is used to obtain information on blood flow velocity and pressure at any location in the coronary artery. From CFD, the pressure drop over a stenosis can be directly extracted and, combined with an estimate of the proximal or distal pressure, the FFR can be computed. Although CFD models provide a detailed approach with high spatial resolution, solving Navier-Stokes equations can be computationally intensive. To decrease computational time, simplified approaches have been proposed that reduce the complexity of the Navier-Stokes equations. Although these approaches allow for faster computation times, they may be less accurate because calculations are based mainly on anatomic characteristics and many assumptions are required.

Apart from geometric information, all models require input regarding the flow in the arterial segment where FFR needs to be computed.[17] At the inlet, boundary conditions for blood flow or pressure are applied. For the pressure at the inlet, either patient-specific measurements or population-averaged data can be used. Blood flow can be modeled as steady or transient flow. However, transient CFD models introduce a higher level of complexity to the model and prolong computational time. The pulsatile nature of blood flow is therefore mostly ignored and a time-averaged value over the cardiac cycle is used for the inflow velocity instead based on either thrombolysis in myocardial infarction (TIMI) frame count or intracoronary Doppler ultrasound. If these patient-specific measurements are not available, scaling laws can be applied that relate lumen diameter to flow rate.[17,20–22] The hyperemic flow rate can be derived by applying a hyperemia-specific scaling law to lumen measurements or by applying a conversion based on physiologic assumptions to the resting flow rate.

At the outlet, a constant pressure boundary can be applied. Alternatively, a lumped parameter model (LPM) representing the coronary microcirculation can be used to couple the inlet and outlet.[23]

CURRENTLY AVAILABLE SOLUTIONS

In **Tables 1** and **2**, the characteristics and diagnostic performance of the currently available intravascular imaging-derived physiologic indices are summarized. The sensitivity and specificity of these indices and their corresponding 95% confidence intervals are displayed graphically in **Fig. 1**.

Optical Coherence Tomography-Derived Fractional Flow Reserve Indices

In recent years, several OCT-derived FFR indices have been developed (**table 1**). A major advantage of OCT over IVUS is its resolution with clear contrast between lumen and vessel wall, allowing for more accurate automatic lumen segmentation.

Pivotal indices use a steady-state CFD analysis to calculate FFR, performing blood flow simulations by solving the Navier-Stokes equations.[23–25] In order to construct a 3D geometric model, lumen contours are delineated using semiautomatic procedures while side-branches are eliminated.

An approach named FFR_{OCT} subsequently applies a population-averaged nonhyperemic mean flow velocity based on TIMI frame count at the inlet and a mean blood pressure of 93.2 mm Hg at the outlet. These averaged values were derived from angiography and pressure measurements of 35 out of the 92 included patients. In the full cohort of 92 patients, FFR_{OCT} correlated well with FFR (r = 0.72, P < .001) and had a diagnostic accuracy of 88.0%, sensitivity of 68.7% and 95.6% specificity in predicting an FFR of 0.80 or less. The AUC of FFR_{OCT} was 0.93, which was similar or better compared with anatomic parameters MLD, percentage diameter stenosis, and MLA. The overall analysis time was less than 10 minutes.[24]

A related methodology, *OCT-FFR*, simulates FFR using an approach that is largely similar to the procedure described above. In this approach, however, FFR is simulated by coupling the 3D CFD model to an LPM representing the coronary microcirculation, based on vessel length extracted from angiography data. In addition, hyperemic flow is simulated by reducing the coronary resistance value to 25% of the normal resistance. In a

simulation of 17 vessels in 13 patients, OCT-FFR showed a good correlation with clinically measured FFR (r = 0.82, P < .001). The methodology proved to be limited by a total computational time of approximately 29 minutes. Additionally, only single stenosis cases were studied and therefore the technique is not validated for serial stenoses.[23]

Jang and colleagues validated 2 different methods, an analytical fluid dynamics (AFD) and a CFD approach. A training set of 9 randomly selected patients was used for parameter fitting to model the capillary microcirculation in both the CFD and AFD approaches. The $FFR-OCT_{CFD}$ study resembles the approaches described above but applies a constant pressure condition to the inlet and outlet and uses a distal porous media model, similar to an LPM, to model the capillary vessels. The $FFR-OCT_{AFD}$ approach, however, does not use a 3D reconstruction but reconstructs coronary arteries as axisymmetric tubes based on the OCT images. FFR is calculated using an LPM for which the resistance values are obtained using Poiseuille's and Ohm's law. Microvascular resistance values were derived from the measured FFR in the training set. In the retrospective validation including 95 patients, both $FFR-OCT_{AFD}$ and $FFR-OCT_{CFD}$ showed a good diagnostic performance of 0.86 in predicting an FFR less than 0.80 and an AUC that was significantly higher compared with angiographic diameter stenosis (DS) (0.88 and 0.86 vs 0.59). In addition, both the AFD and CFD method showed a good linear correlation with measured FFR (r = 0.760, P < .001 and r = 0.707, P < .001, respectively). No data on computation time for both the AFD and CFD approach was reported.[25]

Seike and colleagues validated *OCT-derived FFR* using an original algorithm based on basic fluid dynamics that does not require 3D reconstruction of the vessel. This algorithm is based on the equation for fluid dynamics by Gould and colleagues describing the calculated pressure loss across a stenosis.[26] The parameters describing pressure loss are determined based on anatomic parameters obtained from OCT data. Using a prespecified basal coronary flow velocity of 20 cm/s based on previous studies and a patient-specific stenosis flow reserve (SFR), the hyperemic flow velocity is calculated. The OCT-derived FFR is subsequently calculated based on the SFR and an assumed systolic/diastolic mean blood pressure of 120/60 mm Hg.

In a small retrospective cohort including 31 vessels in 31 patients, OCT-derived FFR showed a strong linear correlation with invasive pressure wire-based FFR measurements (r = 0.889,

Table 1
Features of available methodologies for intravascular imaging-based computation of fractional flow reserve

Method	Fluid Dynamics Solution	Flow Pattern	Side Branch Modeling	Hyperemic Flow Assumption	Total Computational Time
IVUS$_{FR}$	CFD	Steady	Yes	3-fold increase compared with resting blood flow	9.1 h
IVUS-FFR	Simplified fluid dynamics equations	Steady	No	Calculated using prespecified basal coronary flow velocity and patient-specific SFR	*Not reported*
UFR	Simplified fluid dynamics equations	Steady	Yes	Hyperemic volumetric flow rate: proximal reference lumen area multiplied by virtual hyperemic flow of 0.35 m/s	2 min
OFR	Simplified fluid dynamics equations	Steady	Yes	Hyperemic volumetric flow rate: proximal reference lumen area multiplied by virtual hyperemic flow of 0.35 m/s	<1 min
FFR-OCT$_{AFD}$	Simplified fluid dynamics equations	Steady	No	NA	*Not reported*
FFR-OCT$_{CFD}$	CFD	Steady	No	NA	*Not reported*
OCT-FFR	CFD	Steady	No	Hyperemic flow simulated by reducing coronary resistance value to 25% of normal	29 min
OCT-derived FFR	Simplified fluid dynamics equations	Steady	No	Calculated using prespecified basal coronary flow velocity and patient-specific SFR	<10 min

(*continued on next page*)

Table 1
(continued)

Method	Fluid Dynamics Solution	Flow Pattern	Side Branch Modeling	Hyperemic Flow Assumption	Total Computational Time
FFR$_{OCT}$	CFD	Steady	No	NA: population-averaged nonhyperemic flow rate applied	<10 min
AccuFFRivus	Simplified fluid dynamics equations	Steady	No	Flow rate conversion from rest to hyperemic state applied	5 min 20s
OCT-based machine learning FFR	Machine-learning	NA	NA	NA	20 min
IVUS-based machine learning FFR	Machine-learning	NA	NA	NA	*Not reported*

$P < .001$). Furthermore, OCT-derived FFR correlated better with wire-based FFR measurements compared with QCA-based percentage DS and OCT measurements of MLA.[27]

Finally, *Optical flow ratio* (OFR) is the most widely studied OCT-derived FFR index to date. The OCTplus software (Pulse Medical Imaging Technology, Shanghai, China) performs automatic lumen contouring, segmentation and side branch detection in order to create a 3D reconstruction. Bifurcation fractal laws are applied to consider the impact of side branches. A computational approach adapted from angiography-based quantitative flow ratio (QFR) is subsequently applied to compute the OFR value at each position along the vessel. More specifically, the proximal reference lumen area is multiplied by a virtual hyperemic flow of 0.35 m/s applied at the inlet boundary in order to simulate the pressure drop under hyperemic conditions. In case of sequential stenosis requiring multiple pullbacks, the pullbacks can be combined in order to calculate the OFR over the whole length of the lesion.[28]

The algorithm was fine-tuned and validated in retrospective datasets, showing high diagnostic accuracy with wire-based FFR as a reference standard.[28,29] Following these retrospective studies, OFR was recently validated in a prospective series including 55 patients, showing an excellent diagnostic performance (sensitivity 92%, specificity 93%, accuracy 93%, AUC 0.95) in predicting an FFR of 0.80 or less.[30] In this multicenter prospective study, median time required for computation of OFR once the OCT data were loaded into the software was 1.07 minute. The

AUC of OFR was numerically higher than that of QFR (0.91, $P = .115$) and significantly higher than that of OCT-derived MLA (0.64, $P < .001$). Moreover, in a head-to-head comparison, Huang and colleagues found a significantly better agreement with FFR for OFR compared with QFR and proved superiority of OFR to QFR.[29] The diagnostic accuracy of OFR proved to be independent of the coronary vessel analyzed, presence of a bifurcation lesion, sequential stenosis, or history of myocardial infarction. Both the retrospective and prospective validation studies showed excellent intraobserver and interobserver variabilities.

Intravascular Ultrasound-Derived Fractional Flow Reserve Indices

One of the first IVUS-derived FFR indices was developed by Bezerra and colleagues under the name *IVUS$_{FR}$*. The method uses a steady-state CFD model similar to the CFD methods described above. In order to generate a 3D reconstruction of the arterial lumen, gating of IVUS images is performed to retrieve the end-diastolic phase from the IVUS dataset. Lumen and external elastic lamina (EEL) contours are traced offline, making it a time-consuming process, although the approach was standardized to generate a model that only requires determination of a few lumen areas per patient. A 3D reconstruction, including the side branches, is made by placing the IVUS-derived cross-sectional areas along the transducer trajectory that is reconstructed from 2 orthogonal angiographic images. The hyperemic flow rate is calculated assuming a 3-fold increase compared

Table 2
Studies investigating diagnostic performance of intravascular imaging derived fractional flow reserve indices in predicting an FFR of 0.80 or less

Study/Author	Method	Modality	Year	Study Design	Number of Vessels (Patients)	Correlation with Wire-based FFR	AUC (95% CI)	Sensitivity, (95% CI)	Specificity, (95% CI)	PPV, (95% CI)	NPV, (95% CI)	Accuracy, (95% CI)	Intraobserver Variability	Interobserver Variability
FFR derived from IVUS														
Bezerra et al,[31] 2019	IVUS$_{FR}$	IVUS	2018	Prospective, single center	34 (24)	0.79	0.93 (0.83–1.00)	0.89 (0.68–1.00)	0.92 (0.81–1.00)	0.80 (0.55–1.00)	0.96 (0.89–1.00)	0.91 (0.82–1.00)	–	–
Seike et al,[27] 2017	IVUS-FFR	IVUS	2018	Retrospective, single center	50 (48)	0.78	–	–	–	–	–	–	–	–
Yu et al,[28] 2017	UFR	IVUS	2021	Retrospective, single center	97 (94)	0.87	0.97 (0.93–0.99)	0.91 (0.82–0.96)	0.96 (0.90–0.99)	0.96 (0.89–0.99)	0.91 (0.93–0.96)	0.92 (0.87–0.96)	0.0 ± 0.03	0.01 ± 0.03
FFR derived from OCT														
Yu et al,[28] 2017	OFR	OCT	2019	Retrospective, multicenter	125 (118)	0.70	0.93 (0.87–0.97)	0.87 (0.77–0.94)	0.92 (0.82–0.97)	0.92 (0.82–0.97)	0.88 (0.77–0.95)	0.90 (0.84–0.95)	0.00 ± 0.02	0.00 ± 0.03
Huang et al,[29] 2020	OFR	OCT	2020	Retrospective, single center	212 (181)	0.87	0.97 (0.93–0.99)	0.86 (0.77–0.93)	0.95 (0.90–0.98)	0.92 (0.84–0.97)	0.91 (0.85–0.95)	0.92 (0.88–0.95)	–	–
Gutiérrez-Chico et al,[30] 2020	OFR	OCT	2020	Prospective, multicenter	69 (55)	0.83	0.95 (0.86–0.99)	0.92 (0.73–0.99)	0.93 (0.82–0.99)	0.88 (0.69–0.98)	0.96 (0.85–0.99)	0.93 (0.86–0.99)	ICCa 0.97	ICCa 0.95
Jang et al,[25] 2017	FFR-OCT$_{AFD}$	OCT	2017	Retrospective, single center	95 (95)	0.76	0.88 (0.76–0.94)	0.65 (0.44–0.82)	0.94 (0.85–0.98)	0.81 (0.57–0.94)	0.88 (0.78–0.94)	0.86	–	–
	FFR-OCT$_{CFD}$	OCT	2017	Retrospective, single center	95 (95)	0.71	0.86 (0.74–0.93)	0.73 (0.52–0.88)	0.91 (0.81–0.96)	0.76 (0.55–0.90)	0.90 (0.80–0.96)	0.86	–	–
Lee et al,[23] 2017	OCT-FFR	OCT	2017	Retrospective, single center	17 (13)	0.82	–	–	–	–	–	–	–	–
Seike et al,[27] 2017	OCT-derived FFR	OCT	2017	Retrospective, multicenter	31 (31)	0.89	–	–	–	–	–	–	–	–
Ha et al,[24] 2016	FFR$_{OCT}$	OCT	2016	Retrospective, single center	92 (92)	0.72	0.93	0.69	0.96	0.84	0.89	0.88	ICCa 0.94	ICCa 0.94
FFR derived from fusion of IVUS and Angiography														
Jiang et al,[32] 2021	AccuFFRivus	OCT & 3D-QCA	2021	Retrospective, single center	32 (31)	0.86	0.98 (0.86–1.00)	0.93 (0.66–1.00)	0.94 (0.72–1.00)	0.93 (0.66–0.99)	0.94 (0.72–0.99)	0.94 (0.79–0.99)	–	–

Machine-learning–based FFR

Study	FFR	Modality	Year	Design	N								
Cha et al,[36] 2021	OCT-based machine-learning FFR	OCT	2020	Retrospective, single center	125 (125)	0.85	0.98	1.00	0.93	0.88	1.00	0.95	-
Lee et al,[37] 2017	IVUS-based machine-learning FFR	IVUS	2020	Retrospective, single center	1328 (1328)	-	0.87[a]	0.70[a]	0.86[a]	0.70[a]	0.87[a]	0.82[a]	-

[a] Based on the L2-logistic regression model. Several other models were tested.

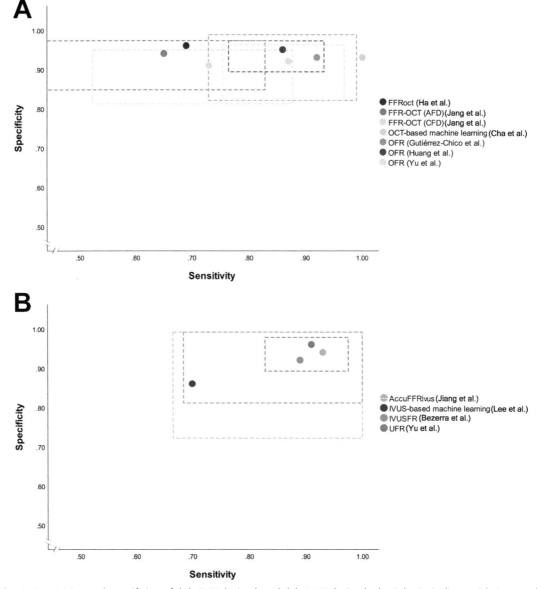

Fig. 1. Sensitivity and specificity of (A) OCT-derived and (B) IVUS-derived physiologic indices with invasively measured FFR as reference. Colored dots represent the sensitivity and specificity of different methods as reported in the validation studies and 95% confidence intervals (if available) are displayed as rectangles in corresponding colors.

with resting blood flow estimated based on the anatomic morphology. In a prospective cohort of 34 patients, $IVUS_{FR}$ had a strong correlation with invasive FFR (r = 0.79, P < .001) and a good diagnostic performance (diagnostic accuracy 0.91, sensitivity 0.89 and specificity 0.92) in predicting an FFR of 0.80 or less. Furthermore, $IVUS_{FR}$ performed better in predicting an invasive FFR of 0.80 or less and had a higher AUC as compared with MLA and %DS (0.93 vs 0.81 and 0.70).

However, an important limitation to this method is the long computational time of 9.1 hours for image processing, reconstruction, and simulation.[31]

AccuFFRivus combines IVUS and CAG images to calculate FFR using a simplified pressure-drop formula. After automatic extraction of the gated diastolic IVUS images, IVUS-derived luminal boundaries are automatically segmented using a deep learning method. IVUS images are subsequently combined with the catheter path to create a 3D reconstruction of the coronary artery. FFR is calculated using TIMI frame count as estimator for average flow rate and hyperemic flow rate is estimated using a flow rate conversion formula.

Jiang and colleagues performed AccuFFRivus calculations on 32 coronary vessels with invasive FFR as reference standard, which showed a good correlation between AccuFFRivus and FFR and a diagnostic accuracy of 93.4% in predicting an FFR of 0.80 or less (sensitivity 92.9%, specificity 94.4%). Furthermore, AccuFFRivus had a higher AUC (0.98) compared with MLA (0.78) and diameter stenosis rate (0.66). The mean time for AccuFFrivus assessment was approximately 5 minutes.[32]

Seike and colleagues developed *IVUS-FFR*, which applies the same methodology described above for OCT-derived FFR to IVUS images. IVUS-FFR correlated well with pressure wire-based FFR (r = 0.78, *P* < .001) and correlated better with pressure wire-based FFR as compared with quantitative CAG and IVUS measurements of MLA and percentage area stenosis (AS). In contrast to the OCT approach, IVUS segmentation was not performed automatically. Although information on computational time was not provided, manual lumen segmentation is expected to make the approach again more time-consuming and less suitable for routine clinical practice.[33]

Ultrasonic flow ratio (UFR) applies the same approach described above for OFR to IVUS images. Using a deep learning method, lumen and EEL areas are semiautomatically delineated and reconstructed in 3D. Besides the imaging modality, the procedure is identical to the OFR approach. UFR was validated in a cohort of 97 vessels in 94 patients and showed a strong correlation with FFR (r = 0.87, *P* < .001) and a diagnostic accuracy of 92% (sensitivity 91%, specificity 96%) in identifying an FFR of 0.80 or less. The AUC was significantly higher for UFR than IVUS-derived MLA (0.97 vs 0.89). Moreover, Sui and colleagues found a strong correlation (r = 0.74) between QFR and UFR in the assessment of left main coronary artery stenosis and found a diagnostic accuracy of 95% (sensitivity 82%, specificity 100%)[34] for UFR in predicting a QFR of 0.80 or less. With a median lumen delineation time through deep learning of 34 seconds per pullback and a median analysis time of 102 seconds, the approach is relatively fast compared with other methodologies.[35]

Machine-learning Approaches

In addition to the CFD and simplified fluid dynamics-based methodologies, 2 machine-learning methods have been developed to predict FFR. Cha and colleagues attempted to derive FFR from OCT by selecting a total of 36 features as inputs for the machine-learning model according to expert opinion and prior literature search. In the testing sample, the Random Forest model obtained the highest performance using the 6 most important features based on weight, namely, MLA, percentage of the stenotic area, lesion length, proximal LA, preprocedural platelet count, and hypertension. The machine-learning–derived FFR was trained and validated in a cohort of 125 patients (training and testing groups partitioned in the ratio of 5:1) with intermediate lesions in the left descending artery, which showed a good correlation with wire-based FFR (r = 0.853, *P* < .001). Furthermore, the method showed a diagnostic accuracy of 0.95 in predicting an FFR of 0.8 or less with a sensitivity of 100% and a specificity of 93%. Overall, the computation time of OCT-derived FFR according to the authors was about 20 minutes due to manual lumen extraction, although the machine-learning FFR only took 2 to 3 minutes to extract key OCT features and analyze FFR.[36] Similarly, Lee and colleagues developed a machine-learning algorithm to predict FFR based on IVUS. Semiautomatic lumen segmentation was performed after which the cross-sectional images were segmented and coded into compartments. A total of 105 features based on IVUS and clinical features were identified and used for the machine-learning algorithm, based on which 6 different algorithms were evaluated. Algorithms were trained in a training set of 1063 lesions and evaluated in a test set of 264 lesions. All algorithms showed an overall accuracy greater than 80% (AUCs 0.84–0.87) in predicting an FFR of 0.80 or less in non-left main coronary lesions.[37]

DISCUSSION

In the past decades, the use of both IVUS-guided and OCT-guided PCIs steadily increased following several randomized trials that demonstrated their superiority as compared with angiography-guided PCI.[12–14] Both modalities allow for tailored lesion preparation, more accurate stent sizing and identification of appropriate landing zones, decreasing the risk of geographic miss.[38–40] Moreover, intravascular imaging enables identification and visualization of high-risk plaques.[41–43] In addition, post-PCI imaging allows for the detection of suboptimal stent implantation and may guide optimization.[40]

IVUS-derived and OCT-derived MLAs have shown only a moderate correlation with physiologic parameters such as FFR. Extension of the standard morphometric IVUS-derived and OCT-derived parameters with a physiologic parameter would therefore be of great value to assess physiologic lesion significance and to assess the relevance of residual disease after stenting. Therefore, various IVUS-based and OCT-based FFR indices have been proposed that show a good diagnostic performance and an improved predictive ability compared with MLA only. A major advantage of IVUS-based and OCT-based approaches is that they enable accurate assessment of lumen geometry and are not dependent on obtaining suitable angiographic projections, which can be challenging in patients with more complex anatomy. However, several challenges need to be overcome before these methods will be embraced in routine clinical setting. First, most of the indices described above disregard the impact of side branches. Especially omitting side branches between the location where flow is estimated and the stenosis will overestimate flow rates resulting in lower computed FFR values. When based on scaling laws, flow through the diseased segment should be based on the nearest healthy proximal cross section. Second, as IVUS and OCT provide no direct information on coronary flow, they remain dependent on population-averaged values and thereby disregard the interindividual differences in hyperemic response.

Third, from a clinical perspective, the relatively long computational times of most indices preclude uptake in clinical practice (see **table 1**). The latter limitation mostly relates to the IVUS-derived indices in which there is a need for manual correction of lumen contours. New-generation high-definition IVUS systems might open the door to better semiautomatic contour detection algorithms. Thanks to its higher resolution, OCT-based physiologic lesion assessment is at present a more appealing option with respect to feasibility in routine clinical practice. However, OCT with the most widely used OCT system (ILLUMIEN, Abbott, St. Paul, Minnesota, USA) is still limited by a maximum pullback length of 75 mm. Ideally, the imaging catheter should be pulled back to the ostium of the vessel to include the pressure drop along the entire vessel. In longer or more distal lesions, this may not always be feasible using an OCT catheter, although a methodology to combine 2 OCT pullbacks was described for the computation of OFR.

Fourth, most of the proposed methodologies have only been validated in retrospective cohorts, with the exception of OFR, which was validated in a prospective series.[30] Most studies assessed the diagnostic performance in predicting significant FFR. However, prospective clinical outcome studies demonstrating the noninferiority as compared with conventional physiologic lesion assessment and superiority as compared with angiography-guided PCI are lacking. Dedicated prospective trials are needed to demonstrate the feasibility of these approaches in a clinical setting and to define optimal cutoffs for a significant gradient.

Finally, to date, the uptake of routine intracoronary imaging to guide coronary revascularization remains limited. The latter directly limits the premise of invasive imaging-derived physiologic parameters, especially in an era where angiography-based FFR is emerging with multiple indices that demonstrated to have excellent diagnostic accuracy and even demonstrated to improve clinical outcome as compared with angiography-guided PCI.[9–11,44,45]

Acknowledging the fact that both intracoronary imaging and physiology (using both conventional pressure wire systems and angiography-based indices) demonstrated to improve clinical outcome in a continuously growing number of studies, the potential of merging imaging and physiology into a single procedure, enhanced by artificial intelligence and deep learning algorithms that minimize the need for manual input, seems imperative. When aforementioned limitations can be overcome, imaging-derived physiology would allow functional and morphologic assessment using one catheter, saving time and costs.

SUMMARY

Intravascular imaging-derived physiology is a promising alternative to conventional pressure-wire–based FFR. Recently, several OCT-based and IVUS-based FFR indices have been developed that compute FFR through CFD, fluid dynamics equations, or machine-learning methods. Although the first validation studies have shown favorable results, the body of evidence is still limited and is built mainly on small, retrospective studies. Prospective validation and randomized trials are needed to prove the clinical value of intravascular imaging-derived FFR.

CLINICS CARE POINTS

- IVUS-derived and OCT-derived MLAs have a moderate correlation with invasively measured FFR.
- Currently available indices have shown a good diagnostic performance in predicting an FFR of 0.80 or less in (mostly retrospective) validation studies.

- Dedicated prospective trials are required to demonstrate the feasibility of these approaches in a clinical setting, to define optimal cutoffs for a significant gradient and to evaluate the effect of IVUS or OCT-based physiology-guided PCI on clinical outcomes.

DISCLOSURE

Joost Daemen received institutional grant/research support from AstraZeneca, Abbott Vascular, Boston Scientific, ACIST Medical Systems, Medtronic, Pie Medical, and ReCor Medical. Gijs van Soest is an advisor to, and holds equity in, Kaminari Medical BV. He is the principal investigator of projects at Erasmus MC that receive research support from Terumo.

REFERENCES

1. De Bruyne B, Pijls NH, Kalesan B, et al. Fractional flow reserve-guided PCI versus medical therapy in stable coronary disease. N Engl J Med 2012; 367(11):991–1001.

2. Tonino PA, De Bruyne B, Pijls NH, et al. Fractional flow reserve versus angiography for guiding percutaneous coronary intervention. N Engl J Med 2009; 360(3):213–24.

3. Zimmermann FM, Ferrara A, Johnson NP, et al. Deferral vs. performance of percutaneous coronary intervention of functionally non-significant coronary stenosis: 15-year follow-up of the DEFER trial. Eur Heart J 2015;36(45):3182–8.

4. Neumann FJ, Sousa-Uva M, Ahlsson A, et al. 2018 ESC/EACTS Guidelines on myocardial revascularization. Eur Heart J 2019;40(2):87–165.

5. Writing Committee M, Lawton JS, Tamis-Holland JE, et al. 2021 ACC/AHA/SCAI Guideline for Coronary Artery Revascularization: Executive Summary: A Report of the American College of Cardiology/American Heart Association Joint Committee on Clinical Practice Guidelines. J Am Coll Cardiol 2022;79(2): 197–215.

6. Pijls NH, Tonino PA. The crux of maximum hyperemia: the last remaining barrier for routine use of fractional flow reserve. JACC Cardiovasc Interv 2011;4(10):1093–5.

7. Tebaldi M, Biscaglia S, Fineschi M, et al. Evolving Routine Standards in Invasive Hemodynamic Assessment of Coronary Stenosis: The Nationwide Italian SICI-GISE Cross-Sectional ERIS Study. JACC Cardiovasc Interv 2018;11(15):1482–91.

8. De Maria GL, Garcia-Garcia HM, Scarsini R, et al. Novel Indices of Coronary Physiology: Do We Need Alternatives to Fractional Flow Reserve? Circ Cardiovasc Interv 2020;13(4):e008487.

9. Masdjedi K, Tanaka N, Van Belle E, et al. Vessel fractional flow reserve (vFFR) for the assessment of stenosis severity: the FAST II study. EuroIntervention 2022;17(18):1498–505.

10. Westra J, Tu S, Campo G, et al. Diagnostic performance of quantitative flow ratio in prospectively enrolled patients: An individual patient-data meta-analysis. Catheter Cardiovasc Interv 2019;94(5): 693–701.

11. Fearon WF, Achenbach S, Engstrom T, et al. Accuracy of Fractional Flow Reserve Derived From Coronary Angiography. Circulation 2019;139(4):477–84.

12. Bavishi C, Sardar P, Chatterjee S, et al. Intravascular ultrasound-guided vs angiography-guided drug-eluting stent implantation in complex coronary lesions: Meta-analysis of randomized trials. Am Heart J 2017;185:26–34.

13. Groenland FTW, Neleman T, Kakar H, et al. Intravascular ultrasound-guided versus coronary angiography-guided percutaneous coronary intervention in patients with acute myocardial infarction: A systematic review and meta-analysis. Int J Cardiol 2022;353:35–42.

14. Kuku KO, Ekanem E, Azizi V, et al. Optical coherence tomography-guided percutaneous coronary intervention compared with other imaging guidance: a meta-analysis. Int J Cardiovasc Imaging 2018; 34(4):503–13.

15. Gonzalo N, Escaned J, Alfonso F, et al. Morphometric assessment of coronary stenosis relevance with optical coherence tomography: a comparison with fractional flow reserve and intravascular ultrasound. J Am Coll Cardiol 2012;59(12):1080–9. https://doi.org/10.1016/j.jacc.2011.09.078.

16. Chu M, Dai N, Yang J, et al. A systematic review of imaging anatomy in predicting functional significance of coronary stenoses determined by fractional flow reserve. Int J Cardiovasc Imaging 2017; 33(7):975–90.

17. Gijsen F, Katagiri Y, Barlis P, et al. Expert recommendations on the assessment of wall shear stress in human coronary arteries: existing methodologies, technical considerations, and clinical applications. Eur Heart J 2019;40(41):3421–33.

18. Tu S, Echavarria-Pinto M, von Birgelen C, et al. Fractional flow reserve and coronary bifurcation anatomy: a novel quantitative model to assess and report the stenosis severity of bifurcation lesions. JACC Cardiovasc Interv 2015;8(4):564–74.

19. Li Y, Gutiérrez-Chico JL, Holm NR, et al. Impact of Side Branch Modeling on Computation of Endothelial Shear Stress in Coronary Artery Disease: Coronary Tree Reconstruction by Fusion of 3D Angiography and OCT. J Am Coll Cardiol 2015;66(2):125–35.

20. Dodge JT Jr, Rizzo M, Nykiel M, et al. Impact of injection rate on the Thrombolysis in Myocardial Infarction (TIMI) trial frame count. Am J Cardiol 1998;81(10):1268–70.

21. Tanedo JS, Kelly RF, Marquez M, et al. Assessing coronary blood flow dynamics with the TIMI frame count method: comparison with simultaneous intracoronary Doppler and ultrasound. Catheter Cardiovasc Interv 2001;53(4):459–63.

22. Kassab GS. Scaling laws of vascular trees: of form and function. Am J Physiol Heart Circ Physiol 2006;290(2):H894–903.

23. Lee KE, Lee SH, Shin ES, et al. A vessel length-based method to compute coronary fractional flow reserve from optical coherence tomography images. Biomed Eng Online 2017;16(1):83.

24. Ha J, Kim JS, Lim J, et al. Assessing Computational Fractional Flow Reserve From Optical Coherence Tomography in Patients With Intermediate Coronary Stenosis in the Left Anterior Descending Artery. Circ Cardiovasc Interv 2016;9(8).

25. Jang SJ, Ahn JM, Kim B, et al. Comparison of Accuracy of One-Use Methods for Calculating Fractional Flow Reserve by Intravascular Optical Coherence Tomography to That Determined by the Pressure-Wire Method. Am J Cardiol 2017;120(11):1920–5.

26. Gould KL, Kelley KO, Bolson EL. Experimental validation of quantitative coronary arteriography for determining pressure-flow characteristics of coronary stenosis. Circulation 1982;66(5):930–7.

27. Seike F, Uetani T, Nishimura K, et al. Intracoronary Optical Coherence Tomography-Derived Virtual Fractional Flow Reserve for the Assessment of Coronary Artery Disease. Am J Cardiol 2017;120(10):1772–9.

28. Yu W, Huang J, Jia D, et al. Diagnostic accuracy of intracoronary optical coherence tomography-derived fractional flow reserve for assessment of coronary stenosis severity. EuroIntervention 2019;15(2):189–97.

29. Huang J, Emori H, Ding D, et al. Diagnostic performance of intracoronary optical coherence tomography-based versus angiography-based fractional flow reserve for the evaluation of coronary lesions. EuroIntervention 2020;16(7):568–76.

30. Gutiérrez-Chico JL, Chen Y, Yu W, et al. Diagnostic accuracy and reproducibility of optical flow ratio for functional evaluation of coronary stenosis in a prospective series. Cardiol J 2020;27(4):350–61.

31. Bezerra CG, Hideo-Kajita A, Bulant CA, et al. Coronary fractional flow reserve derived from intravascular ultrasound imaging: Validation of a new computational method of fusion between anatomy and physiology. Catheter Cardiovasc Interv 2019;93(2):266–74.

32. Jiang J, Feng L, Li C, et al. Fractional flow reserve for coronary stenosis assessment derived from fusion of intravascular ultrasound and X-ray angiography. Quant Imaging Med Surg Nov 2021;11(11):4543–55.

33. Seike F, Uetani T, Nishimura K, et al. Intravascular Ultrasound-Derived Virtual Fractional Flow Reserve for the Assessment of Myocardial Ischemia. Circ J 2018;82(3):815–23.

34. Sui Y, Yang M, Xu Y, et al. Diagnostic performance of intravascular ultrasound-based fractional flow reserve versus angiography-based quantitative flow ratio measurements for evaluating left main coronary artery stenosis. Catheter Cardiovasc Interv 2022 May;99 Suppl 1:1403–9. https://doi.org/10.1002/ccd.30078. Epub 2022 Feb 7. PMID: 35129284.

35. Yu W, Tanigaki T, Ding D, et al. Accuracy of Intravascular Ultrasound-Based Fractional Flow Reserve in Identifying Hemodynamic Significance of Coronary Stenosis. Circ Cardiovasc Interv 2021;14(2):e009840.

36. Cha JJ, Son TD, Ha J, et al. Optical coherence tomography-based machine learning for predicting fractional flow reserve in intermediate coronary stenosis: a feasibility study. Sci Rep 2020;10(1):20421.

37. Lee JG, Ko J, Hae H, et al. Intravascular ultrasound-based machine learning for predicting fractional flow reserve in intermediate coronary artery lesions. Atherosclerosis 2020;292:171–7.

38. de Jaegere P, Mudra H, Figulla H, et al. Intravascular ultrasound-guided optimized stent deployment. Immediate and 6 months clinical and angiographic results from the Multicenter Ultrasound Stenting in Coronaries Study (MUSIC Study). Eur Heart J 1998;19(8):1214–23.

39. Ahn JM, Kang SJ, Yoon SH, et al. Meta-analysis of outcomes after intravascular ultrasound-guided versus angiography-guided drug-eluting stent implantation in 26,503 patients enrolled in three randomized trials and 14 observational studies. Am J Cardiol 2014;113(8):1338–47.

40. Ali ZA, Maehara A, Généreux P, et al. Optical coherence tomography compared with intravascular ultrasound and with angiography to guide coronary stent implantation (ILUMIEN III: OPTIMIZE PCI): a randomised controlled trial. Lancet 2016;388(10060):2618–28.

41. Prati F, Romagnoli E, Gatto L, et al. Relationship between coronary plaque morphology of the left anterior descending artery and 12 months clinical outcome: the CLIMA study. Eur Heart J 2020;41(3):383–91.

42. Xing L, Higuma T, Wang Z, et al. Clinical Significance of Lipid-Rich Plaque Detected by Optical Coherence Tomography: A 4-Year Follow-Up Study. J Am Coll Cardiol 2017;69(20):2502–13.

43. Stone GW, Maehara A, Lansky AJ, et al. A prospective natural-history study of coronary atherosclerosis. N Engl J Med 2011;364(3):226–35.

44. Masdjedi K, van Zandvoort LJC, Balbi MM, et al. Validation of a three-dimensional quantitative coronary angiography-based software to calculate fractional flow reserve: the FAST study. EuroIntervention 2020;16(7):591–9.

45. Xu B, Tu S, Song L, et al. Angiographic quantitative flow ratio-guided coronary intervention (FAVOR III China): a multicentre, randomised, sham-controlled trial. Lancet 2021;398(10317):2149–59.

Computed Tomography-Derived Physiology Assessment: State-of-the-Art Review

Robert D. Safian, MD, MSCAI, FACC, FSCCT

KEYWORDS

- Coronary computed tomography angiography • Fractional flow reserve • Coronary artery disease
- Myocardial ischemia • Plaque characterization • Planning revascularization

KEY POINTS

- Cardiac computed tomography (CT) angiography is the best noninvasive technique to identify coronary artery disease (CAD) and characterize atherosclerotic plaque.
- Fractional flow reserve can be measured noninvasively using coronary CT angiography (CCTA)-derived techniques (CT-derived FFR [FFRCT]) and provides physiologic information about lesion-specific ischemia that is similar to invasive techniques.
- CCTA and FFRCT have broad applications including simple and complex plaque characterization, assessment of ischemia in patients with stable CAD and with acute chest pain in the emergency department, preoperative evaluation, and planning revascularization strategies.
- CCTA and FFRCT will likely become the gatekeeper to the cardiac catheterization laboratory.

INTRODUCTION

Techniques for the diagnosis of coronary artery disease (CAD) and the assessment of myocardial ischemia have been evolving for more than five decades. "Functional" testing has dominated the noninvasive landscape in the United States, including exercise and pharmacologic techniques relying on radionuclide scintigraphy, echocardiography, and MRI, whereas physiology has dominated the invasive landscape (**Fig. 1**). In the last decade or more, there is increasing evidence that such functional studies have limited accuracy for adjudicating symptomatic status, identifying obstructive CAD, determining the need for (and site of) myocardial revascularization, and predicting cardiac events,[1–3] raising concerns that "stress tests" are overutilized and frequently not-actionable.

In contrast, coronary computed tomography angiography (CCTA) is a noninvasive technique that provides direct anatomic imaging of the coronary arteries (**Fig. 2**) and is more accurate than invasive coronary angiography (ICA) for plaque characterization, assessment of plaque burden, and determining the extent of CAD (**Fig. 3**). Studies of anatomic versus functional testing for CAD suggest similar clinical outcomes at 2 years, but better outcomes for CCTA at 5 years are not related to more frequent revascularization.[4,5] CCTA enhances the ability to clarify the diagnosis of CAD in patients with chest pain and leads to more effective utilization of medications for primary prevention.[6]

At this time, there is no doubt that CCTA is the best noninvasive imaging study to "rule-in" or "rule-out" CAD (see **Fig. 3**). However, all noninvasive imaging studies, including CCTA, lose specificity for identifying myocardial ischemia (ie, false positive results), often leading to unnecessary ICA[7] (**Fig. 4**). Furthermore, interventional societal guidelines, expert consensus documents, and appropriate use criteria have established recommendations for

This article originally appeared in *Interventional Cardiology Clinics*, Volume 12 Issue 1, January 2023.

The Lucia Zurkowski Endowed Chair, Center for Innovation & Research in Cardiovascular Diseases (CIRC), Department of Cardiovascular Medicine, Oakland University, William Beaumont School of Medicine, William Beaumont University Hospital, Royal Oak, MI 48073, USA

E-mail address: robert.safian@beaumont.edu

Cardiol Clin 42 (2024) 101–123
https://doi.org/10.1016/j.ccl.2023.07.004

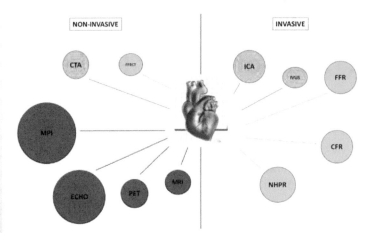

Fig. 1. Schematic representation of noninvasive and invasive tests for evaluation of CAD. Anatomical imaging (blue); functional imaging (red); physiological imaging (green). CCTA, coronary computed tomography angiography; CFR, coronary flow reserve; ECHO, echocardiography; FFRINV, invasive fractional flow reserve; FFRCT, CCTA-derived fractional flow reserve; ICA, invasive coronary angiography; IVUS, intravascular ultrasound; MPI, myocardial perfusion imaging; NHPR, non-hyperemic pressure ratios.

invasive pressure measurements for the physiologic assessment of 50% to 90% stenosis in CAD patients,[8–11] including invasive fractional flow reserve (FFRINV) and various non-hyperemic pressure measurements (such as instantaneous wave-free ratio [iFR]) (see **Fig. 1**). FFRINV and iFR have been incorporated into European and American guidelines for percutaneous coronary intervention (PCI) to provide objective assessment of myocardial ischemia, reduce unnecessary revascularization, and improve clinical outcomes.[9,10] Just as FFRINV improves the specificity of ICA, CT-derived FFR (FFRCT) improves the specificity of CCTA (**Fig. 5**) and enhances the potential of CCTA to assess myocardial ischemia and to serve as the "gatekeeper" to the cardiac catheterization laboratory.

Principles of Computed Tomography-Derived Fractional Flow Reserve

The principles and requirements for determination of FFRCT have been previously delineated.[12,13]

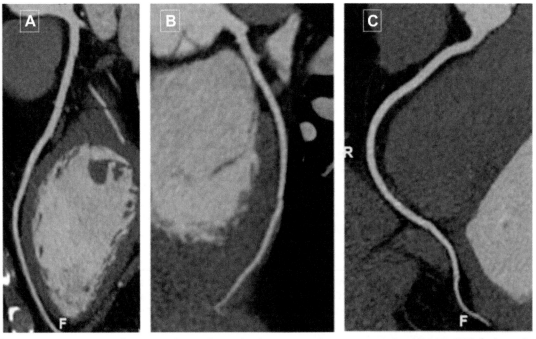

Fig. 2. Coronary computed tomography angiography shows normal coronary arteries. (*A*) LAD. (*B*) left circumflex coronary artery (LCX). (*C*) RCA.

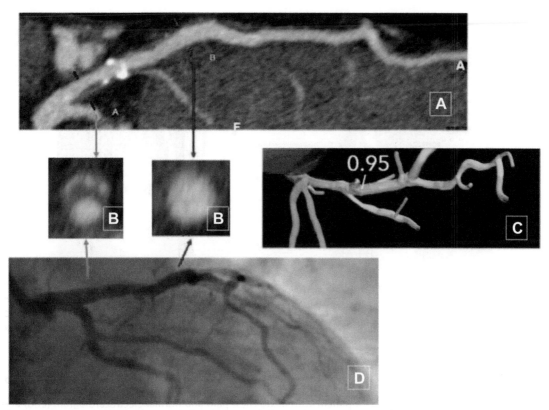

Fig. 3. CCTA shows more anatomic information and plaque characterization than ICA. (*A*) Curved multiplanar reconstruction shows mixed calcified and noncalcified plaque in the proximal LAD. (*B*). Cross-sectional image (*blue arrow*) shows ~50% stenosis compared with the normal reference segment (*red arrow*). (*C*) FFRCT coronary model does not suggest lesion-specific ischemia. (*D*) ICA does not show any disease or calcification in the proximal LAD.

CCTA protocol and image acquisition are identical to standard CCTA, including the requirements for beta blockers for heart rate control and sublingual nitroglycerin to achieve maximal coronary vasodilation. CCTA images should be identified by the reader and sent to the remote DICOM server for analysis (**Fig. 6**). Our institution uses a standardized template for ordering FFRCT that identifies the vessel(s) and lesion(s) of interest and the indication for FFRCT (**Fig. 7**). The computational fluid dynamics (CFD) model (HeartFlow, Inc; Redwood City, CA) can assess FFRCT in all coronary artery segments without the need for additional instrumentation, adenosine administration, or radiation exposure (**Fig. 8**). The CCTA data are uploaded to a cloud-based server, where artificial intelligence (AI) and deep learning (DL) algorithms are applied to generate a 3-dimensional (3D) anatomic model of the aortic root and coronary arteries. The anatomic model undergoes inspection and correction at a workstation, and the anatomic data are returned to the cloud for construction of a patient-specific physiologic model. The physiologic model is based on three assumptions: that there is a direct relationship between resting coronary blood flow and left ventricular myocardial mass; an inverse relationship between microvascular resistance and coronary artery diameter; and that there is a predictable reduction in microvascular resistance in response to maximal hyperemia. Computation of coronary flow and pressure is accomplished by supercomputers which solve the Navier–Stokes equations governing fluid dynamics. The final product seen on the HeartFlow Web site as a 3D color-coded model of FFRCT of the coronary arteries. This model is fully interactive and can be displayed on a desktop computer, mobile phone, or tablet (**Fig. 9**). The data from the coronary model are returned to the cloud, which allows further training of the DL algorithm, and are reported in the patients' medical record. From a clinical perspective, the time span from submission of the raw CCTA data set to reporting of FFRCT results is approximately 4 hours, although studies from the emergency department are usually available within 1 hour.

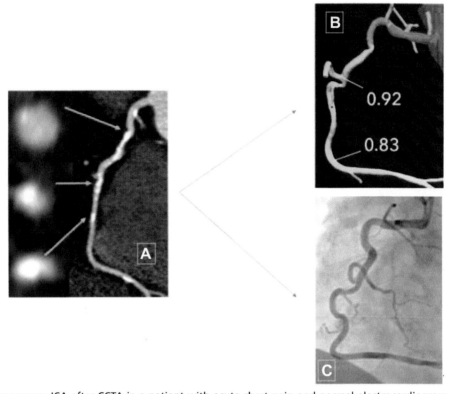

Fig. 4. Unnecessary ICA after CCTA in a patient with acute chest pain and normal electrocardiogram (ECG) and biomarkers. (*A*) CCTA shows sequential calcified plaques in the RCA, but blooming artifact precludes further assessment of stenosis severity. (*B*) FFRCT is negative for lesion-specific ischemia. (*C*) The referring physician decides not to wait for FFRCT results. ICA was unnecessary and did not identify obstructive disease.

On-Site Computed Tomography-Derived Fractional Flow Reserve

HeartFlow FFRCT is the only CCTA-based FFRCT solution that has Conformite Europeene marking in Europe, National Institute for Health and Care Excellence endorsement in the United Kingdom, and Food and Drug Administration (FDA) clearance in the United States. However, the need for off-site supercomputers and the temporal delay in reporting FFRCT results has led to interest in the development of various reduce-order models, simplifying the equations to compute flow dynamics, and permitting on-site determination of FFRCT using dedicated software and standard workstations. Although there are several reports of the feasibility of on-site FFRCT in small numbers of patients,[14–16] there are limited data to validate these with standard invasive or noninvasive measures of ischemia, and none demonstrate the breadth of FFRCT clinical applications that will be detailed below. These point-of-care solutions may offer convenience at the expense of quality assurance, reproducibility, and scope.

Interpretation and Reporting of Computed Tomography-Derived Fractional Flow Reserve

Broad adoption of FFRCT standards for interpretation and reporting is essential for clinical implementation and research.[17] Expertise is required in CCTA and coronary artery anatomy, and an appropriate interpretation of FFRCT mandates an understanding of the clinical context, patient symptoms, and CCTA findings. FFRINV and FFRCT share similar thresholds for hemodynamically significant stenoses; values $\leq$ 0.80 are considered hemodynamically significant. Some centers identify borderline hemodynamic significance as FFRCT values 0.76 to 0.80, although it seems that most of these will require ICA and FFRINV for further adjudication. The incremental value of ΔFFRCT compared with absolute FFRCT values is uncertain.

The site of measurement of FFRCT is important; lesion-specific ischemia is best assessed by sampling values 1 to 2 cm distal to the lesion, rather than from the terminal vessel. FFR values decline from the ostium to the terminal vessel, regardless of FFR technique, even in normal coronary

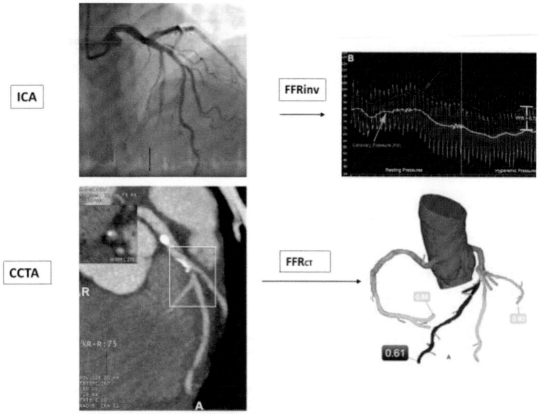

Fig. 5. One of the major goals of invasive and noninvasive imaging is to assess lesion-specific ischemia. Anatomic imaging by ICA and CCTA share similar limitations, and more precise information about lesion-specific ischemia is provided by physiologic assessment with FFRINV and FFRCT. CCTA, coronary computed tomography angiography; FFRCT, CCTA-derived fractional flow reserve; FFRINV, invasive, fractional flow reserve; ICA, invasive coronary angiography.

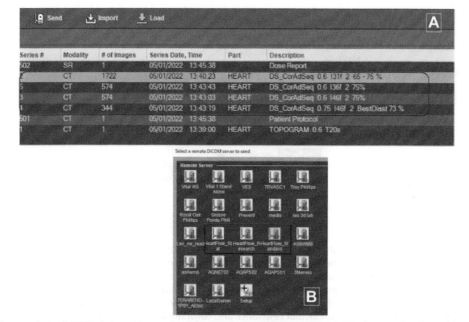

Fig. 6. Screen shot of CCTA data set to send to HeartFlow for FFRCT. (*A*) The CCTA data set is selected (outlined in red), which includes the appropriate phase and kernel. (*B*) The CCTA data set is sent to the remote DICOM server after selecting the appropriate node for STAT (emergency department), research, or standard (outpatient) FFRCT analysis.

FFR_{CT} ORDER ADDENDUM

FFR_{CT} Coronary Analysis (HeartFlow, Inc*) was ordered to define the extent of lesion-specific ischemia in the {FFRCTORDER_CORONARY ARTERY:17097} coronary artery. Results will be available in 12–24 hours if technical quality is sufficient for analysis (Emergency Department FFRCT study results will be available in 2–3 hours).

Indication for request of FFR_{CT} analysis (check all that apply):

☐ Mild coronary artery stenosis (26–50% stenosis) in selected patients who may benefit from FFRCT
☐ Moderate coronary artery stenosis (51–70% stenosis)
☐ Severe coronary artery stenosis (>70% stenosis) of uncertain significance
☐ Uncertain stenosis severity due to calcified plaque in the coronary artery
☐ Presence of high risk plaque features
☐ Other

Coronary CT Angiography IMAGE INSERT

* FFRCT is an FDA-approved noninvasive technique for defining lesion-specific ischemia that correlates with invasive FFR. The overall assessment requires integration of the CTA findings, FFRCT model and clinical correlation.

Fig. 7. Suggested template for ordering FFRCT, identifying the vessel(s) and lesion(s) of interest and the indication for FFRCT.

arteries.[18,19] Values obtained from the terminal vessel may overestimate lesion-specific ischemia and should be avoided. FFRCT measured distal-to-the-lesion improves the diagnostic performance of FFRCT relative to FFRINV, ensures that FFRCT values are due to lesion-specific ischemia, and could reduce the risk and cost of unnecessary invasive procedures.[20] Our institution uses a standardized template for reporting FFRCT results, including the FFRCT value(s), assessment of lesion-specific ischemia, and images that depict the CCTA and FFRCT coronary model (**Fig. 10**).

Diagnostic Performance of Computed Tomography-Derived Fractional Flow Reserve

Several prospective and retrospective studies have been performed to evaluate the diagnostic performance of FFRCT compared with CCTA alone and with FFRINV. Three prospective studies

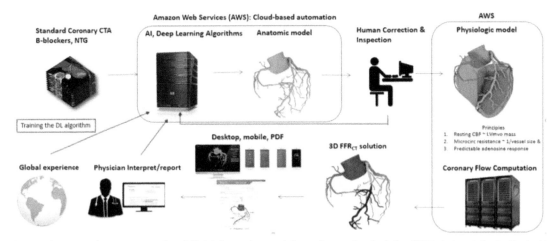

Fig. 8. The HeartFlow computational fluid dynamics model requires upload of the CCTA data set (as indicated in **Fig. 6**) to a cloud-based server, where artificial intelligence (AI) and deep learning algorithms are used to generate a 3D anatomic model of the aortic root and coronary arteries. The anatomic model is inspected and corrected at a workstation, and uploaded to the cloud for construction of a 3D physiologic model, based on three assumptions: there is direct relationship between resting coronary blood flow and left ventricular mass; there is an inverse relationship between microvascular resistance and coronary artery diameter; and there is a predictable reduction in microvascular resistance in response to maximal hyperemia. Computation of coronary flow and pressure is accomplished by supercomputers. The final color-coded 3D FFRCT coronary model is displayed on the HeartFlow Web site; various data points are returned to the cloud to train the deep learning algorithm.

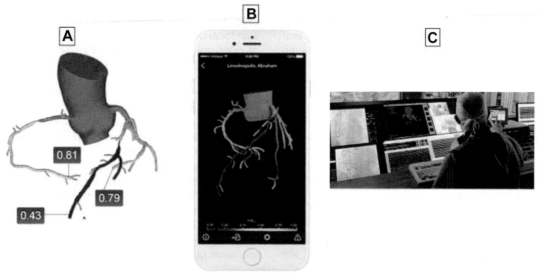

Fig. 9. The FFRCT model (*A*) is fully interactive and can be displayed on a mobile phone or tablet (*B*) or on a desktop computer (*C*).

show that FFRCT has better specificity than CCTA alone for the assessment of ischemia, without compromising sensitivity.[21–24] These studies also showed the importance of beta blockers to achieve heart rate control and sublingual nitroglycerin to achieve maximum coronary vasodilation; failure to adhere to "best practices" for CCTA acquisition is associated with lower diagnostic performance of FFRCT. When compared with measured FFRINV, FFRCT shows excellent correlation, manifested by area under the receiver-operator curve (AUC) of 0.90 and 0.93 on a per-patient and per-vessel analysis, respectively.[24] In a large retrospective analysis of FFRCT compared with FFRINV, there is marked improvement in diagnostic performance when FFRCT is measured distal-to-the-lesion rather than from the terminal vessel, including statistically significant improvements in specificity (50% to 86%), accuracy (65% to 85%), and AUC (0.83–0.91).[20]

FFRcT CORONARY ANALYSIS

FFRcT values were evaluated corresponding to CTA identified lesions, as illustrated below in original CTA report (see "Indication for request for FFRCT analysis").

Interpretation:
1. The *** % stenosis in the *** coronary artery *** segment has a {FFRCT_LOWHIGH:17101} likelihood of lesion-specific ischemia with an FFRCT value of ***.|
2. ***

FFRcT IMAGE INSERT
(Include FFRcT values distal to all segments with stenosis >50% or stenosis >25% in the left main, proximal LAD or when high risk plaque features present)

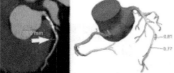

Interpreting Physician: Date/Time: 5:35 AM

Summary of FFRcT Values		
a. >0.80 (distal to the stenosis): Low likelihood of lesion-specific ischemia		
b. ≤0.80 (distal to the stenosis): High likelihood of lesion-specific ischemia		
c. Assessment of lesion-specific ischemia by FFRcT should rely on FFRcT values measured approximately 10-15 mm distal to the lesion of interest, rather than from the terminal vessel. FFRcT values <0.80 measured from the terminal vessel do not necessarily indicate lesion-specific ischemia, particularly if there is only mild disease in the more proximal segments of the vessel.		

Fig. 10. Suggested template for reporting FFRCT results, including the FFRCT value(s), assessment of lesion-specific ischemia, and images that depict the CCTA and FFRCT coronary model.

Although many cardiologists believe that FFRINV is the gold standard for assessment of hemodynamic significance, it is important to realize that FFRINV values are influenced by stenosis severity, site of measurement, and errors in interpretation related to pressure drift and dampening.[19]

Limitations of Computed Tomography-Derived Fractional Flow Reserve

As previously mentioned, essential aspects of the HeartFlow coronary digital model include segmentation to identify the lumen boundaries and estimation of myocardial mass; both are dependent on CTA spatial resolution and image quality. FFRCT cannot be determined when the myocardium is not fully included in the field of view (**Fig. 11**) and when coronary artery lumen boundaries are obscured by motion, streak artifact, or low contrast resolution (**Fig. 12**). The quality of segmentation has improved with each software upgrade: Versions 1.0 to 1.3 were preclinical software (never commercially available); version 1.4 is approved by the FDA and was used in the studies of FFR_{CT} mentioned above. Improvements in lumen segmentation by sub-voxel analysis and DL methods of AI have led to the development of version 2.0+, resulting in marked improvement in detection of lumen boundaries. HeartFlow also recommends vendor-specific acquisition and reconstruction protocols to further enhance spatial resolution and edge detection. These protocols are especially important in patients with coronary artery calcification and low contrast resolution, where blooming and beam-hardening artifacts and reduced contrast-to-noise ratio may significantly degrade CCTA image quality.

The loss of specificity of CCTA in assessing ischemia can be significantly improved by FFRCT, particularly in patients with coronary artery calcification. The use of sharp kernels for CCTA reconstruction has significantly improved the ability to identify lumen boundaries and enhance the accuracy of FFRCT in calcified lesions (**Fig. 13**). FFRCT is readily performed in coronary arteries with focal dense calcification, even in the presence of extensive blooming artifact (**Fig. 14**).

Many of the technical limitations of FFRCT are related to technical limitations of CCTA, as delineated above. Accordingly, many solutions rely on technical improvements in CCTA technology, such as spatial and temporal resolution, image reconstruction, postprocessing, and field of view. These technical improvements heavily influence CCTA image quality in patients with obesity, heart rate variability, and vessel calcification. At present, FFRCT cannot be performed in patients with prior coronary stenting or coronary artery bypass surgery (CABG), which account for greater than 25% of patients referred for ICA at our institution (personal communication, Amy Mertens, DO).

Clinical Applications of Computed Tomography-Derived Fractional Flow Reserve

Guideline recommendations for coronary computed tomography angiography and computed tomography-derived fractional flow reserve

The 2021 Chest Pain Guidelines provide the most contemporary recommendations for evaluating patients with stable and acute chest pain (or equivalent).[25] These guidelines incorporate an evidence-based approach to risk stratification and the diagnostic evaluation of chest pain, value-based considerations, and shared decision-making with patients. In patients with intermediate risk of CAD, CCTA has a class I recommendation for evaluation of chest pain; FFRCT has a IIa recommendation for patients with 40% to 90% stenosis in the proximal or mid-coronary artery.

Lesion-specific ischemia and cardiovascular outcome

In contemporary practice, the most important application of FFRCT is the assessment of lesion-specific ischemia. In 584 symptomatic

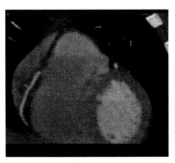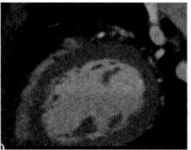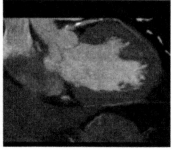

Fig. 11. Determination of myocardial mass relies on inclusion of the entire myocardium in the field of view. Otherwise, FFRCT cannot be calculated.

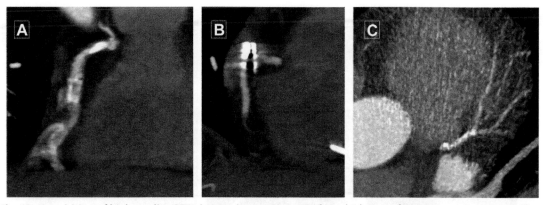

Fig. 12. Acquisition of high-quality CCTA images is a requirement for calculation of FFRCT; some imaging artifacts can degrade CCTA image quality, precluding computation of FFRCT. (*A*) Excessive cardiac motion. (*B*) Severe streak artifact. (*C*) Very low contrast resolution (contrast-to-noise ratio).

patients with stable CAD in the Prospective Longitudinal Trial of FFRCT: Outcome and Resources Impacts (PLATFORM) trial, obstructive disease was identified in 88% of patients when guided by CCTA/FFRCT compared with 27% of patients when guided by usual care (*P* < 0.0001).[26] The use of the CCTA/FFRCT strategy led to the cancellation of ICA in 61% of patients who were initially referred for ICA from the usual care strategy.[27] In PLATFORM, the CCTA/FFRCT strategy was associated with a 32% reduction in cost at 90 days compared with usual care, driven primarily by reduction in the need for ICA, and an improvement in quality-of-life scores.[28] PLATFORM was

severely underpowered to assess clinical outcomes, but 1248 stable CAD patients in Denmark had no major adverse cardiovascular events (MACE) events at 1 year when FFRCT was greater than 0.80.[29] Among 5083 stable CAD patients followed for 1 year in the international Assessing Diagnostic Value of Noninvasive FFRCT in Coronary Care Registry, patients with FFRCT greater than 0.80 were less likely to require revascularization (5.6% vs 38.4%, *P* < 0.001) and experience MACE (relative risk 0.55, *P* = 0.06) compared with patients with FFRCT ≤ 0.80.[30] Among 555 patients with acute chest pain syndromes in the emergency department, there was no difference

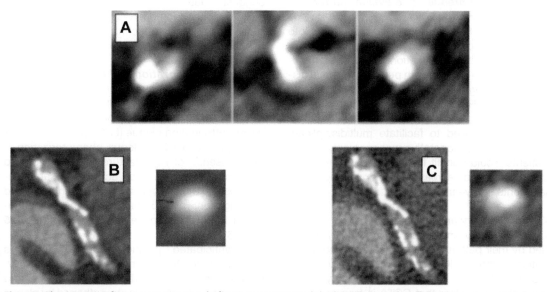

Fig. 13. The impact of coronary artery calcification on FFRCT. (*A*) Blooming artifact from calcium can adversely impact CCTA quality. (*B*) Standard "soft" kernels may be associated with image blur and limit edge detection required for FFRCT. (*C*) "Sharp" kernels are routinely recommended by HeartFlow, to significantly improve edge detection and facilitate FFRCT.

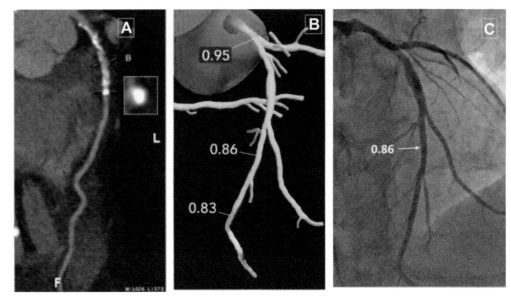

Fig. 14. FFRCT can improve the specificity of CCTA even when calcification and blooming artifact obscure the lumen and preclude assessment of stenosis severity. (*A*) CCTA for chest pain shows dense calcified plaque and blooming artifact in the proximal LAD, precluding assessment of stenosis severity. (*B*) FFRCT was 0.86 distal-to-the-lesion, but the referring physician was concerned about disease in the proximal LAD. (*C*) ICA-confirmed calcified plaque in the proximal LAD and FFRINV was 0.86, identical to FFRCT. The patient was managed with medical therapy; ICA could have been avoided.

in 90-day MACE and overall cost between patients evaluated with CCTA/FFRCT compared with CCTA alone; there were no MACE in patients with FFRCT greater than 0.80 when revascularization was deferred.[31]

Screening and preoperative evaluation for coronary artery disease

CCTA and FFRCT have been incorporated into standardized protocols in some institutions for preoperative risk stratification before liver transplantation.[32] In patients with peripheral arterial disease requiring vascular surgery, preoperative CCTA and FFRCT were used to identify high-risk patients with silent myocardial ischemia.[33] This strategy was used to facilitate multidisciplinary care, improve perioperative management, identify patients would benefit from postoperative revascularization, and decrease the risk of cardiovascular events at 1 year.

Coronary artery anomalies

Coronary artery anomalies are frequently classified by their patterns of origin, course, and termination. Although ICA was considered the gold standard for the diagnosis of coronary artery anomalies, it is clear that CCTA is far superior to ICA.[34,35] A large international registry is currently underway to study CCTA and FFRCT in patients with anomalous coronary arteries (FFRCT of

Anomalous Coronary Arteries by Computed Tomography Study [FACTs], personal communication, Michael J. Gallagher MD). The optimal noninvasive and invasive strategies for evaluation of ischemia are the subject of ongoing debate, but there are several observational studies that suggest value of FFRCT.[36,37] Further study of FFRCT is needed, but CCTA and FFRCT may prove to be the best techniques to evaluate patients with coronary anomalies.

Plaque characterization and ischemia

CCTA is widely acknowledged as the best noninvasive imaging tool for simple (calcified plaque) and advanced (high-risk plaque [HRP] defined as low-attenuation plaque [LAP], positive remodeling, plaque burden) plaque characterization.[38] The presence of HRP features, the relationship to ischemia, and risk of acute coronary syndromes (ACS) are topics of intense interest and investigation, and partially explain the enthusiasm for CCTA in patients with CAD (**Figs. 15** and **16**).

As anticipated, plaque volume by CCTA is strongly related to ischemia by FFRCT or FFRINV, irrespective of measured diameter stenosis, and assessment of ischemia is strengthened by plaque characterization by CCTA and FFRCT. LAP is also a strong predictor of ischemia, independent of other plaque characteristics.[39] By multivariable

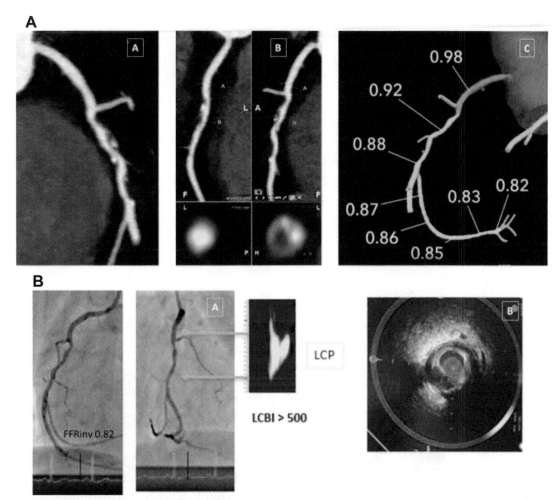

Fig. 15. Case 1 (See text for details). High-risk plaque without lesion-specific ischemia. (15A). Noninvasive imaging with CCTA and FFRCT. (*A*) CCTA shows a long segment of irregular mixed plaque in the mid-RCA, with focal ulceration. (*B*) CCTA and cross-sectional imaging show positive remodeling, contrast penetration, and low attenuation plaque, consistent with high-risk plaque. (*C*) The FFRCT is 0.86, suggesting the absence of lesion-specific ischemia. (15B) Invasive imaging with ICA, near-infrared spectroscopy/intravascuar ultrasound (NIRS-IVUS), and FFRINV. (*A*) ICA shows a long segment of disease but the vessel contour appears less disturbing compared with CCTA. NIRS-IVUS demonstrates a bulky lipid-core plaque and LCBI 4 mm > 500, consistent with highly vulnerable plaque. FFRINV is 0.82, suggesting the absence of lesion-specific ischemia. (*B*) The cross-sectional image shows that the lipid-core plaque corresponds to the location of the low attenuation plaque by CCTA (**). FFRINV, invasive fractional flow reserve; LCBI, lipid-core burden index within 4 mm; LCP, lipid-core plaque.

analysis, the likelihood of ischemia by FFRCT increases more than 3-fold in the presence of 1 versus ≥ 2 HRP features.[40] Although it is easy to understand the relationship between abnormal FFR and lesion-specific ischemia, the relationship between abnormal FFR, HRP, and the risk of ACS is not so intuitive. A recently published review suggests that LAP may be associated the diminished vasodilator capacity of the arterial wall, leading to an abnormal FFR.[41] Stated another way, normal FFR may suggest the absence of lesion-specific ischemia and the presence of normal vasodilator capacity.

Biomechanical forces and the impact on plaque progression and instability

There are a variety of biomechanical forces resulting from the influence of pressure and flow that act within blood vessels, including effects on atherosclerotic plaque. Most of our understanding of fluid dynamics in the coronary arteries has been derived from invasive data, but CTA and CFD have provided additional insight into the relationship between shear stress and CAD.[42] Wall shear stress (WSS) is the tangential stress exerted on the vascular wall and is determined by blood viscosity and the gradient of blood velocity at the

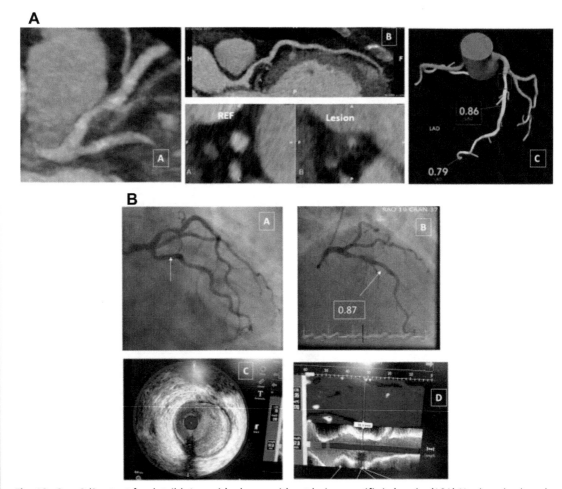

Fig. 16. Case 2 (See text for details). Low-risk plaque without lesion-specific ischemia. (16A) Noninvasive imaging with CCTA and FFRCT. (*A*) CCTA shows bulky noncalcified eccentric plaque in the proximal LAD, with positive remodeling and 50% to 70% stenosis. (*B*) Curved multiplanar reconstruction and cross-sectional imaging did not suggest high-risk plaque. (*C*) FFRCT is 0.86, suggesting the absence of lesion-specific ischemia. (16B) Invasive imaging with NIRS-IVUS. (*A*) ICA shows ~ 50% stenosis (AP caudal projection). (*B*) ICA shows ~ 50% stenosis (AP cranial projection). FFRINV is 0.87, consistent with the absence of lesion-specific ischemia. (*C*) NIRS-IVUS (cross-section) shows bulky noncalcified plaque, positive remodeling, and minimal cross-sectional area 5.4 mm². (*D*) NIRS-IVUS (long view) shows low-risk plaque and no LCP.

lumen surface. WSS influences normal and abnormal endothelial function and is an important determinant of plaque localization and progression. The application of CFD-derived WSS improved the identification of HRP.[43] In contrast, axial plaque stress (APS) is the axial component of stress on the atherosclerotic plaque and plays a more direct role on plaque rupture, particularly in more focal areas of disease.[44] In Exploring the Mechanism of Plaque Rupture in Acute Coronary Syndrome Using Coronary CT Angiography and Computational Fluid Dynamic, 72 patients had CCTA within 1 to 24 months before documented ACS.[45] The addition of FFRCT, ΔFFRCT, WSS, and APS was more predictive of subsequent ACS when compared with diameter stenosis alone or diameter stenosis plus HRP features.

Insights into anatomy-physiology mismatch

There are several potential explanations for the observation that some patients with abnormal FFR do not have significant stenosis by angiography. First, diffuse nonobstructive coronary atherosclerosis could induce a graded, continuous fall in pressure along the length of a coronary artery, creating resistance to flow and abnormal FFRINV.[46] Second, a CCTA and FFRCT study reports a gradual decline in FFRCT in completely normal arteries, not just in vessels with nonobstructive atherosclerosis,[18] suggesting a relationship between changes in pressure, vessel length, and vessel diameter as defined by Poiseulle's equation. Third, there seems to be a dynamic relationship between serial FFRCT and the development of positive and negative arterial remodeling that influence vessel lumen area.[47] Finally, as mentioned above, abnormal FFR in the absence of significant epicardial CAD could reflect underlying abnormalities in coronary vasodilator reserve of any cause.[48]

Myocardial infarction and myocardial ischemia in the absence of obstructive coronary artery disease

Myocardial infarction in the absence of obstructive CAD (MINOCA) and ischemia with nonobstructive CAD (INOCA) are clinical entities on the spectrum of ischemic heart diseases that occur in patients with minimal or no CAD. In patients with MINOCA, potential etiologies include plaque instability, spontaneous coronary dissection, Takotsubo syndrome, myocarditis, coronary artery vasospasm, microvascular dysfunction, and supply-demand mismatch (often classified as a type 2 MI).[49] For many of these patients, ICA and invasive coronary imaging may be the appropriate initial strategy, but in others, CCTA and FFRCT may be useful to exclude obstructive CAD and identify non-atherosclerotic causes of MI (such as spontaneous coronary dissection). In contrast to patients with MINOCA, patients with INOCA do not have elevated cardiac biomarkers, and ischemic symptoms may often be misdiagnosed as noncardiac conditions. Potential etiologies include coronary vasospasm and microvascular dysfunction, and CCTA and FFRCT are highly reliable for excluding obstructive disease without ICA.[50]

In addition to providing FFRCT values, Heart-Flow has the capability of calculating the ratio of the coronary artery lumen volume to left ventricular myocardial mass (volume to mass ratio [V/M] ratio), by using the 3D anatomic model of the coronary arteries to measure the total coronary artery lumen volume, and by calculating myocardial mass from the volume of myocardium extracted from the CCTA data set.[51] V/M ratio can identify patients with microvascular angina and with supply-demand mismatch,[52,53] suggesting a potential incremental role when applying CCTA and FFRCT to patients with MINOCA and INOCA.

Comprehensive Planning of Myocardial Revascularization

For decades, ICA has been the mainstay of decision-making regarding the need for, and the type of, myocardial revascularization. In the last 15 years or so, there have been several paradigm shifts that have resulted in profound impact on revascularization decisions and cardiovascular outcomes. The first was a shift away from ICA alone to the incorporation of FFRINV, iFR, and other objective physiologic measures into routine decision-making about the need for revascularization.[54,55] The second was a shift away from ICA to assess vessel and lesion morphology to the utilization of risk prediction models as defined by the Synergy Between Percutaneous Coronary Intervention with Taxus and Cardiac Surgery (SYNTAX) score.[56] The anatomic SYNTAX score was later modified by the addition of clinical factors to create the SYNTAX score II[57] and by incorporating FFRINV values to create the functional SYNTAX score.[58] The third was a shift away from unilateral decision-making by a cardiologist to a shared decision model incorporating a heart team, other key stakeholders, and the patient and family.

We are now in the midst of another paradigm shift, which is gaining momentum in Europe, Asia, and North America: integration of noninvasive anatomic and functional assessment using CCTA and FFRCT for calculation of CT-derived anatomic and functional SYNTAX scores.[59–61] Direct comparisons between ICA- and CCTA-derived anatomic SYNTAX scores demonstrate a strong correlation in patients with single and multi-vessel CAD,[62,63] suggesting that a heart team consensus might be achievable before ICA. Early observations suggested the feasibility of calculating functional SYNTAX scores based on CCTA and FFRCT. CCTA and FFRCT were later incorporated into the design of the SYNTAX III Revolution Trial,[64] which was designed to determine the impact of CCTA and FFRCT on the heart teams' decisions regarding PCI or CABG in 223 patients with three-vessel CAD and to compare decisions based on the calculation of anatomic and functional SYNTAX scores derived from ICA versus CTA. The functional SYNTAX score based on FFRCT resulted in[1]: reclassification of 14% of patients with intermediate–high to low SYNTAX score tertile[2]; change in plans for CABG or PCI in 7% of patients; and[3] modification of vessels selected for revascularization in 12% of patients.

It is evident that CCTA and FFRCT are no longer used to simply rule out CAD; the newest applications include a HeartFlow planning tool for PCI or CABG, allowing the cardiologist to assess lesion-specific ischemia, plan stent location and sizing, and use virtual remodeling of the lumen to assess the functional impact of PCI.[65] Early studies of the planning tool in small numbers of patients report the feasibility of determination of FFRCT before and after virtual remodeling and the correlation between FFRCT and FFRINV before and after PCI.[66,67] In a prospective multicenter observational study in 120 patients, the HeartFlow Planner is highly accurate and precise relative to FFRINV and to minimal stent area by optical coherence tomography, even in vessels with diffuse disease and calcification.[68]

Coronary Computed Tomography Angiography and Computed Tomography-Derived Fractional Flow Reserve Case Studies

Case 1: Acute chest pain in the emergency department, high-risk plaque. A 53-year-old woman presents to the emergency department with ischemic chest pain (see **Fig. 15**). The initial electrocardiogram (ECG) and cardiac biomarkers are normal. She has hypertension, hyperlipidemia, and a strong family history for premature CAD. CCTA shows bulky calcified and noncalcified plaque in the mid-RCA, 50% to 70% stenosis, and HRP features including LAP, contrast penetration, and a signet-ring sign. The FFRCT distal-to-the-lesion is 0.83 (see **Fig. 15**A). The patient is referred for ICA due to the combination of symptoms and HRP features, despite FFRCT greater than 0.80. ICA demonstrates a tubular 50% stenosis in the mid-RCA, and the FFRINV is 0.82. However, near-infrared spectroscopy-intravascular ultrasound (NIRS-IVUS) demonstrates minimal calcification and a prominent lipid-core plaque (LCP) with a lipid-core burden index-4 mm (LCBI) greater than 500, consistent with a very HRP (see **Fig. 15**B). PCI is performed without complication.

Case 2: Acute chest pain in the emergency department, low-risk plaque. A 45-year-old woman presents to the emergency department with possible ischemic chest pain (see **Fig. 16**). The initial ECG and cardiac biomarkers are normal. She has hypertension and hyperlipidemia. CCTA shows eccentric bulky noncalcified plaque in the proximal LAD, 50% to 70% stenosis, and positive remodeling. The FFRCT is 0.86 measured 20 mm distal-to-the-lesion (see **Fig. 16**A). The patient is referred for ICA due to the symptoms and plaque location in the proximal LAD, which confirms bulky plaque in the proximal LAD and FFRINV 0.87. NIRS-IVUS demonstrates noncalcified plaque, positive remodeling, and minimal cross-sectional area 4.5 mm^2; there is no LCP, so the patient is managed conservatively without revascularization (see **Fig. 16**B).

Case 3: Acute chest pain equivalent in the emergency department, normal stress test. A 56-year-old woman presents to the emergency department with dyspnea on exertion (**Fig. 17**). The initial ECG and cardiac biomarkers are normal. She has hypertension, hyperlipidemia, and obesity. She is referred for stress myocardial perfusion imaging and achieves 8.3 METS and 78% of age-predicted maximum heart rate. The test is negative for symptoms, and the ECG and perfusion scan are normal. CCTA shows 50% to 70% stenosis in the proximal RCA; FFRCT is 0.63, consistent with severe ischemia. ICA shows subtotal occlusion of the RCA, managed by PCI.

Case 4: Outpatient chest pain, possible pseudo-artifact. An 80-year-old man experiences exertional chest pain (**Fig. 18**). CCTA shows calcified plaque and nonobstructive stenosis in the proximal LAD, and ambiguous disease in the mid-LAD just distal to the diagonal branch, "likely due to misalignment artifact." Other coronary artery segments are normal. FFRCT is 0.66, consistent with severe anterior ischemia. ICA confirms 90% stenosis in the mid-LAD, managed by PCI. FFRCT correctly identifies misalignment artifact as a "pseudo-artifact," leading to appropriate ICA and PCI.

Case 5: Exertional chest pain, marathon runner, normal stress test. A 47-year-old man is a competitive marathon runner (**Fig. 19**). He trains daily and experiences mild exertional chest pain after running 5 miles per day, relieved spontaneously. He has hypertension, hyperlipidemia, and a strong family history of premature CAD. He undergoes a stress perfusion study and exercises for 15 minutes and achieves 98% of age-predicted maximum heart rate. He does not experience chest pain, and the stress ECG and perfusion scan are normal. He is "cleared" to run in the marathon, but before race day he is advised to seek a second opinion. Another cardiologist orders a CCTA, which shows calcified plaques and blooming artifacts in the proximal and mid-LAD, precluding assessment of stenosis severity. FFRCT in the mid-LAD is 0.69, consistent with lesion-specific ischemia. ICA shows hazy calcification in the proximal LAD, and FFRINV is 0.77. After further discussion and shared-decision making, the patient undergoes successful PCI and is advised against entering the marathon.

Case 6: Planning percutaneous coronary intervention using coronary computed tomography angiography. A 55-year-old man develops typical low-threshold exertional angina about 18 months after mechanical aortic valve replacement (**Fig. 20**). CCTA shows severe disease in the proximal LAD and FFRCT of 0.69, consistent with significant ischemia. Other coronary arteries are normal. The CCTA suggests a proximal and distal reference diameter of 4.5 and 3.5 mm, respectively, and a lesion length of 30 mm (see **Fig. 20**A). ICA confirms severe proximal LAD stenosis, managed by implantation of a

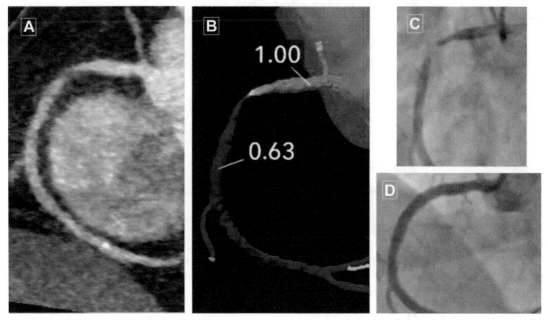

Fig. 17. Case 3 (See text for details). Exertional dyspnea, normal exercise MPI, and abnormal CCTA requiring PCI. (*A*) CCTA shows single vessel disease and high-grade stenosis in the proximal RCA. (*B*) FFRCT was 0.63, consistent with severe lesion-specific ischemia. (*C*) ICA confirms severe stenosis in the proximal RCA. (*D*) PCI is performed with an excellent result.

3.5 × 28 mm drug-eluting stent (DES), dilated with a 3.5-mm noncompliant balloon distally and a 4.0-mm noncompliant balloon proximally. Final ICA shows an excellent result (see **Fig. 20**B).

Case 7: Planning percutaneous coronary intervention using the HeartFlow Planner, single-vessel coronary artery disease. A 55-year-old man presents to the emergency department with exertional chest pain at a low workload (**Fig. 21**). CCTA shows severe stenosis in the proximal RCA due to noncalcified plaque (see **Fig. 21**A); other coronary arteries are normal. The FFRCT coronary model indicates severe ischemia and FFRCT less than 0.50. Application of the

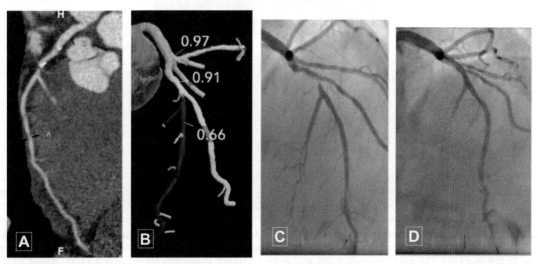

Fig. 18. Case 4 (See text for details). Exertional chest pain, pseudo-artifact, and severe ischemia by FFRCT. (*A*) CCTA shows non-obstructive disease in the proximal LAD and calcified plaque in the mid-LAD that was interpreted as "likely due to misalignment artifact". (*B*) FFRCT was 0.66, consistent with severe lesion-specific ischemia. The abnormal FFRCT suggests that the artifact is a "pseudo-artifact". (*C*) ICA confirms severe stenosis in the mid-LAD distal to the diagonal branch. (*D*) Successful PCI is performed.

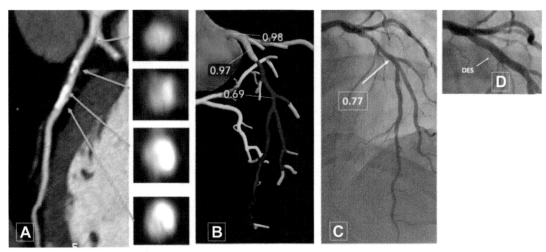

Fig. 19. Case 5 (See text for details). Exertional chest pain, normal exercise MPI, calcified plaque in LAD, and positive FFRCT. (*A*) CCTA identifies calcified plaque and blooming artifacts in the proximal and mid-LAD, precluding assessment of stenosis severity. (*B*) FFRCT is 0.69, consistent with severe ischemia. (*C*) ICA and FFRINV confirms anterior ischemia. (*D*) Successful PCI of LAD. DES, drug-eluting stent.

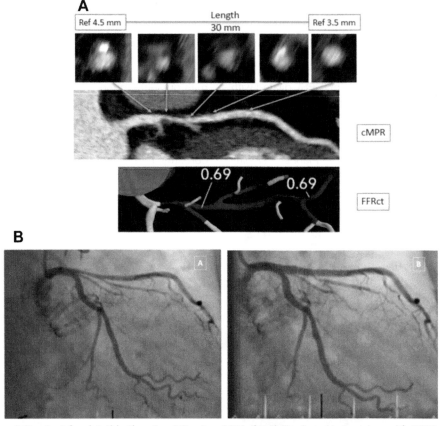

Fig. 20. Case 6 (See text for details). Planning PCI using CCTA. (20A) Noninvasive imaging with CCTA and FFRCT. (*A*) CCTA showed mixed plaque and severe ostial LAD stenosis extending over a length of 30 mm from the left main to the mid-LAD. The proximal (left main) and distal reference diameters are 4.5 and 3.5 mm, respectively. (*B*) FFRCT is 0.69, consistent with severe lesion-specific ischemia. (20B) Invasive coronary angiography. (*A*) Baseline ICA shows severe disease in the proximal and mid-LAD, similar to CCTA. (*B*) Final ICA after PCI using a 3.5 × 28 mm drug-eluting stent, dilated at high pressure with a 3.5 × 20 noncompliant balloon in the distal half of the stent and a 4.0 × 15 mm noncompliant balloon in the proximal half of the stent. IVUS-confirmed optimal stent sizing and lesion coverage.

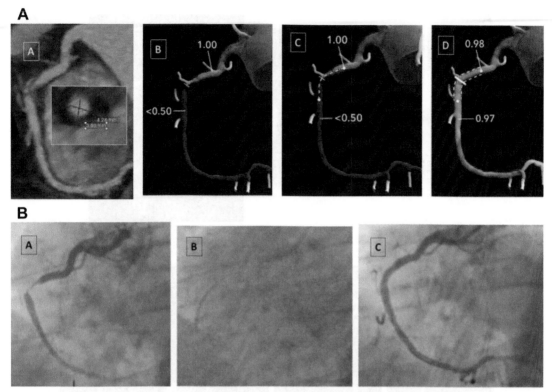

Fig. 21. Case 7 (See text for details). Planning PCI using the HeartFlow Planner, single-vessel disease. (21A) CCTA and Heartflow Planner. (*A*) CCTA shows severe stenosis in the proximal RCA. (*B*) The baseline FFRCT is < 0.50, consistent with severe lesion-specific ischemia. (*C*) The HeartFlow Planner suggests that a 4.0 × 23 mm stent will cover the entire lesion. (*D*) The 4.0 × 23 mm stent will normalize the FFRCT to 0.97. (21B) ICA and FFRINV. (*A*) ICA shows severe stenosis in the proximal RCA, identical to the CCTA. (*B*) A 4.0 × 24 mm stent covers the entire lesion, as anticipated from the HeartFlow Planner. (*C*) Final ICA shows an excellent result. The post-PCI FFRINV is 0.96.

HeartFlow Planner suggests that a 4 × 23 mm DES will cover the entire lesion, and normalize the FFRCT distal to the stent. ICA shows severe stenosis in the proximal RCA, managed by implantation of a 4 × 24 mm DES (see **Fig. 21**B). FFRINV is 0.96 at the end of PCI.

Case 8: Planning percutaneous coronary intervention using the HeartFlow Planner, left main and multivessel coronary artery disease. A 53-year-old woman undergoes outpatient evaluation for progressive exertional chest discomfort and dyspnea (**Fig. 22**). She had prior radiation treatment of left breast cancer and is being evaluated for metastatic disease. CCTA shows sequential mixed calcified and noncalcified plaque causing greater than 70% stenoses in the distal left main coronary artery and proximal LAD, nonobstructive disease in the LCX, and greater than 70% stenosis in the distal RCA (see **Fig. 22**A). The FFRCT coronary model shows significant ischemia in the proximal LAD and proximal LCX due to severe left main stenosis, in the mid LAD and large diagonal branch due to severe proximal LAD stenosis, and in the distal RCA due to distal RCA stenosis. The

HeartFlow Planner is used to examine several scenarios for DES of the left main, LAD, LCX, and RCA. Virtual remodeling indicates that placement of a 4 × 12 mm DES from the left main to the proximal LAD will normalize FFRCT in the proximal LAD and LCX, indicating correction of ischemia due to the left main stenosis, but there is significant residual ischemia due to the proximal LAD stenosis. Virtual remodeling of the proximal LAD after deployment of an additional 3.5 × 21 mm DES will normalize FFRCT in the left main, LAD, diagonal branch, and LCX (see **Fig. 22**B). ICA is performed, with a plan to deploy a 3.5 × 32 mm DES in the left main and LAD, dilate the LAD with a 3.5 × 20 noncompliant balloon, and dilate the left main with a 4.0 × 12 mm noncompliant balloon. After the first two injections, the patient develops unremitting chest pain, global ST-segment depression, and cardiogenic shock. A test injection shows occlusion of the left main, so a 0.014″ guidewire is immediately passed into the distal LAD, and a 3.5 × 32 mm DES is deployed in the left main and LAD, as planned. High-pressure percutaneous transluminal coronary

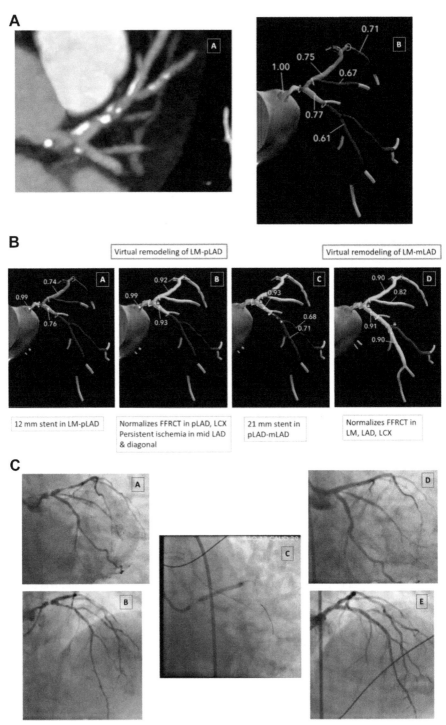

Fig. 22. Case 8 (See text for details). Planning PCI using the HeartFlow Planner, left main and two-vessel disease. (22A). Noninvasive imaging with CCTA and FFRCT. (*A*) CCTA shows mixed plaque and severe disease in the distal left main coronary artery and mid-LAD. There is nonobstructive disease in the LCX and severe disease in the RCA (not shown). (*B*) The FFRCT coronary model shows ischemia in the proximal LAD (FFRCT 0.77) and proximal LCX (FFRCT 0.75), consistent with severe left main stenosis. There is marked decline in FFRCT in the mid-LAD (0.61), consistent with severe stenosis in the proximal LAD. (22B) The HeartFlow Planner is used to evaluate several potential stent strategies for PCI of the left coronary artery. (*A*) A 12-mm-long stent is considered for deployment in the left main and proximal LAD. (*B*) Virtual remodeling of the lumen in the left main and proximal LAD lumen

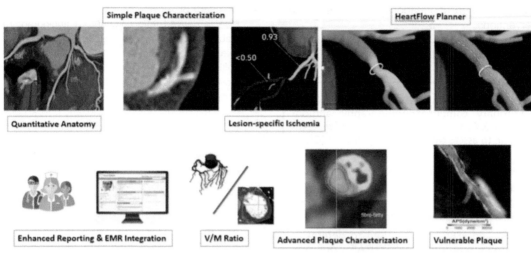

Fig. 23. CCTA and FFRCT as the gatekeeper to the cardiac catheterization laboratory. CCTA and FFRCT can provide essential information about coronary artery anatomy, simple and advanced plaque characterization, lesion-specific ischemia, vessel and plaque wall stress, and V/M ratio. CCTA and FFRCT also allow derivation of anatomic and functional SYNTAX scores, and provide tools for PCI planning. HeartFlow will provide enhanced reporting and EMR integration, which will allow unique opportunities for data collection and sharing. EMR, electronic medical record; V/M ratio, volume to mass ratio.

angioplasty (PTCA) is performed with sequential 3.5 and 4.0 mm noncompliant balloons, and optimal stent sizing is confirmed with IVUS and ICA (see **Fig. 22**C). The duration of left main occlusion was less than 90 seconds; chest pain, ECG changes, and hypotension resolve.

Coronary Computed Tomography Angiography and Computed Tomography-Derived Fractional Flow Reserve as the Gatekeeper to the Cardiac Catheterization Laboratory

Based on the content presented herein, it is reasonable to consider CCTA and FFRCT as the gatekeeper to the cardiac catheterization laboratory. CCTA and FFRCT provide unique information and a degree of empowerment that is not available with any other noninvasive technique, by providing essential data about coronary artery anatomy, lesion-specific ischemia, simple and advanced plaque characterization, vessel and plaque wall stress, and V/M ratio (**Fig. 23**). Furthermore, the ability to calculate anatomic and functional SYNTAX scores and provide tools for PCI planning signals a dramatic shift of CCTA and FFRCT as a diagnostic tool to a therapeutic tool. If we can overcome the limitations of FFRCT in patients with prior stents and CABG, CCTA may replace ICA as a diagnostic tool for CAD, and enrich the

---

shows that this strategy will normalize the FFRCT in the LCX, but result in persistent ischemia in the mid-LAD (FFRCT 0.71). This observation indicates that planned stenting of the LCX is not necessary, but that additional stenting is required for the LAD. (C) The Planner indicates that an additional 21 mm of stent is required to treat the remaining disease in the proximal and mid-LAD. (D) Virtual remodeling of the lumen in the proximal and mid-LAD will normalize the FFRCT in the distal LAD (FFRCT 0.90). Based on the Planner, the decision is made to deploy a 3.5 × 32 mm drug-eluting stent in the LAD and left main, and then dilate the LAD with 3.5 mm × 20 noncompliant balloon and dilate with left main with a 4.0-mm noncompliant balloons at high pressure. (22C) ICA and PCI of the left coronary artery. (A) ICA confirms severe stenosis in the distal left main and the proximal LAD (AP caudal projection). (B) ICA shows the landing zone for the stent in the vicinity of the diagonal branch (AP cranial projection). (C) After these two injections, the patient develops chest pain and cardiogenic shock, and a limited test injection shows acute occlusion of the left main. After passing a 0.014-inch guidewire into the LAD, the left main and LAD are immediately stented with a 3.5 × 32 mm drug-eluting stent, and dilated at high pressure with 3.5 and 4.0 mm noncompliant balloons, as indicated by the HeartFlow Planner. (D) Final ICA shows an excellent angiographic result (AP caudal projection). (E) ICA shows an excellent result and no injury to the diagonal branch. The adequacy of stent deployment is confirmed by IVUS. The duration of left main occlusion is < 90 seconds. FFRCT, fractional flow reserve derived from CCTA; LM, left main coronary artery; mLAD, mid-LAD; pLAD, proximal LAD.

cardiac catheterization laboratory for therapeutic interventions.

CLINICS CARE POINTS

- Coronary computed tomography angiography (CCTA) is the best non-invasive technique to assess coronary artery disease (CAD).
- CCTA-derived fractional flow reserve (FFRCT) is the best non-invasive technique to assess myocardial ischemia.
- CCTA is the best non-invasive technique to assess plaque characteristics.
- CCTA and FFRCT can be used to determine anatomic and functional SYNTAX scores and to plan the approach to myocardial revascularization.

SOURCE OF FUNDING

None.

CONFLICT OF INTEREST

None.

REFERENCES

1. Patel MR, Peterson ED, Dai D, et al. Low diagnostic yield of elective coronary angiography. N Engl J Med 2010;362:886–95.
2. Patel MR, Dai D, Hernandez AF, et al. Prevalence and predictors of nonobstructive coronary artery disease identified with coronary angiography in contemporary clinical practice. Am Heart J 2014; 167:846–52.
3. Vavalle JP, Shen L, Broderick S, et al. Effect of the presence and type of angina on cardiovascular events in patients without known coronary artery disease referred for elective coronary angiography. JAMA Cardiol 2016;1:232–4.
4. Douglas PS, Hoffman U, Patel MR, et al. Outcomes of anatomical versus functional testing for coronary artery disease. N Engl J Med 2015;372:1291–300.
5. The SCOT-HEART investigators. CT coronary angiography in patients with suspected angina due to coronary heart disease (SCOT-HEART): an open-label, parallel-group, multicentre trial. Lancet 2015; 385:2383–91.
6. Williams MC, Hunter A, Shah ASV, et al. Use of coronary computer tomographic angiography to guide management of patients with coronary disease. J Am Coll Cardiol 2016;67:1759–68.
7. Nørgaard BL, ensen JM, Leipsic J. Fractional flow reserve derived from coronary CT angiography in stable coronary disease: a new study in non-invasive testing? Eur Radiol 2015;25:2282–90.
8. Lofti A, Jeremias A, Fearon WF, et al. Society of Cardiovascular Angiography and Interventions. Expert consensus statement on the use of fractional flow reserve, intravascular ultrasound, and optical coherence tomography: a consensus statement of the Society of Cardiovascular Angiography and Interventions. Catheter Cardiovasc Interv 2014;83: 509–18.
9. Patel MR, Calhoon JH, Dehmer GJ, et al. ACC/AATS/ABA/ASE/ASNC/SCAI/SCCT/STS 2016 appropriate use criteria for coronary revascularization in patients with acute coronary syndromes: a report of the American College of Cardiology Appropriate Use Criteria Task Force, American Association for Thoracic Surgery, American Heart Association, American Society of Echocardiography, American Society of Nuclear Cardiology, Society for Cardiovascular Angiography and Interventions, Society of Cardiovascular Computed Tomography, and the Society of Thoracic Surgeons. J Nucl Cardiol 2017;24: 439–63.
10. Kohl P, Windecker s, Alfonso F, et al. European Society of Cardiology Committee for Practice Guidelines; EACTS Clinical Guidelines Committee; Task Force on Myocardial Revascularization of the European Society of Cardiology and the European Association for Cardio-Thoracic Surgery; European Association of Percutaneous Coronary Interventions. Eur J Cardiothorac Surg 2014;2014:517–92.
11. Levine GN, Bates ER, Blankenship JC, et al. 2011 ACCF/AHA/SCAI guideline for percutaneous coronary intervention: executive summary. Circulation 2011;124:2574–609.
12. Taylor CA, Fonte TA, Min JK. Computational fluid dynamics applied to cardiac computed tomography for noninvasive quantification of fractional flow reserve. J Am Coll Cardiol 2013;61:2233–41.
13. Min JK, Taylor CA, Achenback S, et al. Noninvasive fractional flow reserve derived from coronary CT angiography: clinical data and scientific principles. J Am Coll Cardiol Img 2015;81:1209–22.
14. Kruk M, Wardziak L, Demkow M, et al. Workstation-based calculation of CTA-based FFR for intermediate stenosis. J Am Coll Cardiol Img 2016;9:690–9.
15. Coenen A, Lubbers MM, Kurata A, et al. Fractional flow reserve computed from noninvasive CT angiography data: diagnostic performance of an on-site clinician-operated computational fluid dynamics algorithm. Radiology 2015;274:674–83.
16. Tang CX, Liu CY, Lu MJ, et al. CT FFR for ischemia-specific CAD with a new computational fluid dynamics algorithm. J Am Coll Cardiol Img 2020;13: 980–90.

17. Norgaard BL, Fairbairn TA, Safian RD, et al. Coronary CT angiography-derived fractional flow reserve testing in patients with stable coronary artery disease: recommendations on interpretation and reporting. Radiol:Cardiothorac Img 2019;1:e190050.

18. Cami E, Tagami T, Raff G, et al. Assessment of lesion-specific ischemia using fractional flow reserve (FFR) profiles derived from coronary computed tomography angiography (FFRCT) and invasive pressure measurements (FFRINV): importance of the site of measurement and implications for patient referral for invasive coronary angiography and percutaneous coronary interventions. J Cardiovasc Comput Tomog 2018;12:480–92.

19. Renard BM, Cami E, Jiddou-Patros MR, et al. Optimizing the technique for invasive fractional flow reserve to assess lesion-specific ischemia. Circ Cardiovasc Interv 2019;12:e0077939.

20. Cami E, Tagami T, Raff G, et al. Importance of measurement site on assessment of lesion-specific ischemia and diagnostic performance by coronary computed tomography angiography-derived fractional flow reserve. J Cardiovasc Comput Tomog 2021;15:114–20.

21. Koo BK, Erglis A, Doh JH, et al. Diagnosis of ischemia-causing coronary stenoses by noninvasive fractional flow reserve computed from coronary computed tomographic angiograms. Results from the prospective multicenter DISCOVER-FLOW (Diagnosis of Ischemia-Causing Stenoses Obtained Via Noninvasive Fractional Flow Reserve) study. J Am Coll Cardiol 2011;58:1989–97.

22. Kin JK, Leipsic J, Pencina MJ, et al. Diagnostic accuracy of fractional flow reserve from anatomic CT angiography. JAMA 2012;308:1237–45.

23. Min JK, Berman DS, Budoff MJ, et al. Rationale and design of the DeFACTO (Determination of Fractional Flow Reserve by Anatomic Computed Tomographic Angiography) study. J Cardiovasc Comput Tomog 2011;5:301–9.

24. Norgaard BL, Leipsic J, Gaur S, et al. Diagnostic performance of noninvasive fractional flow reserve derived from coronary computed tomography angiography in suspected coronary artery disease: the NXT Trial (Analysis of Coronary Blood Flow Using CT Angiography: Next Steps). J Am Coll Cardiol 2014;63:1145–55.

25. Gulati M, Levy PD, Mukherjee D, et al. 2021 AHA/ACC/ASE/CHEST/SAEM/SCCT/SCMR guideline for the evaluation and diagnosis of chest pain: a report of the American College of Cardiology/American Heart Association joint committee on clinical practice guidelines. Circulation 2021;144:e368–454.

26. Douglas PS, De Bruyne B, Pontone G, et al. 1-Year outcomes of FFRCT-guided care in patients with suspected coronary disease. The PLATFORM study. J Am Coll Cardiol 2016;68:435–45.

27. Douglas PS, Pontone G, Hlatky MA, et al. Clinical outcomes of fractional flow reserve by computed tomographic angiography-guided diagnostic strategies vs usual care in patients with suspected coronary artery disease: the prospective longitudinal trial of FFRCT: outcome and resource impacts study. Eur Heart J 2015;36:3359–67.

28. Hlatky MA, De Bruyne B, Pontone G, et al. Quality-of-life and economic outcomes of assessing fractional flow reserve with computed tomography angiography (PLATFORM). J Am Coll Cardiol 2015;66:2315–23.

29. Norgaard BL, Hjort J, Gaur S, et al. Clinical use of coronary CTA-derived FFR for decision-making in stable CAD. J Am Coll Cardiol Img 2017;10:541–50.

30. Patel MR, Norgaard BL, Fairbairn TA, et al. 1-Year impact on medical practice and clinical outcomes of FFRCT. The ADVANCE registry. J Am Coll Cardiol Img 2020;13:97–105.

31. Chinnaiyan KM, Safian RD, Gallagher MJ, et al. Clinical use of CT-derived fractional flow reserve in the emergency department. J Am Coll Cardiol Img 2020;13:452–61.

32. McCarthy KJ, Motta-Calderon D, Estrada-Roman A, et al. Introduction of a standardized protocol for cardiac risk assessment in candidates for liver transplant – A retrospective cohort analysis. Ann Hepatol 2021;27:100582.

33. Krievins D, Zellans E, Latkovskis G, et al. Pre-operative diagnosis of silent coronary ischaemia may reduce post-operative death and myocardial infarction and improve survival of patients undergoing lower extremity surgical revascularization. Eur J Vasc Endovasc Surg 2020;60:411–20.

34. Gräni C, Buechel R, Kaufmann PA, et al. Multimodality imaging in individuals with anomalous coronary arteries. J Am Coll Cardiol Img 2017;10:471–81.

35. Gentile F, Castiglione V, De Caterina R. Coronary artery anomalies. Circulation 2021;144:983–96.

36. Tang CX, Lu MJ, Schoepf JU, et al. Coronary computed tomography angiography-derived fractional flow reserve in patients with anomalous origin of the right coronary artery from the left coronary sinus. Korean J Radiol 2020;21:192–202.

37. Adjedj J, Hyafil F, du Fretay, et al. Physiological evaluation of anomalous aortic origin of a coronary artery using computed tomography-derived fractional flow reserve. J Am Heart Assoc 2021;10:e018593.

38. Motoyama S, Ito H, Sarai M, et al. Plaque characterization by coronary computed tomography angiography and the likelihood of acute coronary events in mid-term follow-up. J Am Coll Cardiol 2015;66:337–46.

39. Gaur S, Øvrehus KA, Dey D, et al. Coronary plaque quantification and fractional flow reserve by coronary computed tomography angiography identify

ischaemia-causing lesions. Eur Heart J 2016;37: 1220–7.

40. Park HB, Heo R, Hartaigh B, et al. Atherosclerotic plaque characteristics by CT angiography identify coronary lesions that cause ischemia. A direct comparison to fractional flow reserve. J Am Coll Cardiol Img 2015;8:1–10.

41. Ahmadi A, Stone GW, Leipsic J, et al. Association of coronary stenosis and plaque morphology with fractional flow reserve and outcomes. JAMA Cardiol 2016;1:350–7.

42. Nørgaard BL, Leipsic J, Koo BK, et al. Coronary computed tomography angiography derived fractional flow reserve and plaque stress. Curr Cardiovasc Imaging Rep 2016;9:1–12.

43. Park JB, Choi G, Chun EJ, et al. Computational fluid dynamic measures of wall shear stress are related to coronary lesion characteristics. Heart 2016;102: 1655–61.

44. Choi G, Lee JM, Kim HJ, et al. Coronary artery axial plaque stress and its relationship with lesion geometry. Application of computational fluid dynamics to coronary CT angiography. J Am Coll Cardiol Img 2015;8:1156–66.

45. Lee JM, Choi G, Koo BK, et al. Identification of high-risk plaques destined to cause acute coronary syndrome using coronary computed tomographic angiography and computational fluid dynamics. J Am Coll Cardiol Img 2019;12:1032–43.

46. De Bruyne B, Hersbach F, Pijls NHJ, et al. Abnormal epicardial coronary resistance in patients with diffuse atherosclerosis but "normal" coronary angiography. Circulation 2001;104:2401–6.

47. Collet C, Katagiri Y, Miyazaki Y, et al. Impact of coronary remodeling on fractional flow reserve. Circulation 2018;137:747–9.

48. Imai S, Kondo T, Stone GW, et al. Abnormal fractional flow reserve in nonobstructive coronary artery disease. The relationship with plaque characteristics. Circ Cardiovasc Interv 2019;12:e006961.

49. Tamis-Holland J, Jneid H, Reynolds HR, et al. Contemporary diagnosis and management of patients with myocardial infarction in the absence of obstructive coronary artery disease. A scientific statement from the American Heart Association. Circulation 2019;139:e891–908.

50. Kunadian V, Chieffo A, Camici PG, et al. An EAPCI expert consensus document on ischaemia with non-obstructive coronary arteries in collaboration with European society of cardiology working group on coronary pathophysiology & microcirculation endorsed by coronary vasomotor disorders international study group. Eur Heart J 2020;41: 3504–20.

51. Taylor CA, Gaur S, Leipsic J, et al. Effect of the ratio of coronary arterial lumen volume to left ventricle myocardial mass derived from coronary CT angiography on fractional flow reserve. J Cardiovasc Comput Tomog 2017;11:429–36.

52. Grover R, Leipsic JA, Mooney J, et al. Coronary lumen volume to myocardial mass ratio in primary microvascular angina. J Cardiovasc Comput Tomog 2017;11:423–8.

53. Kuneman JH, El Mahdiui M, van Rosendael AR, et al. Coronary volume to left ventricular mass ratio in patients with diabetes mellitus. J Cardiovasc Comput Tomog 2022;01:0004.

54. De Bruyne B, Pijls NHJ, Kalesan B, et al. Fractional flow reserve-guided PCI versus medical therapy in stable coronary disease. N Engl J Med 2012;367: 991–1001.

55. Tonino PAL, De Bruyne B, Pijls NHJ, et al. Fractional flow reserve versus angiography for guiding percutaneous coronary intervention. N Engl J Med 2009; 360:213–24.

56. Sianos G, Morel MA, Kappetein AP, et al. The SYNTAX score: an angiographic tool grading the complexity of coronary artery disease. EuroIntervention 2005;1:219–27.

57. Farooq V, van Klaveren D, Steyerberg EW, et al. Anatomical and clinical characteristics to guide decision making between coronary artery bypass surgery and percutaneous coronary intervention for individual patients: development and validation of SYNTAX score II. Lancet 2013;381:639–50.

58. Nam CW, Mangiacapra F, Entjes R, et al. Functional SYNTAX score for risk assessment in multivessel coronary artery disease. J Am Coll Cardiol 2011; 58:1211–8.

59. Papadopoulou SL, Girasis C, Dharampal A, et al. CT-SYNTAX score. J Am Coll Cardiol Img 2013;6: 413–5.

60. Collet C, Miyazaki Y, Ryan N, et al. Fractional flow reserve derived from computed tomographic angiography in patients with multivessel CAD. J Am Coll Cardiol 2018;71:2756–69.

61. Collet C, Onuma Y, Miyazaki Y, et al. Integration of non-invasive functional assessments with anatomical risk stratification n complex coronary artery disease: the non-invasive functional SYNTAX score. Cardiovasc Diagn Ther 2017;7:151–8.

62. Kerner S, Abadi S, Abergel E, et al. Direct comparison between coronary computed tomography and invasive angiography for calculation of SYNTAX score. EuroIntervention 2013;8:1428–34.

63. Yüceler Z, Kantarci M, Tanboğa I, et al. Coronary lesion complexity assessed by SYNTAX score in 256-slice dual-source MDCT angiography. Diagn Interv Radiol 2016;22:334–40.

64. Andreini D, Modolo R, Katagiri Y, et al. Impact of fractional flow reserve derived from coronary computed tomography angiography on heart team treatment decision-making in patients with multivessel coronary artery disease. Insights from the

SYNTAX III REVOLUTION trial. Circ Cardiovasc Interv 2019;12:e007607.

65. Feldmann K, Cami E, Safian RD. Planning percutaneous coronary interventions using computed tomography angiography and fractional flow reserve-derived from computed tomography: a state-of-the-art review. Catheter Cardiovasc Interv 2019;93:298–304.

66. Kim KH, Doh JH, Koo BK, et al. A novel noninvasive technology for treatment planning using virtual coronary stenting and computed tomography-derived computed fractional flow reserve. J Am Coll Cardiol Intv 2014;7:72–8.

67. Bom MJ, Schumacher SP, Driessen RS, et al. Noninvasive procedural planning using computed tomography-derived fractional flow reserve. Catheter Cardiovasc Interv 2021;97:614–22.

68. Sonck J, Nagumo S, Norgaard BL, et al. Clinical validation of a virtual planner for coronary interventions based on coronary CT angiography. J Am Coll Cardiol Img 2022;15(7):1242–55.

Beyond Coronary Artery Disease
Assessing the Microcirculation

Sonal Pruthi, MD[a], Emaad Siddiqui, MD[a],
Nathaniel R. Smilowitz, MD, MS[a,b,c],*

KEYWORDS

- Coronary flow reserve • Coronary microvascular disease • Coronary microvascular dysfunction
- Coronary physiology • Hyperemic microvascular resistance • Index of microcirculatory resistance
- Ischemia with nonobstructive coronary arteries • INOCA

KEY POINTS

- Coronary microvascular dysfunction (CMD) is an important cause of ischemia with nonobstructive coronary arteries (INOCA).
- The pathophysiology of CMD is not well established.
- Coronary flow reserve, the index of microcirculatory resistance, hyperemic microvascular resistance, and resistive reserve ratio are invasively measured indices to evaluate the microcirculation.
- CMD is associated with clinical outcomes in patients with INOCA and obstructive coronary artery disease.

BACKGROUND

Ischemic heart disease (IHD) affects more than 20 million adults in the United States and is a leading cause of death.[1] Stable IHD is associated with angina, decreased exercise tolerance, and adverse health-related quality of life. Although angina is classically attributed to atherosclerosis of the epicardial coronary arteries, recent evidence suggests that nearly half of patients who undergo invasive coronary angiography for the evaluation of angina do not have obstructive coronary disease.[2,3] This perplexing clinical scenario, first described in 1967 and later termed *cardiac Syndrome X*, is now referred to as ischemia with nonobstructive coronary arteries (INOCA).[4] Underlying mechanisms of INOCA include microvascular angina with coronary microvascular dysfunction (CMD), epicardial coronary spasm, and noncardiac chest pain.[5,6] Recent

American and European clinical practice guidelines recognize the impact of INOCA and recommend functional assessment of the coronary microcirculation to determine mechanisms of ischemia and guide pharmacologic therapy.[7–9] The objective of this review is to (1) outline the anatomy of the coronary circulation and the pathophysiology of CMD, (2) describe current approaches to assess the coronary microcirculation in the cardiac catheterization laboratory, and (3) examine the clinical implications of CMD in INOCA and other cardiovascular disorders.

Anatomy and Physiology of the Coronary Microcirculation

Anatomy

From the epicardial vessels to the myocardium, the coronary circulation can be divided into 3

This article originally appeared in *Interventional Cardiology Clinics*, Volume 12 Issue 1, January 2023.

[a] Division of Cardiology, Department of Medicine, NYU Langone Health, 550 First Avenue, New York, NY 10016, USA; [b] Cardiology Section, Department of Medicine, VA New York Harbor Healthcare System, 423 East 23rd Street, New York, NY 10010, USA; [c] The Leon H. Charney Division of Cardiology, NYU Langone Health, NYU School of Medicine, 423 East 23rd Street, 12-West, New York, NY 10010, USA

* Corresponding author. The Leon H. Charney Division of Cardiology, NYU Langone Health, NYU School of Medicine, 423 East 23rd Street, 12-West, New York, NY 10010.

E-mail address: nathaniel.smilowitz@nyulangone.org

distinct "compartments" (**Fig. 1**). Blood enters the coronary circulation via the major epicardial coronary arteries, vessels 500 μm to 5 mm in size that course predominantly along the surface of the myocardium and can be easily visualized by coronary angiography. Epicardial coronary arteries have been the focus of coronary interventions for more than half a century. Despite their important role as proximal conduit vessels, the epicardial coronaries only directly supply 5% to 10% of the myocardium. In normal physiologic conditions, epicardial coronary arteries offer little resistance to blood flow due to their relatively large diameters. Nitric oxide-mediated vasodilation of the epicardial coronaries accommodates increased blood flow in times of high metabolic demand. Atherosclerotic plaques in the epicardial coronaries can lead to dramatic increases in resistance to flow.[10] The epicardial coronary arteries branch and taper into a vast network of arterioles to supply the myocardium.

Extramyocardial prearteriolar vessels, which range in diameter from 100 to 500 μm, form the intermediate compartment of the coronary circulation. These prearteriolar vessels run in parallel, leading to physiologic drops in pressures.[11] Proximal prearterioles in this compartment are most sensitive to changes in intravascular flow, whereas distal vessels are sensitive to changes in pressure. Vasoconstriction and vasodilation of the prearterioles maintains constant arteriolar pressures.[12] This compartment may be responsible for CMD in patients with INOCA.

The third and final compartment of the coronary circulation consists of innumerable intramural arterioles less than 100 μm in diameter. These vessels directly supply low-pressure myocardial capillary beds that serve as the site for nutrient and gas exchange. Arterioles in the coronary circulation have a high resting tone and dilate in response to local metabolites produced by the surrounding myocardium, including adenosine, nitric oxide, and prostaglandins.[11] Thus, arterioles are responsible for the metabolic regulation of myocardial blood flow.

In normal circumstances, the 3 compartments of the coronary circulation work in concert to regulate myocardial blood flow in response to metabolic demands. Once maximal myocardial oxygen extraction (~75%) has been reached, additional metabolic demands must be met with increases in myocardial blood flow.[13] Increases in heart rate and contractility can augment cardiac output, and vasodilatory metabolites from the myocardium decrease microcirculatory arteriolar resistance to enhance coronary blood flow (CBF).[13] Thus, the microcirculation plays a pivotal role to ensure coronary perfusion matches myocardial oxygen demand.

Pathobiology of Coronary Microvascular Disease

Coronary microvascular disease has been broadly classified as microvascular dysfunction (1) in the absence of obstructive coronary artery disease (CAD) or myocardial diseases, (2) in the presence of myocardial disease, (3) in the presence of obstructive CAD, or (4) from an iatrogenic cause.[14] A variety of mechanisms can contribute to structural or functional abnormalities of the microcirculation.[15,16] In patients without obstructive atherosclerosis or myocardial diseases, the pathogenesis of microvascular disease may include arteriolar remodeling and fibrosis, intimal proliferation, smooth muscle hypertrophy, or vessel rarefaction. Small vessel atherosclerosis, platelet activation and plugging,[17] or microembolization of thrombotic material in the setting of epicardial atherosclerotic disease may also contribute.[18] In the setting of myocardial disease, such as left ventricular hypertrophy, increased intramyocardial, left ventricular diastolic, and coronary venous pressures may also lead to increased resistance to microcirculatory flow.[19]

In addition to structural disorders of the microcirculation, functional abnormalities associated with impairment to the normal responses to neurohormonal and metabolic signaling can lead to impaired microcirculatory flow. This may include attenuated responses to or decreased synthesis of vasodilators such as nitric oxide.[20,21] Coronary microvascular spasm, with episodic increases in microvascular resistance and provocation of myocardial ischemia can also occur.[22]

Although the exact pathophysiology of CMD is uncertain, risk factors include older age, hypertension, dyslipidemia, diabetes mellitus, cigarette smoking, and chronic inflammatory disorders, including systemic lupus erythematosus and rheumatoid arthritis.[23–28] Additional investigation is needed to identify modifiable risk factors to prevent development of microcirculatory disease.

Assessing the Microcirculation in the Catheterization Laboratory

Unlike the epicardial coronary arteries, coronary microcirculation cannot be directly visualized. Thus, assessments are largely based on parameters of microcirculatory flow. Coronary flow reserve (CFR), the original integrated measure of coronary epicardial flow and microvascular function, is defined as the ratio of hyperemic CBF to

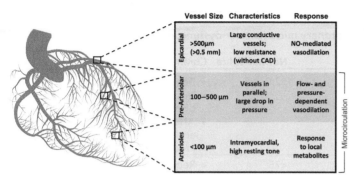

Vessel Size	Characteristics	Response
Epicardial >500μm (>0.5 mm)	Large conductive vessels; low resistance (without CAD)	NO-mediated vasodilation
Pre-Arteriolar 100–500 μm	Vessels in parallel; large drop in pressure	Flow- and pressure-dependent vasodilation
Arterioles <100 μm	Intramyocardial, high resting tone	Response to local metabolites

Microcirculation

Fig. 1. Anatomy of the compartments of the coronary circulation. CAD, coronary artery disease; NO, nitric oxide.

CBF at rest. Normal coronary arteries can augment blood flow greater than 4-fold at maximal hyperemia, whereas a CFR less than 2 to less than 2.5 in the absence of epicardial coronary disease is abnormal and reflects microvascular dysfunction (**Table 1**).[5,6]

Invasive evaluation of CFR can be performed in the catheterization laboratory using thermodilution or Doppler-based assessment of CBF. The intracoronary Doppler guidewire, first developed in the late 1980s, contains a piezoelectric ultrasound transducer mounted at the tip to measure CBF velocity.[29] The current generation of wire (FloWire or ComboWire XT, Phillips, Amsterdam, Netherlands) can measure the average peak velocity (APV) of CBF at a specific location using a commercially available console with dedicated software (ComboMap, Philips Volcano). Coronary APV is typically measured at rest, and then again after induction of hyperemia with the administration of a nonendothelial-dependent vasodilator such as adenosine. Doppler-derived CFR is typically simplified as the ratio of the hyperemic APV to the APV measured at rest. To estimate CBF, the vessel diameter (D) at the site of APV measurement can be determined using quantitative coronary angiography, and flow can then be calculated by the formula: $CBF = 0.5 \times APV \times (D2 \pi)/4$.[29] In response to an infusion of acetylcholine, an endothelial-dependent vasodilator, CBF typically increases substantially. Augmentation of CBF by less than 50% in the presence of acetylcholine is abnormal and in the absence of significant epicardial coronary constriction indicates that endothelial dependent microvascular dysfunction may be present.[30,31]

In contrast to Doppler-based measures that measure coronary velocity at a single location, coronary thermodilution techniques assesses flow based on temperature changes across the vessel. This technique requires 3 mL bolus injections of room temperature saline through the guide catheter, with a distal thermistor on a coronary

pressure-wire recording temperatures in the coronary artery (PressureWire X, Abbott Vascular, Abbott Park, IL USA). The shaft of this wire acts as a proximal thermistor. The speed of change of the distal temperature (relative to the proximal temperature) is used to calculate the mean transit time (T_{mn}), which is inversely proportional to coronary flow according to the principles of indicator dilution theory.

Doppler and thermodilution approaches to measurement of coronary flow each have limitations. Doppler-derived measures of coronary flow velocity assume that flow at the transducer is parallel, laminar, and parabolic, and may not remain constant at different wire positions.[32] Indeed, animal and human studies have demonstrated significant variability in Doppler wire measurements,[33] and Doppler measurements tend to be technically more challenging, require more time for data acquisition, and have a steeper learning curve.[34,35] Although coronary thermodilution is somewhat easier to obtain, it can be significantly impacted by changes in guide catheter position during administration of saline boluses. In an early porcine model, thermodilution-derived CFR correlated better with absolute flow measured by an external coronary flow probe than did the Doppler wire-derived CFR.[36] However, in a study of 98 vessels in 40 consecutive patients, Doppler-derived CFR correlated more closely with PET-derived CFR than thermodilution-derived CFR.[37] Ultimately, both techniques are considered to be valid in the assessment of the coronary microcirculation (see **Table 1**).

Unfortunately, CFR is not specific to microcirculation and is affected by epicardial coronary stenosis and resting hemodynamics. In the absence of obstructive epicardial disease, a reduced CFR can reflect increased microcirculatory resistance to flow, an abnormal response to the standard vasodilatory stimulus, or increased resting coronary flow before vasodilator administration. Among patients with INOCA, high resting flow is

Table 1
Invasively derived measures to assess coronary microvascular dysfunction

Technique	Measurement Method	Normal Value	Comments
CFR	Doppler or Thermodilution	>2.0–2.5	• Requires hyperemia • Not specific for microvascular disease • Affected by resting hemodynamics and coronary epicardial stenosis • Predicts long-term MACE
IMR	Thermodilution (Bolus dose)	<25	• Requires hyperemia • Specific to the coronary microcirculation • Less variable than CFR despite change in hemodynamics • Requires correction (Yong) in the presence of significant epicardial stenosis • Predicts long-term death and heart failure readmissions in patients with STEMI • May predict graft dysfunction early after orthotopic heart transplant
hMR	Doppler	≤2	• Specific to the coronary microcirculation • Technical challenges of optimal Doppler signal acquisition
RRR	Doppler or thermodilution	<1.7–3.5	• Superior to CFR for prognosis
mMR	Doppler	Not defined	• Measured during wave-free period window of diastole and does not require hyperemia • Limited data on prognostic value
R_{micro}	Thermodilution (continuous infusion)	< 500 WU	• Strong agreement with PET-derived coronary flow • Saline infusion induces hyperemia • Accuracy in obstructive coronary artery disease is not well defined • Equipment not available in the United States
MRR	Thermodilution (continuous infusion)	Not defined	• Novel index • Specific to microvasculature; corrected for epicardial conductance • Independent of autoregulation and myocardial mass • Requires validation

more common in women, younger patients, and patients with fewer cardiovascular risk factors, and may represent a distinct pathologic condition.[38]

Microvascular resistance indices offer an alternative method to interrogate the microcirculation.[39] The index of microcirculatory resistance (IMR), first reported in 2003, is a thermodilution-based measure that reflects the minimal achievable resistance of the microcirculation with endothelial-independent vasodilators (see **Table 1**).[32] IMR is based on Ohm's law, which states that the potential difference across an ideal conductor is proportional to the current through the conductor (Voltage = current × resistance). Applying this to coronary physiology, the microcirculation acts as a conductor, the voltage is analogous to the difference in pressure across the microvasculature (mean distal coronary pressure $[P_d]$ – coronary venous pressure $[P_v]$), and current is myocardial flow $(1/T_{mn})$. Because P_v is usually negligible, IMR may be calculated by the formula: $IMR = P_d \times T_{mn}$. A normal value of IMR has been reported to be lesser than 25,[40–42] with higher values reported in the right coronary artery (RCA), perhaps due to longer vessel length and larger diameters accounting for a somewhat prolonged T_{mn}.[42]

Yet, there are some situations in which IMR must be interpreted with caution. In the presence of a significant coronary stenosis, collateral flow to the vessel of interest may increase the coronary wedge pressure (Pw). Thus, coronary thermodilution may underestimate flow and IMR may overestimate resistance.[43] To account for collateral flow, the following formula has been proposed: $IMR = Pa \times T_{mn} \times ([P_d - P_w]/[P_a - P_w])$.[43] Because P_w are not routinely measured, a correction factor for IMR has been derived and validated from experimental data with P_w measured during proximal vessel balloon occlusions.[44,45] Corrected IMR can be calculated using Yong's modification (corrected $IMR = Pa \times T_{mn} \times [(1.35 \times Pd/Pa) - 0.32]$) during hyperemia.

There are several benefits to IMR, which remains stable in the presence of increasing epicardial stenosis,[43] and is relatively independent of resting hemodynamics.[46] Variability in IMR is lower than that of CFR, despite changes in heart rate, blood pressure, and contractility.[46] Finally, IMR is a highly reproducible measure over time, with low interobserver variability despite manual injection of saline boluses.[47,48]

Microcirculatory resistance can also be determined using a guidewire with a Doppler ultrasound transducer and simultaneous distal coronary pressure monitoring. The Doppler-derived hyperemic microvascular resistance (hMR) is analogous to IMR and is defined as the ratio of mean distal pressure to the Doppler-derived APV (see **Table 1**).[49] An hMR of 2 or greater is generally considered to be abnormal. In patients with INOCA, hMR less than 1.9 predicted recurrent chest pain in one study, although in another, a threshold of 2.5 or greater provided the highest sensitivity and specificity to detect CMR-determined microvascular disease or abnormal invasive CFR.[34,50] A related measure, the minimal microvascular resistance (mMR), was proposed as the ratio of hyperemic distal coronary pressure and hyperemic APV measured during wave-free period window of diastole, when microvascular resistance is at its lowest.[51] Although conceptually attractive, mMR requires further study.

The resistive reserve ratio (RRR), another recently developed microcirculatory parameter, is calculated as the ratio of baseline microvascular resistance to hMR, with higher values indicating greater vasodilatory capacity of the microcirculation (see **Table 1**).[52,53] Thresholds for abnormal RRR are not well established but have been proposed between less than 1.7 and 3.5 in various populations and with both Doppler and Thermodilution-derived resistance measures.[54–56] In a study of 1692 patients with INOCA, Doppler-derived RRR of less than 2.62 was associated with mortality and was superior to CFR to predict long-term survival.[57] Low RRR was also associated with long-term outcomes in cohorts with acute MI and CAD undergoing revascularization.[55,56]

Continuous thermodilution is another emerging technique to assess the microcirculation.[58] Temperature changes associated with intracoronary saline infusion, administered at a known rate through a dedicated monorail infusion catheter, can be measured in the distal coronary with a thermistor on a pressure-sensing coronary wire to calculate absolute coronary flow (Q). Q can be derived as $Q = 1.08 \times T_i/T \times Q_i$, where T_i is the temperature of saline as it exits the catheter, T is the temperature of the blood in the distal coronary during the steady-state infusion, and Q_i is the saline infusion rate (in milliliter per minute).[59,60] Based on Ohm's law, absolute microvascular resistance ($R = P_d/Q$), measured in Woods units (WU), can be obtained. Slow coronary infusions of saline (typically 8–10 mL/min) are used to assess baseline resistance at rest, whereas hyperemia is induced at higher saline infusion rates (15–25 mL/min).[61] Continuous thermodilution Q has strong agreement with PET-derived coronary flow,[62] absolute resistance greater than 500 WU is the optimal threshold to identify patients with an IMR of 25 or greater,[63] and both absolute flow and resistance are associated with angina.[64]

Based on absolute flow from continuous thermodilution measures, the microvascular resistance reserve (MRR) has been proposed as an index specific for the microvasculature, independent of autoregulation and myocardial mass, and corrected for epicardial conductance. MRR can be defined as the ratio of the pure microvascular resistance at rest because it would exist in the absence of epicardial disease affecting microcirculatory autoregulation, to the mMR measured during hyperemia. Although the derivation of the formula for MRR is beyond the scope of this review, in practice, MRR can be calculated as the CFR divided by fractional flow reserve (FFR), corrected for coronary driving pressures as follows: $MRR = (CFR/FFR) \times (P_{a\ at\ rest}/P_{a\ at\ hyperemia})$.[65] This conceptually elegant and promising new measure of microcirculatory function requires additional validation.

Practical Approach to Invasive Microcirculatory Assessment

Before testing, patients should be advised to abstain from caffeine intake to ensure appropriate responses to hyperemic agents. When combined with acetylcholine or ergonovine reactivity testing, patients should also withhold long-acting nitrates, calcium channel blockers, and beta-blockers for 48 hours before testing. Coronary angiography should be performed to assess for epicardial coronary stenosis and myocardial bridges. Coronary microvascular testing should be performed using a guiding catheter (preferably 6 or greater French) that is stably engaged in the coronary ostium, after administration of intracoronary nitroglycerin and systemic anticoagulation.

To measure thermodilution-based CFR and IMR, a coronary pressure–temperature sensor guidewire (Pressure Wire, Abbott Vascular) should be introduced into the guide, and residual contrast media flushed with saline. Pressure waveforms should be equalized with the pressure sensor at the tip of the guide catheter. Next, the temperature and pressure sensor should be advanced to the distal two-thirds of the left anterior descending (LAD) artery, approximately 8 to 10 cm into the circumflex and placed in a large obtuse marginal branch or dominant distal vessel, or in the distal RCA before the bifurcation of the posterior descending artery. A 3-way stopcock and a 3-mL syringe should be connected to the manifold. Next, 3 mL boluses of room-temperature saline should be briskly injected through the guide catheter to determine T_{mn} at rest. Measurements are performed in triplicate. If there is less than 30% variability between the measurements, the T_{mn} value that deviates most significantly from the mean value should be replaced. Once assessment of baseline flow has been completed, hyperemia is induced with intravenous adenosine (140 mcg/kg/min), or with a bolus of intracoronary papaverine (10–20 mg). Once maximal hyperemia has been achieved, typically ~2 minutes after initiation of intravenous adenosine, 3 mL boluses of room temperature saline should again be briskly injected through the guide. CFR can be calculated as the ratio of T_{mn} at rest to T_{mn} at hyperemia; IMR is the product of T_{mn} and P_d at hyperemia. Nonhyperemic pressure ratios and FFR should also be assessed to determine significance of any angiographically intermediate epicardial lesions. RRR can be calculated as the ratio of baseline to hMR $(T_{mn\ at\ rest} \times P_{d\ at\ rest})$/IMR.

Doppler-based measurements of CFR and hMR follow a similar sequence. After intracoronary nitroglycerin, a 0.014″ coronary guidewire with a pressure sensor and Doppler crystal (ComboWire XT, Philips Volcano) should be positioned parallel to the vessel, away from the vessel wall, and manipulated to obtain a stable maximal Doppler flow signal. APV is measured at rest and again with maximal hyperemia, as previously described. The CFR is calculated as the ratio of hyperemic APV to resting APV. The hMR is calculated as the hyperemic P_d divided by the hyperemic APV. To assess endothelial dependent microvascular function, CBF at rest and during acetylcholine infusions can be estimated from Doppler-derived APV and luminal dimensions from quantitative coronary angiography.

Clinical Implications of Microcirculatory Disease

Microvascular disease in ischemia with nonobstructive coronary arteries

Nearly 50% of patients who present with chest pain have angiographically normal or nonobstructive epicardial coronary arteries (<50% stenosis) by angiography.[2,3,66] A comprehensive approach to the diagnosis of INOCA, including testing for microvascular disease, can improve the care of these patients (**Fig. 2**). In the Coronary Microvascular Angina (CorMicA) trial, 151 patients underwent blinded assessment of coronary microvascular function and provocative testing for coronary artery spasm; participants were randomly assigned to disclosure of the results or usual care.[6] Overall, microvascular angina was identified in 52% of patients, coronary spasm was identified in 20%, and mixed microvascular and spasm diagnosis was present in 17%, with no discernible cause identified in the remaining 11%.[67] Although noncardiac chest pain was presumed in 60% to 65% of participants before randomization, the results of testing improved diagnostic certainty, reduced the number of patients inappropriately diagnosed with noncardiac chest pain, and impacted therapy in the overwhelming majority of patients in the intervention group. Although similar at baseline, patients assigned to disclosure of coronary functional testing had significantly better Angina Summary Scores and quality of life at 6 months and 1 year compared with the control group.[6,68] This trial provides compelling data in support of invasive microvascular testing to guide therapy and improve symptoms in INOCA (see **Fig. 2**). Additional studies to evaluate the clinical benefit of microvascular testing without coronary spasm testing are currently underway (iCorMICA NCT04674449).

Although outcomes are more favorable than patients with obstructive disease, INOCA is associated

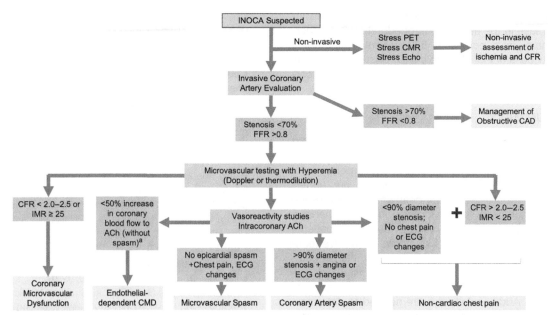

Fig. 2. Diagnostic pathway for the invasive assessment of patients with INOCA. [a]Assessed with Doppler APV and coronary diameter via quantitative coronary angiography to determine coronary blood flow at rest and with ACh. Ach, acetylcholine; CAD, coronary artery disease; CFR, coronary flow reserve; CFVR, coronary flow velocity reserve; CMD, coronary microvascular disease; CMR, cardiovascular magnetic resonance; ECG, electrocardiogram; FFR, fractional flow reserve; IMR, index for microvascular resistance; INOCA, ischemia with nonobstructive coronary arteries; PET, positron emission tomography.

with excess major adverse cardiovascular events compared with reference populations without IHD.[69] Data from Women's Ischemia Syndrome Evaluation registry indicate that CFR of less than 2.3 is associated with increased risks of major adverse cardiovascular events (MACE) in patients with INOCA.[31,70] In a multicenter international study of INOCA patients with microvascular angina, the annual incidence of the composite of MACE was 7.7%.[71] In a study-level meta-analysis, CMD was associated with 5-fold greater odds for major adverse cardiovascular events compared with patients without CMD.[72] Thus, novel therapies to reduce the risk of MACE in patients with microvascular disease are urgently needed.

Impact of Coronary Microvascular Dysfunction in Myocardial Infarction and Percutaneous Coronary Intervention

In patients with acute myocardial infarction (MI), distal embolization of thrombotic material can lead to the "no-reflow phenomenon," characterized by myocardial tissue hypoperfusion in the presence of a patent epicardial coronary artery. No-reflow, mediated by microvascular disease, is a strong predictor for adverse outcomes post-MI.[73] Quantitative assessment of the coronary

microcirculation provides additional insights into MI severity and outcomes. In patients with ST segment elevation MI (STEMI), IMR postpercutaneous coronary intervention (PCI) correlates with myocardial injury, echocardiographic wall motion abnormalities,[74] myocardial viability by PET,[75] and myocardial salvage by cardiac magnetic resonance (CMR).[48] Although IMR correlates with microvascular obstruction by CMR imaging overall,[76] discordances between the 2 measures are reported in up to a third of cases.[77] Yet, in a cohort of 253 patients undergoing primary PCI for STEMI with a median follow-up of 2.8 years, elevated IMR of 40 or greater immediately after revascularization was associated with a 2-fold excess hazard of long-term death or rehospitalization for heart failure, and a 4-fold excess hazard of mortality.[78] The Doppler-derived resistance index, hMR, has also been associated with outcomes after STEMI.[35] Similarly, in patients who presented with NSTEMI and underwent PCI, post-PCI elevated IMR greater than 27 was an independent predictor of MACE over a median follow-up of 21 months.[79]

Even in stable patients undergoing PCI, a high baseline IMR is an independent risk factor for periprocedural MI. Among patients undergoing PCI of simple LAD lesions, pre-PCI IMR of 27 or greater, was independently associated with a 23-fold increase in the risk of periprocedural MI.[80] Furthermore, in a cohort of 572 patients undergoing successful PCI for stable IHD, post-PCI IMR was independently associated with major adverse cardiovascular events at follow-up.[81]

SUMMARY

The coronary microcirculation represents the next frontier in the diagnosis and treatment of coronary artery disease. Recognition of the importance of coronary physiology has expanded our understanding of IHD and European and American societal guidelines now recommend comprehensive assessment of microvascular function in patients with INOCA.[7,8] Recent advances in invasive techniques and technologies to quantify microcirculatory CBF and resistance are vital to the comprehensive evaluation of coronary artery disease. Additional studies are needed to determine optimal therapies for patients with coronary microcirculatory disease in various cardiac disease states.

CLINICS CARE POINTS

- Coronary microvascular dysfunction is an important, and often under-appreciated, cause of angina and ischemia that can be diagnosed invasively based on an abnormally low coronary flow reserve (CFR) and/or an elevated index of microcirculatory resistance (IMR).

ACKNOWLEDGMENTS

Dr N.R. Smilowitz is supported, in part, by the National Heart, Lung, And Blood Institute of the National Institutes of Health, United States under Award Number K23HL150315.

DISCLOSURE

Dr N.R. Smilowitz serves on an advisory board for Abbott Vascular. The remainder of the authors report no financial relationships or conflicts of interest regarding the content herein.

REFERENCES

1. Tsao CW, Aday AW, Almarzooq ZI, et al. Heart Disease and Stroke Statistics-2022 Update: A Report From the American Heart Association. Circulation 2022. https://doi.org/10.1161/CIR. 0000000000001052. CIR0000000000001052.
2. Patel MR, Peterson ED, Dai D, et al. Low diagnostic yield of elective coronary angiography. N Engl J Med 2010;362(10):886–95.
3. Shaw LJ, Shaw RE, Merz CN, et al. Impact of ethnicity and gender differences on angiographic coronary artery disease prevalence and in-hospital mortality in the American College of Cardiology-National Cardiovascular Data Registry. Circulation 2008;117(14):1787–801.
4. Bairey Merz CN, Pepine CJ, Walsh MN, et al. Ischemia and No Obstructive Coronary Artery Disease (INOCA): Developing Evidence-Based Therapies and Research Agenda for the Next Decade. Circulation 2017;135(11):1075–92.
5. Ong P, Camici PG, Beltrame JF, et al. International standardization of diagnostic criteria for microvascular angina. Int J Cardiol 2018;250:16–20.
6. Ford TJ, Stanley B, Good R, et al. Stratified Medical Therapy Using Invasive Coronary Function Testing in Angina: The CorMicA Trial. J Am Coll Cardiol 2018; 72(23 Pt A):2841–55.
7. Gulati M, Levy PD, Mukherjee D, et al. 2021 AHA/ACC/ASE/CHEST/SAEM/SCCT/SCMR Guideline for the Evaluation and Diagnosis of Chest Pain: A Report of the American College of Cardiology/American Heart Association Joint Committee on Clinical Practice Guidelines. Circulation 2021;144(22):e368–454.
8. Kunadian V, Chieffo A, Camici PG, et al. An EAPCI Expert Consensus Document on Ischaemia with Non-Obstructive Coronary Arteries in Collaboration with European Society of Cardiology Working Group on Coronary Pathophysiology & Microcirculation Endorsed by Coronary Vasomotor Disorders International Study Group. Eur Heart J 2020;41(37): 3504–20.
9. Padro T, Manfrini O, Bugiardini R, et al. ESC Working Group on Coronary Pathophysiology and Microcirculation position paper on 'coronary microvascular dysfunction in cardiovascular disease. Cardiovasc Res 2020;116(4):741–55.
10. Wilson RF, Marcus ML, White CW. Prediction of the physiologic significance of coronary arterial lesions by quantitative lesion geometry in patients with limited coronary artery disease. Circulation 1987; 75(4):723–32.
11. Camici PG, d'Amati G, Rimoldi O. Coronary microvascular dysfunction: mechanisms and functional assessment. Nat Rev Cardiol 2015;12(1):48–62.
12. Diez-Delhoyo F, Gutierrez-Ibanes E, Loughlin G, et al. Coronary physiology assessment in the catheterization laboratory. World J Cardiol 2015;7(9): 525–38.
13. Duncker DJ, Bache RJ. Regulation of coronary blood flow during exercise. Physiol Rev 2008; 88(3):1009–86.

14. Camici PG, Crea F. Coronary microvascular dysfunction. N Engl J Med 2007;356(8):830–40.

15. Crea F, Camici PG, Bairey Merz CN. Coronary microvascular dysfunction: an update. *Eur Heart J* May 2014;35(17):1101–11.

16. Lanza GA, Crea F. Primary coronary microvascular dysfunction: clinical presentation, pathophysiology, and management. Circulation 2010;121(21): 2317–25.

17. Lanza GA, Andreotti F, Sestito A, et al. Platelet aggregability in cardiac syndrome X. Eur Heart J 2001;22(20):1924–30.

18. Kleinbongard P, Heusch G. A fresh look at coronary microembolization. Nat Rev Cardiol 2021. https://doi.org/10.1038/s41569-021-00632-2.

19. Cecchi F, Olivotto I, Gistri R, et al. Coronary microvascular dysfunction and prognosis in hypertrophic cardiomyopathy. N Engl J Med 2003;349(11): 1027–35.

20. Mills I, Fallon JT, Wrenn D, et al. Adaptive responses of coronary circulation and myocardium to chronic reduction in perfusion pressure and flow. Am J Physiol 1994;266(2 Pt 2):H447–57.

21. Egashira K, Inou T, Hirooka Y, et al. Impaired coronary blood flow response to acetylcholine in patients with coronary risk factors and proximal atherosclerotic lesions. J Clin Invest 1993;91(1):29–37.

22. Ong P, Athanasiadis A, Borgulya G, et al. Clinical usefulness, angiographic characteristics, and safety evaluation of intracoronary acetylcholine provocation testing among 921 consecutive white patients with unobstructed coronary arteries. Circulation 2014;129(17):1723–30.

23. Recio-Mayoral A, Mason JC, Kaski JC, et al. Chronic inflammation and coronary microvascular dysfunction in patients without risk factors for coronary artery disease. Eur Heart J 2009;30(15):1837–43.

24. Hirata K, Kadirvelu A, Kinjo M, et al. Altered coronary vasomotor function in young patients with systemic lupus erythematosus. Arthritis Rheumatism 2007;56(6):1904–9.

25. Di Carli MF, Charytan D, McMahon GT, et al. Coronary circulatory function in patients with the metabolic syndrome. J Nucl Med 2011;52(9):1369–77.

26. Dayanikli F, Grambow D, Muzik O, et al. Early detection of abnormal coronary flow reserve in asymptomatic men at high risk for coronary artery disease using positron emission tomography. Circulation 1994;90(2):808–17.

27. Laine H, Raitakari OT, Niinikoski H, et al. Early impairment of coronary flow reserve in young men with borderline hypertension. J Am Coll Cardiol 1998;32(1):147–53.

28. Lee BK, Lim HS, Fearon WF, et al. Invasive evaluation of patients with angina in the absence of obstructive coronary artery disease. Circulation 2015;131(12):1054–60.

29. Doucette JW, Corl PD, Payne HM, et al. Validation of a Doppler guide wire for intravascular measurement of coronary artery flow velocity. Circulation 1992; 85(5):1899–911.

30. Sara JD, Widmer RJ, Matsuzawa Y, et al. Prevalence of Coronary Microvascular Dysfunction Among Patients With Chest Pain and Nonobstructive Coronary Artery Disease. JACC Cardiovasc Interv 2015;8(11): 1445–53.

31. AlBadri A, Bairey Merz CN, Johnson BD, et al. Impact of Abnormal Coronary Reactivity on Long-Term Clinical Outcomes in Women. J Am Coll Cardiol 2019;73(6):684–93.

32. Fearon WF, Balsam LB, Farouque HM, et al. Novel index for invasively assessing the coronary microcirculation. Circulation 2003;107(25):3129–32.

33. Barbato E, Aarnoudse W, Aengevaeren WR, et al. Validation of coronary flow reserve measurements by thermodilution in clinical practice. Eur Heart J 2004;25(3):219–23.

34. Williams RP, de Waard GA, De Silva K, et al. Doppler Versus Thermodilution-Derived Coronary Microvascular Resistance to Predict Coronary Microvascular Dysfunction in Patients With Acute Myocardial Infarction or Stable Angina Pectoris. Am J Cardiol 2018;121(1):1–8.

35. de Waard GA, Fahrni G, de Wit D, et al. Hyperaemic microvascular resistance predicts clinical outcome and microvascular injury after myocardial infarction. Heart 2018;104(2):127–34.

36. Fearon WF, Farouque HM, Balsam LB, et al. Comparison of coronary thermodilution and Doppler velocity for assessing coronary flow reserve. Circulation 2003;108(18):2198–200.

37. Everaars H, de Waard GA, Driessen RS, et al. Doppler Flow Velocity and Thermodilution to Assess Coronary Flow Reserve: A Head-to-Head Comparison With [(15)O]H2O PET. JACC Cardiovasc Interv 2018;11(20):2044–54.

38. Nardone M, McCarthy M, Ardern CI, et al. Concurrently Low Coronary Flow Reserve and Low Index of Microvascular Resistance Are Associated With Elevated Resting Coronary Flow in Patients With Chest Pain and Nonobstructive Coronary Arteries. Circ Cardiovasc Interv 2022. https://doi.org/10.1161/CIRCINTERVENTIONS.121.011323.

39. Wilson RF, Wyche K, Christensen BV, et al. Effects of adenosine on human coronary arterial circulation. Circulation 1990;82(5):1595–606.

40. Luo C, Long M, Hu X, et al. Thermodilution-derived coronary microvascular resistance and flow reserve in patients with cardiac syndrome X. Circ Cardiovasc Interv 2014;7(1):43–8.

41. Solberg OG, Ragnarsson A, Kvarsnes A, et al. Reference interval for the index of coronary microvascular resistance. Eurointervention 2014;9(9): 1069–75.

42. Lee JM, Layland J, Jung JH, et al. Integrated physiologic assessment of ischemic heart disease in real-world practice using index of microcirculatory resistance and fractional flow reserve: insights from the International Index of Microcirculatory Resistance Registry. Circ Cardiovasc Interv 2015; 8(11):e002857.

43. Aarnoudse W, Fearon WF, Manoharan G, et al. Epicardial stenosis severity does not affect minimal microcirculatory resistance. Circulation 2004; 110(15):2137–42.

44. Yong AS, Layland J, Fearon WF, et al. Calculation of the index of microcirculatory resistance without coronary wedge pressure measurement in the presence of epicardial stenosis. JACC Cardiovasc Interv 2013;6(1):53–8.

45. Layland J, MacIsaac AI, Burns AT, et al. When collateral supply is accounted for epicardial stenosis does not increase microvascular resistance. Circ Cardiovasc Interv 2012;5(1):97–102.

46. Ng MK, Yeung AC, Fearon WF. Invasive assessment of the coronary microcirculation: superior reproducibility and less hemodynamic dependence of index of microcirculatory resistance compared with coronary flow reserve. Circulation 2006;113(17): 2054–61.

47. Pagonas N, Gross CM, Li M, et al. Influence of epicardial stenosis severity and central venous pressure on the index of microcirculatory resistance in a follow-up study. Eurointervention 2014;9(9): 1063–8.

48. Payne AR, Berry C, Doolin O, et al. Microvascular Resistance Predicts Myocardial Salvage and Infarct Characteristics in ST-Elevation Myocardial Infarction. J Am Heart Assoc 2012;1(4):e002246.

49. Chamuleau SA, Siebes M, Meuwissen M, et al. Association between coronary lesion severity and distal microvascular resistance in patients with coronary artery disease. American Journal of Physiology Heart and Circulatory Physiology 2003;285(5): H2194–200.

50. Sheikh AR, Zeitz CJ, Rajendran S, et al. Clinical and coronary haemodynamic determinants of recurrent chest pain in patients without obstructive coronary artery disease - A pilot study. Int J Cardiol 2018; 267:16–21.

51. de Waard GA, Nijjer SS, van Lavieren MA, et al. Invasive minimal Microvascular Resistance Is a New Index to Assess Microcirculatory Function Independent of Obstructive Coronary Artery Disease. J Am Heart Assoc 2016;5(12). https://doi.org/10. 1161/JAHA.116.004482.

52. Scarsini R, De Maria GL, Borlotti A, et al. Incremental Value of Coronary Microcirculation Resistive Reserve Ratio in Predicting the Extent of Myocardial Infarction in Patients with STEMI. Insights from the Oxford Acute Myocardial Infarction (OxAMI) Study.

Cardiovasc revascularization Med : including Mol interventions 2019;20(12):1148–55.

53. Layland J, Carrick D, McEntegart M, et al. Vasodilatory capacity of the coronary microcirculation is preserved in selected patients with non-ST-segment-elevation myocardial infarction. Circ Cardiovasc Interv 2013;6(3):231–6.

54. Corcoran D, Young R, Adlam D, et al. Coronary microvascular dysfunction in patients with stable coronary artery disease: The CE-MARC 2 coronary physiology sub-study. Int J Cardiol 2018;266:7–14.

55. Maznyczka AM, Oldroyd KG, Greenwood JP, et al. Comparative Significance of Invasive Measures of Microvascular Injury in Acute Myocardial Infarction. Circ Cardiovasc Interv 2020;13(5):e008505.

56. Lee SH, Lee JM, Park J, et al. Prognostic Implications of Resistive Reserve Ratio in Patients With Coronary Artery Disease. J Am Heart Assoc 2020;9(8): e015846.

57. Toya T, Ahmad A, Corban MT, et al. Risk Stratification of Patients With NonObstructive Coronary Artery Disease Using Resistive Reserve Ratio. J Am Heart Assoc 2021;10(11):e020464.

58. Aarnoudse W, Van't Veer M, Pijls NH, et al. Direct volumetric blood flow measurement in coronary arteries by thermodilution. J Am Coll Cardiol 2007; 50(24):2294–304.

59. Jansen TPJ, Konst RE, Elias-Smale SE, et al. Assessing Microvascular Dysfunction in Angina With Unobstructed Coronary Arteries: JACC Review Topic of the Week. J Am Coll Cardiol 2021;78(14): 1471–9.

60. Xaplanteris P, Fournier S, Keulards DCJ, et al. Catheter-Based Measurements of Absolute Coronary Blood Flow and Microvascular Resistance: Feasibility, Safety, and Reproducibility in Humans. Circ Cardiovasc Interv 2018;11(3):e006194.

61. De Bruyne B, Adjedj J, Xaplanteris P, et al. Saline-Induced Coronary Hyperemia: Mechanisms and Effects on Left Ventricular Function. Circ Cardiovasc Interv 2017;10(4). https://doi.org/10.1161/CIRCINTE RVENTIONS.116.004719.

62. Everaars H, de Waard GA, Schumacher SP, et al. Continuous thermodilution to assess absolute flow and microvascular resistance: validation in humans using [15O]H2O positron emission tomography. Eur Heart J 2019;40(28):2350–9.

63. Rivero F, Gutierrez-Barrios A, Gomez-Lara J, et al. Coronary microvascular dysfunction assessed by continuous intracoronary thermodilution: A comparative study with index of microvascular resistance. Int J Cardiol 2021;333:1–7.

64. Konst RE, Elias-Smale SE, Pellegrini D, et al. Absolute Coronary Blood Flow Measured by Continuous Thermodilution in Patients With Ischemia and Nonobstructive Disease. J Am Coll Cardiol 2021;77(6): 728–41.

65. De Bruyne B, Pijls NHJ, Gallinoro E, et al. Microvascular Resistance Reserve for Assessment of Coronary Microvascular Function: JACC Technology Corner. J Am Coll Cardiol 2021;78(15):1541–9.

66. Patel MR, Dai D, Hernandez AF, et al. Prevalence and predictors of nonobstructive coronary artery disease identified with coronary angiography in contemporary clinical practice. Am Heart J 2014; 167(6):846–852 e2.

67. Ford TJ, Yii E, Sidik N, et al. Ischemia and No Obstructive Coronary Artery Disease: Prevalence and Correlates of Coronary Vasomotion Disorders. Circ Cardiovasc Interv 2019;12(12):e008126.

68. Ford TJ, Stanley B, Sidik N, et al. 1-Year Outcomes of Angina Management Guided by Invasive Coronary Function Testing (CorMicA). JACC Cardiovasc Interv 2020;13(1):33–45.

69. Jespersen L, Hvelplund A, Abildstrom SZ, et al. Stable angina pectoris with no obstructive coronary artery disease is associated with increased risks of major adverse cardiovascular events. Eur Heart J 2012;33(6):734–44.

70. Pepine CJ, Anderson RD, Sharaf BL, et al. Coronary microvascular reactivity to adenosine predicts adverse outcome in women evaluated for suspected ischemia results from the National Heart, Lung and Blood Institute WISE (Women's Ischemia Syndrome Evaluation) study. J Am Coll Cardiol 2010;55(25): 2825–32.

71. Shimokawa H, Suda A, Takahashi J, et al. Clinical characteristics and prognosis of patients with microvascular angina: an international and prospective cohort study by the Coronary Vasomotor Disorders International Study (COVADIS) Group. Eur Heart J 2021;42(44):4592–600.

72. Gdowski MA, Murthy VL, Doering M, et al. Association of Isolated Coronary Microvascular Dysfunction With Mortality and Major Adverse Cardiac Events: A Systematic Review and Meta-Analysis of Aggregate Data. J Am Heart Assoc 2020;9(9):e014954.

73. Ndrepepa G, Tiroch K, Fusaro M, et al. 5-year prognostic value of no-reflow phenomenon after percutaneous coronary intervention in patients with acute myocardial infarction. J Am Coll Cardiol 2010; 55(21):2383–9.

74. Fearon WF, Shah M, Ng M, et al. Predictive value of the index of microcirculatory resistance in patients with .ST-segment elevation myocardial infarction. J Am Coll Cardiol 2008;51(5):560–5.

75. Lim HS, Yoon MH, Tahk SJ, et al. Usefulness of the index of microcirculatory resistance for invasively assessing myocardial viability immediately after primary angioplasty for anterior myocardial infarction. Eur Heart J 2009;30(23):2854–60.

76. Carrick D, Haig C, Ahmed N, et al. Comparative Prognostic Utility of Indexes of Microvascular Function Alone or in Combination in Patients With an Acute ST-Segment-Elevation Myocardial Infarction. Circulation 2016;134(23):1833–47.

77. De Maria GL, Alkhalil M, Wolfrum M, et al. Index of Microcirculatory Resistance as a Tool to Characterize Microvascular Obstruction and to Predict Infarct Size Regression in Patients With STEMI Undergoing Primary PCI. JACC Cardiovasc Imaging 2019;12(5):837–48.

78. Fearon WF, Low AF, Yong AS, et al. Prognostic value of the Index of Microcirculatory Resistance measured after primary percutaneous coronary intervention. Circulation 2013;127(24):2436–41.

79. Murai T, Yonetsu T, Kanaji Y, et al. Prognostic value of the index of microcirculatory resistance after percutaneous coronary intervention in patients with non-ST-segment elevation acute coronary syndrome. Catheter Cardiovasc Interv 2018;92(6): 1063–74.

80. Ng MK, Yong AS, Ho M, et al. The index of microcirculatory resistance predicts myocardial infarction related to percutaneous coronary intervention. Circ Cardiovasc Interv 2012;5(4):515–22.

81. Nishi T, Murai T, Ciccarelli G, et al. Prognostic Value of Coronary Microvascular Function Measured Immediately After Percutaneous Coronary Intervention in Stable Coronary Artery Disease: An International Multicenter Study. Circ Cardiovasc Interv 2019;12(9):e007889.

Targeted Therapies for Microvascular Disease

Adam Bland, MBBS[a,b], Eunice Chuah, MBBS[a,b], William Meere, MBBS[a,b], Thomas J. Ford, MBChB (Hons), PhD[a,b,c,*]

KEYWORDS

- CMD • INOCA • Angina • Ischemia • Management

KEY POINTS

- Coronary microvascular dysfunction (CMD) is a common cause of ischemia in patients without obstructive coronary artery disease (INOCA). CMD typically results from impaired vasodilation and/or excessive vasoconstriction.
- Invasive assessment of the coronary microcirculation can stratify anti-ischemic therapy to improved patient outcomes. Beta-blockers are the cornerstone of therapy for angina with CMD.
- Management of CMD includes a combination of pharmacological therapy and cardiovascular risk factor modification including lifestyle interventions. Pharmacological treatment may be divided into antiatherosclerotic therapy and antianginal therapy.
- Further randomized clinical trials are required to determine effects of current management strategies, as well as proposed novel therapies.

INTRODUCTION

Coronary artery disease (CAD) is a leading cause of morbidity and mortality affecting 126 million worldwide individuals (approaching 2% of the earth's population).[1] Obstructive epicardial CAD has been the focus of most research in the era of percutaneous coronary intervention (PCI). Patients with ischemia but no obstructive coronary artery disease (INOCA) have largely been overlooked until recently in part related to challenges in diagnosis, poorly understood pathophysiology, and lack of standardised diagnostic criteria.[2] Coronary microvascular dysfunction (CMD) is one endotype of INOCA along with vasospastic angina, mixed INOCA, and noncardiac chest pain.[3] Chest pain with no obstructive CAD previously was under the umbrella term of cardiac syndrome X (CSX); however, INOCA is now a preferred umbrella term replacing the ambiguous term CSX in

recognition of better understanding of the endotypes that may coexist to drive myocardial ischemia.[4,5]

Approximately 50% of diagnostic coronary angiograms for patients at high risk of CAD demonstrate unobstructed coronary arteries. Many of these patients have abnormal stress testing, unstable angina, and non-ST-elevation myocardial infarction.[6,7] Up to two-thirds of INOCA patients undergoing functional coronary angiography are subsequently demonstrated to have CMD, diagnosed by demonstrating reduced coronary flow reserve (CFR), and/or elevated microvascular resistance.[8] Noninvasive testing of these patients often shows reduced myocardial perfusion reserve on cardiac MRI or PET.[8–10] INOCA is a particularly relevant diagnosis in women presenting with angina in whom unobstructed coronary arteries is a more common finding than in their male counterparts.[11] The COVADIS working group has

This article originally appeared in *Interventional Cardiology Clinics*, Volume 12 Issue 1, January 2023.
a Department of Cardiology, Gosford Hospital - Central Coast LHD, 75 Holden Street, Gosford, New South Wales 2250, Australia; b The University of Newcastle, University Dr, Callaghan, New South Wales 2308, Australia; c University of Glasgow, ICAMS, G12 8QQ Glasgow, UK
* Corresponding author. Department of Cardiology, Gosford Hospital - Central Coast LHD, 75 Holden Street, Gosford, New South Wales 2250, Australia.
E-mail address: Tom.ford@health.nsw.gov.au

Cardiol Clin 42 (2024) 137–145
https://doi.org/10.1016/j.ccl.2023.07.002

helped with some unifying definitions including microvascular angina (MVA) which refers to angina patients without flow-limiting CAD but in whom invasive or noninvasive tests show evidence of CMD[12,13] (**Fig. 1**).

Despite the absence of epicardial obstruction, CMD remains associated with higher major adverse cardiovascular events (MACE) including cardiovascular mortality, as well as higher repeat angiography, higher levels of depression and lower quality of life.[2,9,12,14–16] Patients with CMD, however, remain largely undertreated due to difficulties over recent decades in establishing a widely accepted diagnostic criteria, and subsequently large trials and guidelines addressing CMD management are lacking.[9,17,18] This review aims to discuss the evolving management of CMD including the role of targeted therapies.

TREATMENT TARGETS FOR MICROVASCULAR DYSFUNCTION

Coronary blood flow incorporates 3 distinct compartments. Larger epicardial arteries appreciable on diagnostic coronary angiogram range from approximately 500 μm up to 5 mm or greater.[18,19] The microcirculation consists of intermediate pre-arterioles (~100–500 μm diameter), and smaller intramural arterioles (<100 μm in diameter).[18,19] The coronary microcirculation alters blood flow to meet cardiac myocyte metabolic demand, with increased demand and flow causing vasodilation, and decreased demand and flow causing vasoconstriction. Proximal arteriolar stretch receptors or distal arteriolar local metabolites dictate these alterations in arteriolar size.[18]

CMD results from an inability of the microvasculature to meet cardiac myocyte demand, resulting in ischemia and angina. Traditional cardiovascular risk factors remain the same for CMD including hypertension, dyslipidemia, diabetes mellitus, ageing, and smoking.[18] However, CMD also has significant predisposition for women.[3,16,20] Aggressive reversible risk factor modification,

although limited in evidence, is accepted to be fundamental to CMD management.[3,18,21] CMD is also associated with increased mild epicardial atherosclerosis, which may suggest a reason for increased levels of MACE associated with this disorder but further highlights the need for risk factor optimization.[22,23] Other specific disorders predispose to microvascular dysfunction including hypertrophic cardiomyopathy and idiopathic dilated cardiomyopathy. Treatment of these unique situations is outside the scope of this review.

CMD is heterogenous in its pathophysiology, clinical presentation, and response to therapy.[3] The inability of the coronary microcirculation to meet cardiac myocyte demand in CMD can be because of excessive vasoconstriction, or inadequate vasodilation.[24] Invasive angiographic provocation testing can help direct and individualize pharmacological therapy for CMD. Endothelial dysfunction results in vasoconstriction and can be demonstrated with intracoronary acetylcholine during coronary angiography.[24] Epicardial vasoconstriction detected with acetylcholine represents vasospastic angina, which can coexist with CMD, and is best treated with calcium channel blockade.[25] If there is no epicardial vasoconstriction to acetylcholine, but symptoms or electrocardiogram signs of ischemia are reproduced (or to adenosine), this indicates endothelial-dependent CMD and again suggests likely benefit to calcium channel blockade.[24]

CFR is the ratio of coronary blood flow at maximal dilation (commonly after intracoronary adenosine) compared with blood flow at baseline, which is reduced in CMD. It suggests impaired ability of the microvasculature to dilate and accommodate increased coronary flow during demand resulting in angina.[18] This is termed endothelial-independent CMD.[24] Beta-blockers are the recommended first line for CMD, especially when impaired vasodilation is suspected.[21] Subsequently, individuals with mixed endothelial-independent CMD and either endothelial-dependent CMD or vasospastic angina require

Fig. 1. INOCA endotypes.

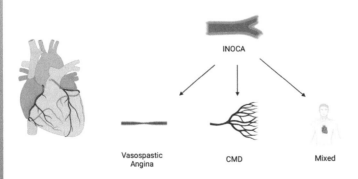

combination therapy.[17] Confirming the diagnosis of CMD at time of angiography and titrating therapy to the endotype of CMD has demonstrated patient benefits including improved angina and quality of life[26] (**Fig. 2**).

Given the lack of large clinical trials, the management of CMD is based on weak evidence and much of the direction for treatment has been made from trials concerning INOCA or CSX. These pathologic conditions do not exclude vasospastic angina and some noncardiac causes of chest pain, rendering them unreliable when applying to CMD.[24] Despite this, widely accepted management principles include a combination of risk factor modification, antiatherosclerotic therapy, and antiangina therapy.[17] Novel therapies are being trialled for this chronic disorder without a cure, particularly as some individuals may have limited benefit to standard care resulting in significant residual morbidity and poor quality of life.

Reversible Risk Factors

Cardiac rehabilitation and physical exercise

Although outside the scope of this review of pharmacological therapy, the role of physical activity and cardiac rehabilitation cannot be emphasized enough. Cardiac rehabilitation may help with illness understanding[27] and alleviate some of the understandable fear that comes with a diagnosis of angina. Neuromodulation in this way may improve symptoms and alleviate anxiety to reduce pain.[28] Cardiac rehabilitation has been shown to have benefit in coronary angina, and exercise has been demonstrated to improve endothelial dysfunction.[29] A small trial of 13 subjects completed a 6-week cardiovascular conditioning program and a low-fat diet, which demonstrated improved myocardial flow reserve through improving vasodilatory capacity and resting blood flow.[30] A systematic review involving 8 trials looking at exercise prescription for angina in individuals with nonobstructive CAD showed improvements in oxygen uptake, angina severity, exercise capacity and quality of life.[31] Although this is not specifically CMD and may include patients with vasospastic angina, it would suggest likely benefit in the CMD population.

Hypertension

Hypertension is associated with lower CFR and subsequent predisposition to CMD.[32] A trial with

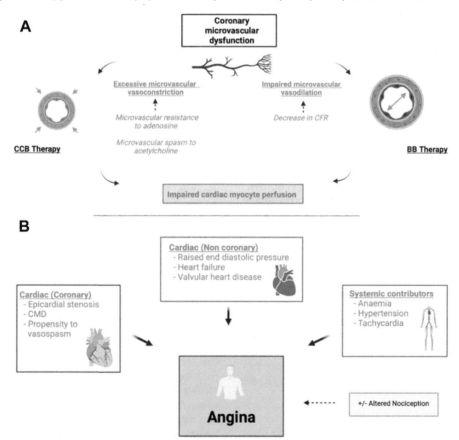

Fig. 2. CMD pathophysiology, therapy, and contributions to angina.

137 subjects demonstrated treatment with antihypertensive therapy down to a normal blood pressure significantly improves CFR suggesting microvascular functional improvement but this data did not capture angina change.[32] Perindopril therapy in 14 hypertensive patients for 12 months has demonstrated regression of periarteriolar fibrosis and improvement in coronary reserve.[33]

Dyslipidemia

Inverse correlations were observed between CFR and total lipid levels including low density lipoprotein (LDL) using PET scanning, suggesting LDL can contribute to CMD.[34] In another study, 25 patients with familial hypercholesterolemia were found to have significant reduction in myocardial blood flow and CFR using PET scanning.[35]

Smoking

In a study with 354 subjects, smoking has been shown to be associated with a significant reduction in transthoracic echocardiogram detected CFR, suggesting microvascular dysfunction.[36] Furthermore, another small trial with 19 subjects demonstrated and average reduced CFR of 21% using PET scan in smokers, which improved following vitamin C to suggest oxidative stress is likely involved in some element of pathogenesis of CMD.[18,37]

Diabetes mellitus

Microvascular dysfunction is a known feature of diabetes resulting in retinopathy, nephropathy, and neuropathy.[18] Type 1 and 2 diabetes mellitus have been shown to have reduced coronary vasodilator function predisposing to CMD.[38] Obesity, which is commonly associated with diabetes, predisposes to coronary atherosclerotic burden.[39] A small randomized trial of 33 subjects with INOCA found significant microvascular function improvement with metformin therapy, suggesting potential improvements of CMD in hyperglycemia reduction.[40]

Antiatherosclerotic Therapy

Aspirin

Aspirin inhibits platelet aggregation but also prevents the vasoconstrictive effects of thromboxane A2. The 2019 European Society of Cardiology guidelines for management of chronic coronary syndromes support at least one antiplatelet agent in diffuse epicardial atherosclerosis but in primary MVA, there is no robust evidence supporting a role of aspirin.[41]

Statin therapy

Statins are associated with anti-inflammatory and antiatherosclerotic effects.[9] Atorvastatin has been demonstrated to improve CFR in patients with slow coronary flow.[42] The 2019 European Society of Cardiology guidelines for management of chronic coronary syndromes suggest using statins in those with MVA.[41]

Angiotensin converting enzyme inhibitors (and angiotensin receptor blockade)

Angiotensin converting enzyme inhibitors act to block the vasoconstrictive effects of angiotensin II, which can reduce vascular tone and promote vasodilation.[23] In a randomized trial on 78 women with confirmed CMD, quinapril therapy was associated with reduction in angina frequency as well as improved CFR in invasive testing.[43] Combination therapy of ramipril and atorvastatin added to diltiazem in a randomized trial with 45 patients was shown to reduce frequency of angina in patients with CSX, suggesting likely some benefit in the CMD population, although CMD was not confirmed.[44]

Antianginal Therapy

Beta-blockers

Beta-blockers reduce myocardial oxygen demand and prolong diastolic filling, improving the chance of coronary flow meeting demand.[9,18] There are limited trials of beta-blocker use in patients with proven CMD. A comparison trial between propranolol and verapamil investigated 16 patients with angina and normal coronary arteries on angiography but no confirmed CMD. It found a significant reduction in angina in the beta-blocker arm compared with placebo but not in verapamil suggesting beta-blockers were superior to calcium channel blockade in this population.[45] A small 10 patient trial comparing atenolol, amlodipine, and nitrate therapy in CSX, showed angina improvement in the beta-blocker population but not in the nitrate or calcium channel blocker (CCB) populations.[46] Beta-blockers are recommended for MVA in the 2019 European Society of Cardiology guidelines for the management of chronic coronary syndromes.[41]

Nitrates

Nitrates act on arteriolar endothelium to cause vasodilation. Although traditionally prescribed for angina, accumulating evidence seem to suggest negligible benefit and even potential harm with the use of long-acting nitrates on MVA.[47,48] Reduced responsiveness from coronary arteries, steal syndrome from redistribution of blood flow to areas of adequate perfusion, and poor medication tolerance and have all been suggested as potential reasons for the lack of nitrate benefit in MVA.[47,48]

Calcium channel blockers

Calcium channel blockers act to cause coronary vasodilation and are particularly effective in coronary vasospasm.[25] Limited trial benefit exists in CMD and diltiazem has been shown to not improve CFR in MVA.[9,49] Verapamil and Nifedipine use have been shown to improve angina symptoms in patients with angina and normal angiographic coronary arteries but this did not remove patients with vasospastic angina.[50] CCB are recommended after beta-blockers in patients with MVA according to 2013 ESC guidelines.[21]

Percutaneous coronary intervention Addressing epicardial coronary obstruction of significant lesions with percutaneous coronary intervention (PCI) when coexistent pathologic conditions exists may be important in the overall management of CMD. PCI should only be performed on physiologically significant stenosis (>90% or lesions with significant Fractional Flow Reserve (FFR) or Non-Hyperemia Pressure Ratio (NHPR).[21] Invasive physiological vessel interrogation allows appraisal of each coronary compartment and may predict improvement in epicardial blood flow after PCI of a coronary stenosis.[47,51] Invasive coronary physiology predicts ischemia relief but is less predictive of angina reduction.[52]

Novel Therapies

Ranolazine

Ranolazine improves myocardial perfusion by decreasing sodium and calcium overload through late sodium channel blockade, promoting myocardial relaxation.[23] Multiple mixed trial results exist where small benefits in CFR have been demonstrated,[53] as well as no benefit in others but benefit in angina symptoms.[54] Therefore, ranolazine requires larger trials to study its benefits.

Ivabradine

Ivabradine reduces heart rate thought I_f channel inhibition at the sinoatrial node. A small trial of 46 patients found symptomatic improvement of angina in ivabradine but no change in microvascular function.[54]

Phosphodiesterase inhibition

Sildenafil has been shown to improve CFR in women with CMD with the significant improvement being in those with a CFR of less than 2.5 but this was not clinically correlated with angina severity.[55]

Rho-kinase inhibition (fasudil)

Endothelin A receptor activates rho-kinase, eventually leading to vasoconstriction. Intracoronary fasudil, a rho-kinase inhibitor, improved angina and features of coronary ischemia in endothelin-dependent CMD.[56]

Zibotentan

Zibotentan is an endothelin A receptor antagonist, preventing the coronary vasoconstrictive effects of endothelin 1, which is often elevated in those with MVA.[57] It is currently undergoing phase 2 trials into its effect on exercise tolerance in MVA.[57]

Coronary sinus occlusion Coronary sinus occlusion can encourage retro filling of blood into the coronary microcirculation.[58,59] One such pressure-controlled intermittent coronary sinus occlusion device has been shown in the ST elevation myocardial infarction population to preserve microvascular function.[58] Another device to narrow the coronary sinus improved symptoms and quality of life in patients with refractory angina who were not candidates for revascularization.[59]

Spinal cord stimulation Electrical stimulation is thought to modulate pain fibers and possibly alter coronary blood flow. A small trial with 8 patients found small benefits in angina frequency in CSX with the use of transcutaneous electrical nerve stimulation.[60] Spinal cord stimulation has been demonstrated in a small trial of 7 subjects to improve angina and exercise tolerance in INOCA patients.[61]

Tricyclic antidepressants (imipramine, amitriptyline)

Tricyclic antidepressants aim to reduce nociceptive stimuli leading to reduced angina severity.[47] TCA's may have a role in treatment resistant MVA where enhanced pain perception is thought to possibly occur.

Hormone replacement Given the predisposition in the postmenopausal women population, estrogen deficiency has been suggested as a cause to CMD.[9] A small trial of 35 women demonstrated a reduction in angina symptoms in postmenopausal women and INOCA but did not alter endothelial dysfunction.[62]

Cognitive behavioral therapy CMD is often associated with anxiety and mood disorders. Autogenic relaxation training in 53 women demonstrated improvements in symptom frequency with CSX.[63] A small systemic review of 6 trials suggested a modest benefit predominately in the first 3 months of psychotherapy in individuals with chest pain and normal coronary arteries mainly focusing on cognitive behavioral framework. However, these patients had no formal CMD diagnosis made, and their pathogenesis could be broad (**Fig. 3**).

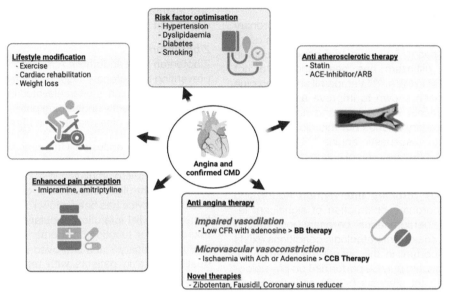

Fig. 3. Management of CMD principles.

SUMMARY

CMD remains a challenging condition to manage due to heterogenous pathophysiology, presentation, and response to therapy. Awareness of CMD is improving but therapeutic randomized trials of therapy are lacking. Invasive assessment of the coronary microcirculation can stratify anti-ischemic therapy to improved patient-centered outcomes. Beta-blockers remain the cornerstone of therapy for angina due to CMD. The role of non-pharmacological interventions including cardiovascular risk factor modification, lifestyle interventions, and cardiac rehabilitation is central to management. Further research is needed to assess traditional and novel pharmacological therapies on symptoms and clinical events in the various CMD endotypes.

CLINICS CARE POINTS

- Functional coronary angiography (coronary provocation testing) may be used to confirm the diagnosis of microvascular angina and tailor patient management.[26]

- Patients with microvascular angina and impaired vasodilator capacity (e.g. low CFR) may benefit from beta blocker therapy. This is the cornerstone of anti-ischaemic therapy in confirmed microvascular angina.[38,42,43]

- Increased microvascular constriction (e.g. microvascular spasm to acetylcholine infusion) often co-exists with epicardial coronary spasm and

should be treated with calcium channel blockade.[21,47]

- Lifestyle modification is essential in managing CMD and should be implemented in all cases including smoking cessation, regular exercise, optimisation of diet and cardiac rehabilitation.[33, 62, 63]

- Hypertension, dyslipidaemia, and diabetes mellitus should all be treated to target as per standard primary prevention guidelines.[30,32,37]

- Statin and ACE Inhibitors are 'disease modifying therapies' for coronary atherosclerosis and may be beneficial in CMD.[41,39,38]

- Novel therapies targeting CMD are being explored in clinical trials including Zybotentan (endothelin A receptor inhibitor[54]).

- Subgroups of INOCA patients with enhanced nociception, altered pain pathways and/or associated depression may benefit from tricyclic antidepressants (amitriptyline 10 mg).[44]

DISCLOSURES

- T.J. Ford: Consultant/speaker/honorarium from Abbott Vascular, Boston Scientific, Boehringer Ingelheim, Biotronik, Bio-Excel, and Novartis.
- All other authors have no relevant disclosures. Funding was not required for the completion of this article.

REFERENCES

1. Khan MA, Hashim MJ, Mustafa H, et al. Global epidemiology of ischemic heart disease: results

from the global burden of disease study. Cureus 2020;12(7):e9349.

2. Herscovici R, Sedlak T, Wei J, et al. Ischemia and no obstructive coronary artery disease (INOCA): what is the risk? J Am Heart Assoc 2018;7(17):e008868.

3. Vancheri F, Longo G, Vancheri S, et al. Coronary microvascular dysfunction. J Clin Med 2020;9(9): 1–36.

4. Lanza GA. Cardiac syndrome X: a critical overview and future perspectives. Heart 2007;93(2):159–66.

5. Beltrame JF, Tavella R, Jones D, et al. Management of ischaemia with non-obstructive coronary arteries (INOCA). BMJ 2021;375:e060602.

6. Ouellette ML, Löffler AI, Beller GA, et al. Clinical characteristics, sex differences, and outcomes in patients with normal or near-normal coronary arteries, non-obstructive or obstructive coronary artery disease. J Am Heart Assoc 2018;7(10):1–13.

7. Patel MR, Peterson ED, Dai D, et al. Low diagnostic yield of elective coronary angiography. N Engl J Med 2010;362(10):886–95.

8. Sara JD, Widmer RJ, Matsuzawa Y, et al. Prevalence of coronary microvascular dysfunction among patients with chest pain and nonobstructive coronary artery disease. JACC Cardiovasc Interv 2015; 8(11):1445–53.

9. Marinescu MA, Löffler AI, Ouellette M, et al. Coronary microvascular dysfunction, microvascular angina, and treatment strategies. JACC Cardiovasc Imaging 2015;8(2):210–20.

10. Ford TJ, Yii E, Sidik N, et al. Ischemia and no obstructive coronary artery disease: prevalence and correlates of coronary vasomotion disorders. Circ Cardiovasc interventions 2019;12(12):e008126.

11. Bugiardini R, Bairey Merz CN. Angina with "normal" coronary arteries: a changing philosophy. JAMA 2005;293(4):477–84.

12. Aribas E, van Lennep JER, Elias-Smale SE, et al. Prevalence of microvascular angina among patients with stable symptoms in the absence of obstructive coronary artery disease: a systematic review. Cardiovasc Res 2021;118(3):763–71.

13. Ong P, Camici PG, Beltrame JF, et al. International standardization of diagnostic criteria for microvascular angina. Int J Cardiol 2018;250:16–20.

14. Jespersen L, Hvelplund A, Abildstrøm SZ, et al. Stable angina pectoris with no obstructive coronary artery disease is associated with increased risks of major adverse cardiovascular events. Eur Heart J 2012;33(6):734–44.

15. Jespersen L, Abildstrøm SZ, Hvelplund A, et al. Persistent angina: highly prevalent and associated with long-term anxiety, depression, low physical functioning, and quality of life in stable angina pectoris. Clin Res Cardiol 2013;102(8):571–81.

16. Shimokawa H, Suda A, Takahashi J, et al. Clinical characteristics and prognosis of patients with microvascular angina: an international and prospective cohort study by the Coronary Vasomotor Disorders International Study (COVADIS) Group. Eur Heart J 2021;42(44):4592–600.

17. Bairey Merz CN, Pepine CJ, Shimokawa H, et al. Treatment of coronary microvascular dysfunction. Cardiovasc Res 2020;116(4):856–70.

18. Chen C, Wei J, AlBadri A, et al. Coronary microvascular dysfunction - epidemiology, pathogenesis, prognosis, diagnosis, risk factors and therapy. Circ J 2016;81(1):3–11.

19. Camici PG, Crea F. Coronary microvascular dysfunction. N Engl J Med 2007;356(8):830–40.

20. Kuruvilla S, Kramer CM. Coronary microvascular dysfunction in women: an overview of diagnostic strategies. Expert Rev Cardiovasc Ther 2013; 11(11):1515–25.

21. Montalescot G, Sechtem U, Achenbach S, et al. 2013 ESC guidelines on the management of stable coronary artery disease: the Task Force on the management of stable coronary artery disease of the European Society of Cardiology. Eur Heart J 2013; 34(38):2949–3003.

22. Gdowski MA, Murthy VL, Doering M, et al. Association of isolated coronary microvascular dysfunction with mortality and major adverse cardiac events: a systematic review and meta-analysis of aggregate data. J Am Heart Assoc 2020;9(9):e014954.

23. Taqueti VR, Di Carli MF. Coronary microvascular disease pathogenic mechanisms and therapeutic options: JACC state-of-the-art review. J Am Coll Cardiol 2018;72(21):2625–41.

24. Shaw J, Anderson T. Coronary endothelial dysfunction in non-obstructive coronary artery disease: risk, pathogenesis, diagnosis and therapy. Vasc Med 2016;21(2):146–55.

25. McIvor ME, Undemir C, Lawson J, et al. Clinical effects and utility of intracoronary diltiazem. Cathet Cardiovasc Diagn 1995;35(4):287–91 [discussion: 292-283].

26. Ford TJ, Stanley B, Sidik N, et al. 1-Year outcomes of angina management guided by invasive coronary function testing (CorMicA). JACC Cardiovasc Interv 2020;13(1):33–45.

27. Ghisi GL, Abdallah F, Grace SL, et al. A systematic review of patient education in cardiac patients: do they increase knowledge and promote health behavior change? Patient Educ Couns 2014;95(2):160–74.

28. den Hollander M, de Jong JR, Volders S, et al. Fear reduction in patients with chronic pain: a learning theory perspective. Expert Rev Neurother 2010;10(11): 1733–45.

29. Beck EB, Erbs S, Möbius-Winkler S, et al. Exercise training restores the endothelial response to vascular growth factors in patients with stable coronary artery disease. Eur J Prev Cardiol 2012;19(3): 412–8.

30. Czernin J, Barnard RJ, Sun KT, et al. Effect of short-term cardiovascular conditioning and low-fat diet on myocardial blood flow and flow reserve. Circulation 1995;92(2):197–204.

31. Kissel CK, Nikoletou D. Cardiac rehabilitation and exercise prescription in symptomatic patients with non-obstructive coronary artery disease-a systematic review. Curr Treat Options Cardiovasc Med 2018;20(9):78.

32. Mizuno R, Fujimoto S, Saito Y, et al. Optimal antihypertensive level for improvement of coronary microvascular dysfunction: the lower, the better? Hypertension 2012;60(2):326–32.

33. Schwartzkopff B, Brehm M, Mundhenke M, et al. Repair of coronary arterioles after treatment with perindopril in hypertensive heart disease. Hypertension 2000;36(2):220–5.

34. Dayanikli F, Grambow D, Muzik O, et al. Early detection of abnormal coronary flow reserve in asymptomatic men at high risk for coronary artery disease using positron emission tomography. Circulation 1994;90(2):808–17.

35. Yokoyama I, Murakami T, Ohtake T, et al. Reduced coronary flow reserve in familial hypercholesterolemia. J Nucl Med 1996;37(12):1937–42.

36. Lee DH, Youn HJ, Choi YS, et al. Coronary flow reserve is a comprehensive indicator of cardiovascular risk factors in subjects with chest pain and normal coronary angiogram. Circ J 2010;74(7):1405–14.

37. Kaufmann PA, Gnecchi-Ruscone T, di Terlizzi M, et al. Coronary heart disease in smokers: vitamin C restores coronary microcirculatory function. Circulation 2000;102(11):1233–8.

38. Di Carli MF, Janisse J, Grunberger G, et al. Role of chronic hyperglycemia in the pathogenesis of coronary microvascular dysfunction in diabetes. J Am Coll Cardiol 2003;41(8):1387–93.

39. Bettencourt N, Toschke AM, Leite D, et al. Epicardial adipose tissue is an independent predictor of coronary atherosclerotic burden. Int J Cardiol 2012;158(1):26–32.

40. Jadhav S, Ferrell W, Greer IA, et al. Effects of metformin on microvascular function and exercise tolerance in women with angina and normal coronary arteries: a randomized, double-blind, placebo-controlled study. J Am Coll Cardiol 2006;48(5):956–63.

41. Knuuti J, Wijns W, Saraste A, et al. 2019 ESC Guidelines for the diagnosis and management of chronic coronary syndromes. Eur Heart J 2020;41(3):407–77.

42. Caliskan M, Erdogan D, Gullu H, et al. Effects of atorvastatin on coronary flow reserve in patients with slow coronary flow. Clin Cardiol 2007;30(9):475–9.

43. Pauly DF, Johnson BD, Anderson RD, et al. In women with symptoms of cardiac ischemia, nonobstructive coronary arteries, and microvascular dysfunction, angiotensin-converting enzyme inhibition is associated with improved microvascular function: a double-blind randomized study from the National Heart, Lung and Blood Institute Women's Ischemia Syndrome Evaluation (WISE). Am Heart J 2011;162(4):678–84.

44. Pizzi C, Manfrini O, Fontana F, et al. Angiotensin-converting enzyme inhibitors and 3-hydroxy-3-methylglutaryl coenzyme A reductase in cardiac Syndrome X: role of superoxide dismutase activity. Circulation 2004;109(1):53–8.

45. Bugiardini R, Borghi A, Biagetti L, et al. Comparison of verapamil versus propranolol therapy in syndrome X. Am J Cardiol 1989;63(5):286–90.

46. Lanza GA, Colonna G, Pasceri V, et al. Atenolol versus amlodipine versus isosorbide-5-mononitrate on anginal symptoms in syndrome X. Am J Cardiol 1999;84(7):854–6. a858.

47. Ford TJ, Berry C. Angina: contemporary diagnosis and management. Heart 2020;106(5):387–98.

48. Beltrame JF, Horowitz JD. Why do nitrates have limited efficacy in coronary microvessels?: Editorial to: "Lack of nitrates on exercise stress test results in patients with microvascular angina" by G. Russo et al. Cardiovasc Drugs Ther 2013;27(3):187–8.

49. Sütsch G, Oechslin E, Mayer I, et al. Effect of diltiazem on coronary flow reserve in patients with microvascular angina. Int J Cardiol 1995;52(2):135–43.

50. Cannon RO 3rd, Watson RM, Rosing DR, et al. Efficacy of calcium channel blocker therapy for angina pectoris resulting from small-vessel coronary artery disease and abnormal vasodilator reserve. Am J Cardiol 1985;56(4):242–6.

51. Ford TJ, Berry C, De Bruyne B, et al. Physiological predictors of acute coronary syndromes: emerging insights from the plaque to the vulnerable patient. JACC Cardiovasc interventions 2017;10(24):2539–47.

52. Al-Lamee R, Howard JP, Shun-Shin MJ, et al. Fractional flow reserve and instantaneous wave-free ratio as predictors of the placebo-controlled response to percutaneous coronary intervention in stable single-vessel coronary artery disease: physiology-stratified analysis of ORBITA. Circulation 2018;138(17):1780–92.

53. Mehta PK, Goykhman P, Thomson LE, et al. Ranolazine improves angina in women with evidence of myocardial ischemia but no obstructive coronary artery disease. JACC Cardiovasc Imaging 2011;4(5):514–22.

54. Villano A, Di Franco A, Nerla R, et al. Effects of ivabradine and ranolazine in patients with microvascular angina pectoris. Am J Cardiol 2013;112(1):8–13.

55. Denardo SJ, Wen X, Handberg EM, et al. Effect of phosphodiesterase type 5 inhibition on microvascular coronary dysfunction in women: a Women's

Ischemia Syndrome Evaluation (WISE) ancillary study. Clin Cardiol 2011;34(8):483–7.

56. Mohri M, Shimokawa H, Hirakawa Y, et al. Rho-kinase inhibition with intracoronary fasudil prevents myocardial ischemia in patients with coronary microvascular spasm. J Am Coll Cardiol 2003;41(1):15–9.

57. Morrow AJ, Ford TJ, Mangion K, et al. Rationale and design of the Medical Research Council's Precision Medicine with Zibotentan in Microvascular Angina (PRIZE) trial. Am Heart J 2020;229:70–80.

58. Scarsini R, Terentes-Printzios D, Shanmuganathan M, et al. Pressure-controlled intermittent coronary sinus occlusion improves the vasodilatory microvascular capacity and reduces myocardial injury in patients with STEMI. Catheter Cardiovasc Interv 2021;99(2): 329–39.

59. Verheye S, Jolicœur EM, Behan MW, et al. Efficacy of a device to narrow the coronary sinus in refractory angina. N Engl J Med 2015;372(6):519–27.

60. Jessurun GA, Hautvast RW, Tio RA, et al. Electrical neuromodulation improves myocardial perfusion and ameliorates refractory angina pectoris in patients with syndrome X: fad or future? Eur J Pain 2003;7(6):507–12.

61. Lanza GA, Sestito A, Sandric S, et al. Spinal cord stimulation in patients with refractory anginal pain and normal coronary arteries. Ital Heart J 2001;2(1):25–30.

62. Merz CN, Olson MB, McClure C, et al. A randomized controlled trial of low-dose hormone therapy on myocardial ischemia in postmenopausal women with no obstructive coronary artery disease: results from the National Institutes of Health/National Heart, Lung, and Blood Institute-sponsored Women's Ischemia Syndrome Evaluation (WISE). Am Heart J 2010;159(6). 987.e981-987.

63. Asbury EA, Kanji N, Ernst E, et al. Autogenic training to manage symptomology in women with chest pain and normal coronary arteries. Menopause 2009; 16(1):60–5.

Coronary Physiology as Part of a State-of-the-Art Percutaneous Coronary Intervention Strategy
Lessons from SYNTAX II and Beyond

Asad Shabbir, MD[a], Alejandro Travieso, MD[a],
Hernán Mejía-Rentería, MD, PhD[a], Carolina Espejo-Paeres, MD[a],
Nieves Gonzalo, MD, PhD[a], Adrian P. Banning, MD[b],
Patrick W. Serruys, MD, PhD[c,d], Javier Escaned, MD, PhD[a,*]

KEYWORDS

• Coronary • Intervention • PCI • Percutaneous • Revascularization • SYNTAX II

KEY POINTS

- The SYNTAX II trial highlights the value of state-of-the-art percutaneous coronary intervention, utilizing coronary physiology in conjunction with precision medicine, prognostic prediction, and probabilistic risk assessment to assist with coronary revascularization.
- The use of pre- and post-percutaneous coronary intervention (PCI) physiology are both key in improving long-term clinical outcomes, and the parametric assessment is prognostically relevant.
- Coronary physiology can assist with the objective grading of lesion severity, beyond that of angiography alone, thereby altering the anatomical SYNTAX score in favor of a functional SYNTAX score and simplifying disease patterns.
- Functional coronary angiography is emerging as a clinically useful armamentarium of tools for the physiological assessment of coronary stenoses, with emerging data supporting the use of these indices pre- and post-PCI, with prognostic guidance.

INTRODUCTION

The widespread implementation of coronary physiology to assist with the planning and guidance of percutaneous coronary intervention (PCI) has initiated a significant quantum change in the manner in which revascularization is performed. Based upon the vast volume of available literature supporting the benefit of the objective assessment of coronary stenoses with physiologic tools, the use of both hyperemic and non-hyperemic pressure ratios (NHPRs) is supported by international clinical guidance recommendations.[1,2]

Although physiology has significantly improved the way in which key decisions are made regarding the appropriateness of PCI at a lesion level, it is also important to consider how to optimally utilize the technique in conjunction with other contemporary technologies and practices. In the SYNTAX II study, physiology formed one part of a holistic approach to perform state-of-the-art PCI,[3] in addition to dedicated experienced operators in treating

This article originally appeared in *Interventional Cardiology Clinics*, Volume 12 Issue 1, January 2023.
[a] Interventional Cardiology Unit, Hospital Clínico San Carlos IDISCC, Complutense University of Madrid, Calle del Prof Martín Lagos, Madrid 28040, Spain; [b] Heart Centre, John Radcliffe Hospital, Oxford University Hospitals NHS Foundation Trust, Oxford, UK; [c] Department of Cardiology, National University of Ireland, Galway, Ireland; [d] National Heart and Lung Institute, Imperial College London, London, UK
* Corresponding author.
E-mail address: escaned@secardiologia.es

Cardiol Clin 42 (2024) 147–158
https://doi.org/10.1016/j.ccl.2023.07.001

complex disease patterns, the use of intravascular imaging to ensure adequate stent deployment and lesion coverage, and the use of contemporary stent platforms with cutting-edge drug eluting kinetics.

In this review, the technical aspects regarding the use of physiology in the SYNTAX II strategy are discussed. In addition, insights into functional coronary angiography (FCA), a summary of the use of physiology in simulation, and the use of physiology in the setting of post-PCI functional assessments are evaluated.

The SYNTAX II Trial

The SYNTAX II trial was a study of state-of-the-art PCI in patients with de-novo three-vessel coronary artery disease (CAD) and clinical equipoise between PCI and coronary artery bypass graft (CABG) revascularization strategies based upon the SYNTAX II score, compared with a matched cohort from the original SYNTAX I trial.[4] The study showed that excellent long-term outcomes are feasible following percutaneous coronary revascularization in this complex patient subset.[3,5] The study epitomizes a model of best practice in the cardiac catheterization laboratory and shows that the integration of diagnostic and therapeutic tools, along with operator expertise, contributes to a sustained positive improvement in survival over long-term follow-up.[6]

The key pillars of the SYNTAX II strategy were; risk stratification for PCI and CABG using the SYNTAX score II, the use of coronary physiology to guide PCI based on ischemia (a hybrid of instantaneous wave-free ratio (iFR) and fractional flow reserve (FFR)), imaging guidance of PCI using intravascular ultrasound (IVUS), involvement of chronic total occlusion (CTO) operators, and use of everolimus eluting SYNERGY (Boston Scientific, USA) drug-eluting stents (DES). The key components of the SYNTAX II study are shown in **Fig. 1**.

The study has been influential in contemporary practice guidelines and highlights that sole angiographic interpretation of coronary stenoses when attempting to comprehensively characterize a lesion is insufficient. Since the original SYNTAX I trial,[7] the tools available to interventional cardiologists have significantly evolved, and now enable the precise interrogation of disease through accurate physiologic metrics and high-fidelity imaging. A key aim of the study was to address one of the criticisms of SYNTAX I; the higher rate of target vessel failure (TVF) in patients treated PCI, compared with surgical revascularization.[8] Unique to the SYNTAX II study, the investigators recognized the potential benefit of a holistic approach to complex PCI when conceptualizing the study, incorporating several complimentary techniques.

The findings of the study were revolutionary, with sustained improvements over 5-year follow-up[3,5,6] when compared with patients treated with PCI from the SYNTAX I study, culminating in a significantly lower rate of major adverse cardiovascular events (MACEs) in the SYNTAX II group compared with the SYNTAX I cohort (21.5% vs 36.4%, $P < 0.001$), lower rates of revascularization (13.8% vs 23.8%, $P < 0.001$), all-cause mortality (8.1% vs 13.8%, $P = 0.013$) and cardiac death (2.8% vs 8.4%, $P = 0.004$). MACE was similar at 5-years between the SYNTAX II PCI and SYNTAX I CABG cohorts (21.5% vs 24.6%, $P = 0.35$). SYNTAX II successfully showed that state-of-the-art PCI can be an effective strategy in some patients with complex disease. Interestingly, it showed that, at a difference with the original SYNTAX study, long-term outcomes of patients with and without diabetes did not differ significantly.[9] Importantly, the techniques used in the study are readily available.

The interventional community must also consider emerging technologies not used in the SYNTAX II study, which have recently been shown to improve the results of PCI. These new physiology concepts, along with the key aspects pertaining to the use of physiology in the SYNTAX II study, are described in greater detail below.

Physiology Guidance in SYNTAX II

Physiology grants additional insight into the functional significance of coronary lesions, and literature supports that physiology-guided revascularization offers improved clinical outcomes for patients with CAD, beyond sole angiographic assessment, as investigated in the FAME and FAME II studies.[10,11] With physiologic assistance, the deferral of non-hemodynamically significant lesions is safe, even over long-term follow-up.[12] It should be noted that although these studies investigated the hyperemic index FFR, the diagnostic and prognostic utility of NHPRs, specifically iFR, is equivalent to that of FFR; a finding recognized by the landmark DEFINE FLAIR[13] and IFR SWEDEHEART[14] trials. An additional practical benefit of NHPR in the assessment of coronary stenosis is the lack of a requirement to administer a hyperemic inducing pharmacotherapeutic, such as adenosine, which can often be uncomfortable for patients and inconvenient in instances where physiologic testing is performed in multiple vessels, as was the case in SYNTAX II, hence the adoption of a hybrid physiologic approach.

Components of the SYNTAX II strategy

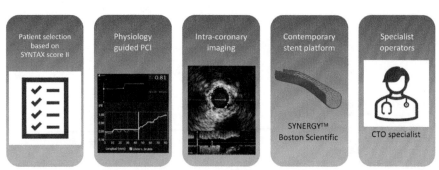

| Patient selection based on SYNTAX score II | Physiology guided PCI | Intra-coronary imaging | Contemporary stent platform | Specialist operators |

SYNERGY™
Boston Scientific

CTO specialist

Fig. 1. Key components of the SYNTAX II study. The key components of the SYNTAX II study are shown. The SYNTAX score II was used to assess patients. PCI was guided by invasive physiology with a hybrid iFR and FFR approach, and the use of post-PCI intracoronary imaging assisted with optimal stent deployment. A contemporary stent platform was deployed, and specialist operators treated chronic total occlusions where possible.

The use of physiology in SYNTAX II was primarily to functionally assess coronary disease such that the physiologic information could be incorporated into the SYNTAX score II,[15] thus determining a functional risk score. As has been previously shown, the use of a functional SYNTAX score often reclassifies the number of vessels and better discriminates patients with multivessel CAD.[16,17] The use of physiology in the grading of vessel stenosis was distinct from the methods used in SYNTAX I, where multivessel coronary disease was diagnosed purely on the visual interpretation of the angiograms. The use of a functional score permitted the safe deferral of disease through the incorporation of physiology. This enabled the simplification of anatomy, with fewer lesions treated on a per-patient basis (2.64 vs 4.02, in SYNTAX II vs SYNTAX I, respectively, $P < 0.001$). As a consequence of this, fewer cases of three-vessel disease in SYNTAX II cohort were observed when compared with the matched SYNTAX I cohort (37.2% vs 83.3%, respectively, $P < 0.001$). Recently, the SYNTAXES (SYNTAX Extended Survival) investigators[18] have revised the SYNTAX score II and formed the SYNTAX score II 2020, using an updated Cox regression analysis model which now offers 10-year all-cause death prediction and 5-year MACE risk modeling.

Based on the results of the ADVISE II trial,[19] SYNTAX II used a combination of iFR and FFR to determine the physiologic significance of stenoses, with the hyperemic index used when equivocal iFR readings were acquired (iFR 0.86–0.93). This hybrid approach ensured that patients with equivocal NHPR underwent sufficiently rigorous physiologic testing to definitively show either a positive or negative lesion. Despite this, 72% of the patients entered into the study were assessed with iFR, with very low levels of repeat revascularization at the 5-year follow-up timepoint, showing the safety of iFR in deferral and supporting the previous studies comparing the index with FFR. With the assistance of the hybrid iFR/FFR approach, whereas the number of anatomic target lesions was found to be 3.49 lesions/patient, the number of treated lesions (guided by physiology) reduced significantly to 2.64 lesions/patient. A case example of how physiology was used in the SYNTAX II study is shown in **Fig. 2**.

Important lesional-level information can also be gained from the pressure pullback. Although not part of the SYNTAX II strategy, a pullback maneuver can be performed to offer insights into the pattern of disease and differentiate between focal, serial, and diffuse lesions; the former being more amenable to PCI. With technological development, lesional-level ischemia patterns can be differentiated and NHPR assessments are more appealing owing to the relative ease of digital integration in computer systems.[20] The pullback pressure curve can also be co-registered with the coronary angiogram to facilitate highly precise interventions.[21] A method aimed at distinguishing focal and diffuse patterns of disease is currently under investigation, using a pressure gradient index derived from the FFR; the pressure pullback gradient (PPG_{index}) (NCT04789317).[22]

Other Components of the SYNTAX II Strategy

Intracoronary imaging

The use of physiology in conjunction with intravascular imaging in the SYNTAX II study was protocolized (84.1% in SYNTAX II vs 4.8% in SYNTAX, P

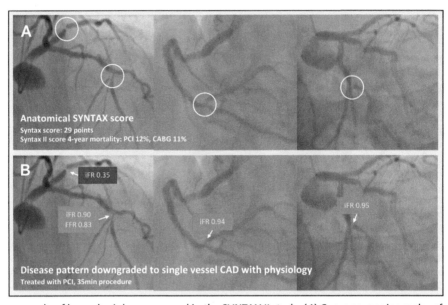

Fig. 2. Case example of how physiology was used in the SYNTAX II study. (*A*) Coronary angiography of an 80-year-old patient with diabetes, dyslipidemia and hypertension showing angiographically significant three-vessel coronary artery disease. Anatomical SYNTAX score calculated as 29 points, with a SYNTAX score II 4-year mortality for PCI and CABG of 12% and 11%, respectively. (*B*) When coronary physiology is used to assess the functional significance of the stenoses in the same patient, the disease pattern is downgraded to single vessel disease. The patient was successfully treated with PCI in a 35-min procedure.

< 0.0001), and one of the key factors for the low rate of stent failure compared with the original SYNTAX I study (0.7% vs 2.7%, respectively, $P = 0.045$).

The clinical benefit of intravascular imaging is well established. In both the IVUS-XPL[23] and UL-TIMATE[24] studies, significant reductions in target vessel revascularization (TVR) were observed, with a combined analysis of the two studies showing a reduction in cardiac death in patients that underwent IVUS-guided stent optimization (1% vs 2.2%, IVUS vs control, respectively, HR 0.43, $P = 0.011$) and reductions in stent thrombosis (0.2% vs 0.7%, IVUS vs control, respectively, HR 0.33, $P = 0.082$).[25,26] Intravascular imaging can also ensure adequate peri-lesion coverage along the length of the vessel, avoid geographic mismatch, and minimize stenting into plaque located at the edge of the stent, resulting in longer stents being deployed in SYNTAX II, compared with the historic cohort (24.4 mm vs 18.8 mm, respectively, $P < 0.001$).[3]

Another use of intravascular imaging is for the identification of calcific disease and the assistance of lesion preparation, as inadequate lesion preparation correlates with negative procedural outcomes.[27] Where possible the use of pre-PCI intracoronary imaging is encouraged to identify highly calcific complex disease, as the distribution of calcification is relevant to the success of the procedure, specifically the angular extent, thickness, and length of the calcification.[28]

Physiology pullback can also allow for longitudinal vessel characterization and assist with the identification of pressure-loss along the length of a vessel which can be performed before and/or after PCI.[29–31] This co-registration can also be conducted with IVUS and offers highly precise longitudinal vessel analysis. The ongoing DEFINE GPS study (NCT04451044) aims to investigate whether co-registration at the time of PCI can influence patient outcome.

Operator competency in complex percutaneous coronary interventions

In SYNTAX II, the success of CTO interventions was significantly higher compared with that found in SYNTAX I, with higher rates of complete revascularization (87% vs 53% success rate, respectively, $P < 0.0001$),[3] and a deliberate consequence of the involvement of specialist CTO operators in complex cases.

CTO PCI has undergone rapid technical development, with the introduction of specialist equipment (guidewires and microcatheters) and techniques.[32] The PROGRESS-CTO[33] and RECHARGE[34] registries have offered insight into CTO PCI. Although an antegrade wire escalation strategy is often sufficient to recanalize the target vessel, skilled operators should be able to switch to antegrade dissection re-entry or retrograde approaches if required. The benefit of imaging in the form of pre-procedure CT or intracoronary imaging to guide the procedure should not be understated. The presence of complex bifurcations, severe calcification, heart failure, vessel tortuosity, multiple CTOs, and cap ambiguity are all contributors to a negative outcome.[35] Clinical guidance documents from the Chronic Total Occlusion Academic Research Consortium (CTO-ARC)[36] and EuroCTO Club[37] have set out comprehensive guidelines on maximizing CTO PCI success and how to manage complications.

Contemporary stent platforms

In the SYNTAX II study, a contemporary stent platform was used. There have been significant refinements in stent technology since the 1990s and the introduction of the first-generation DES. As used in SYNTAX II, the everolimus DES (SYNERGY, Boston Scientific, USA) exerts their anti-inflammatory and anti-proliferative effects through the inhibition of mammalian target of rapamycin (mTOR).[38]

As with most of the latest generation scaffolds, the stent used in the SYNTAX II study presented specific features to improve trackability while maintaining a high radial force; an important characteristic when performing PCI in highly calcific vessels. The stents offer an ultra-thin (74 µm) strut design with abluminal drug coverage to allow for a more physiological stent endothelialization process.[39] Furthermore, the ultra-thin strut design enables improved side branch (SB) access in bifurcation PCI and yet maintains a wide expansile range which is particularly useful when performing PCI in proximal vessels.

FUNCTIONAL CORONARY ANGIOGRAPHY

In the context of a modest uptake of invasive physiology in cardiac catheterization laboratories, there has been significant interest in the development wire-free methods for the assessment of the functional significance of coronary stenoses. Although the risks of complication directly arising from the use of coronary pressure guidewires is low, conventional diagnostic coronary angiography is less time-consuming and safer. Furthermore, the necessity of administering a hyperemic agent when measuring FFR adds a degree of complexity and might hinder cardiac catheterization laboratory workflow. Although not used in the SYNTAX II strategy, these wire-free methods of quantifying the physiologic significance of coronary artery lesions warrant discussion, as their use is likely to be widespread in the near future. FCA largely circumvents many of the drawbacks of the invasive wire-based physiological measurements stated above, providing good estimates of functional stenosis relevance.[40] FCA can be derived from 3D reconstructions of the invasive diagnostic coronary angiogram, and also from noninvasive coronary computed tomography angiography (CCTA).[41]

Quantitative flow ratio (QFR), currently the most widely used FCA tool, relies on invasive angiographic projections to create a 3D reconstruction of the vessel, which is then contoured using quantitative coronary angiography (QCA) in a dedicated software programme.[42] An example of a QFR workflow is shown in **Fig. 3**. The contrast flow rate is assessed from the thrombolysis in myocardial infarction (TIMI) frame count. Unlike other FCA, QFR has been prognostically validated in the FAVOR III China study,[43] and is currently under investigation in the FAVOR III Europe Japan study (NCT0372939) to compare QFR with pressure wire-guided revascularization. Additional angiography-based indices are being developed, including FFR derived from angiography (FFR_{angio}),[44,45] virtual fractional flow reserve $(vFFR)$[46,47] and the virtual functional assessment index (vFAI),[48] but these predominantly remain in the remit of clinical research.

FFR derived from CCTA (FFR_{CT}) is a noninvasive FCA, derived from a computation fluid dynamics (CFD) algorithm of CT coronary artery reconstructions.[49] Although CT is well established to diagnose CAD and identify coronary calcification, the use of FFR_{CT} in clinical practice is less established with limited prognostic data available. However, medium-term outcomes are similar to that of invasive wire-based techniques[50] with good diagnostic accuracy.[51]

There are pitfalls specifically related to the use of FCA, which are not found in invasive diagnostic coronary angiography. QFR is reliant upon high-quality diagnostic angiography and manual vessel contouring which can be time-consuming. Furthermore, the technology is not applicable in some anatomical scenarios, although progress has been made in addressing some of them; such as in coronary bifurcations.[52] As for all the angiography-derived FCA techniques mentioned above, there is a requirement for proprietary software to be used, for which there will be a learning curve and cost, and relatively high-powered hardware to reconstruct the vessels and solve the physics/mathematical problems to compute the CFD. Specifically relating to CT, only the latest generation scanners have the capacity to acquire sufficient imaging quality and avoid step artifacts.

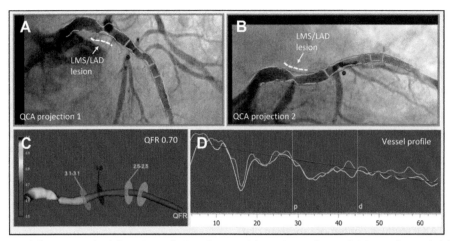

Fig. 3. QFR workflow example. (*A*) LMS/LAD lesion shown with angiography, and QCA performed. (*B*) QCA performed in orthogonal projections. (*C*) Vessel reconstruction with QFR showing QFR value of 0.70. (*D*) Longitudinal vessel profile shown.

PHYSIOLOGY-GUIDED POST-PERCUTANEOUS CORONARY INTERVENTIONS OPTIMIZATION

Physiology can assist with the detection of flow-limiting disease post-PCI and differentiate between residual focal, tandem, and diffuse lesions. It has been established that suboptimal wire-based post-PCI physiological measurements are associated with adverse clinical outcomes.[53,54] Furthermore, FCA also reveals prognostic information of the physiological results of PCI, as shown with QFR in a substudy of the SYNTAX II trial[55] and in other investigations.[56,57] Some of the clinical studies that have investigated the prognostic value of post-PCI physiology are shown in **Table 1**. Although acceptable limits for residual pressure loss remain uncertain, data currently suggests that a post-PCI FFR ≥ 0.90[58] and an iFR ≥ 0.95[53,59] are associated with improved patient outcomes. As identified in the TARGET FFR trial, in which patients were randomized to receive either FFR-guided or angiography-guided post-PCI optimization, the decision to optimize based solely on the final angiographic result was found to be inadequate. Significantly fewer patients with a suboptimal post-procedure FFR were observed in the physiology-guided arm of the study.[60]

In addition to wire-based measurements, data have confirmed the utility of QFR in the post-PCI setting. As shown in the HAWKEYE study, this computational modeling-based tool can also be used with a sufficient degree of confidence to drive prognostic intervention decision-making, with lower post-PCI QFR values accurately predicting adverse clinical outcomes.[57]

If residual disease is identified post-PCI, it is recommended that optimization should also be performed with co-registered intracoronary imaging modalities, such as those highlighted above, to accurately identify the mechanism of the physiologic result and anatomy of the vessel. Such imaging techniques are also indispensable in ensuring adequate stent apposition and lesion coverage. In SYNTAX II, post-PCI IVUS resulted in further optimization in approximately 30% of patients.

PHYSIOLOGY IN SIMULATED PERCUTANEOUS CORONARY INTERVENTIONS

Although the physiologic success of a PCI procedure can be assessed post-PCI with wire-based methods immediately following the deployment of the stent, novel technology also allows for the simulation of functional results to be assessed before embarking on PCI, enabling the interventionalist to plan and refine their plan before undertaking the procedure.

Pre-PCI longitudinal vessel analysis using a pullback in conjunction with NHPR allows for the comprehensive hemodynamic profiling of the vessel and identification of segments of functionally significant disease. The physiological effects of PCI can be calculated using the formula; predicted NHPR ($NHPR_{pred}$) = pre-PCI NHPR (lowest value) + $\sum$intention to treat NHPR gradient(s).[20,61] This principle can be applied to iFR, diastolic pressure ratio (dPR) and resting full-cycle ratio (RFR). With iFR, the software package allows for an automated approach to simulation in conjunction with IVUS co-registration. Examples of PCI simulation using NHPR workflows are shown in **Fig. 4**.

Table 1
Clinical studies that have investigated post-PCI physiology and prognosis

First Author	Index	Title	Study Findings
Pijls et al,[68] 2002	FFR	Coronary pressure measurement after stenting predicts adverse events at follow-up.	Post-PCI FFR <0.80 correlates with MACE at 6 months. Composite MACE outcome OR (adjusted for stent length) 7.35 (95%CI, 3.04–17.73).
Klauss et al,[69] 2005	FFR	Fractional flow reserve for the prediction of cardiac events after coronary stent implantation.	Post-PCI FFR <0.95 (OR 6.22, 95% CI 1.79–21.62) predictor of MACE.
Nam et al,[70] 2011	FFR	Relation of fractional flow reserve after drug-eluting stent implantation to 1-year outcomes.	MACE in group with low-FFR (FFR ≤0.90) driven by TVR compared with high-FFR group (FFR >0.90); 12.5% vs 2.5%, respectively ($P < 0.01$).
Rimac et al,[58] 2017	FFR	Clinical value of post-percutaneous coronary intervention fractional flow reserve value: a systemic review and meta-analysis.	Post-PCI FFR ≥0.90 associated with lower rate of repeat revascularization, OR 0.43 95% CI 0.34–0.56, $P < 0.001$ and MACE.
Li et al,[71] 2017	FFR	Cutoff value and long-term prediction of clinical events by FFR measured immediately after implantation of a drug-eluting stent in patients with coronary artery disease.	FFR ≤0.88 correlates with TVF at 1-year post PCI, which was maintained at 3-year follow-up ($P = 0.002$).
Fournier et al,[72] 2019	FFR	Association of improvement in fractional flow reserve with outcomes, including symptomatic relief, after percutaneous coronary intervention.	Low improvement in post-PCI FFR (ΔFFR ≤0.18) associated with highest VOCE (9.1%), and lowest in high post-PCI FFR improvement (ΔFFR ≥0.31) with VOCE rate of 4.7%, HR 2.01 (95% CI 1.03–3.92) $P = 0.04$.
Hwang et al,[73] 2019	FFR	Influence of target vessel on prognostic relevance of fractional flow reserve after coronary stenting.	Different optimum cutoff values predicting TVF observed in LAD (FFR 0.82) and non-LAD (0.88), respectively. LAD; TVF 10.9% vs 2.5% ($P < 0.001$) in low vs high FFR, respectively. Non-LAD; 8% vs 1.9% ($P = 0.004$) in low vs high FFR, respectively.
Jeremias et al,[59] 2019	iFR	Blinded physiological assessment of residual ischemia after successful angiographic percutaneous coronary intervention: The DEFINE PCI study.	Residual ischemia present in 24% of patients with angiographically adequate PCI. One-year outcome data; Post-PCI iFR correlates with MACE at 1 year. Post-PCI iFR ≥0.95 associated with improved MACE compared with low iFR <0.95, 1.8% vs 5.7%, respectively, $P = 0.04$.[53]

(continued on next page)

Table 1
(continued)

First Author	Index	Title	Study Findings
Biscaglia et al,[57] 2019	QFR	Prognostic value of QFR measured immediately after successful stent implantation: the international multicenter prospective HAWKEYE study.	ROC analysis estimates post-PCI QFR cutoff of ≤0.89, with post-PCI QFR ≤0.89 associated with 3× increase in VOCE (*P* < 0.001).
Kogame et al,[55] 2019	QFR	Clinical implication of quantitative flow ratio after percutaneous coronary intervention for three-vessel disease.	Post-PCI QFR is associated with improved outcomes in de novo three-vessel disease; optimum cutoff value post-PCI QFR in predicting 2-year VOCE was 0.91.

Table summarizing pertinent clinical studies investigating the prognostic impact of post-PCI physiology, and their respective findings.

The concept of *in-silico* simulation can also be applied to FCA, with studies showing the clinical utility of residual post-PCI QFR, derived from pre-intervention angiograms and CFD modeling.[62] Although this shows the potential of QFR PCI simulation, the recently completed QFR-based AQVA study (NCT04664140) aims to assess whether a strategy of pre-PCI QFR-assisted planning might reduce suboptimal post-PCI physiological results.

The performance of FFR_{CT} on the prediction of post-PCI physiological results has been assessed,[63,64] with evidence supporting agreement with invasive wire-based FFR, and it is likely this will form part of an enhanced planning workflow in the near future.[65] The Precise Percutaneous Coronary Intervention Plan (P3) (NCT03782688) study will use the latest generation FFR_{CT} Heart-Flow Planner tool (HeartFlow Inc., CA, USA) and assess its performance with invasive FFR as the comparator.

REFLECTIONS IN THE AFTERMATH OF FAME III

Having discussed the different elements of the SYNTAX II strategy, it is also worthwhile to reflect upon the results of the recently published FAME III study.[66] The study, which randomized 1500 patients with the three-vessel disease to PCI or CABG and implemented FFR as a decision-making tool for revascularization in the PCI arm, failed to show noninferiority of FFR-guided PCI with CABG. In contrast to SYNTAX II, FAME III did not use a clinical risk stratification tool such as the SYNTAX score II. By not doing so, at a difference with SYNTAX II, patients with a predicted better 4-year outcome with CABG than PCI were included in the study, an aspect that may be debatable. By using a risk score that integrates both anatomical and clinical variables, the SYNTAX II showed that outcomes of patients with low (≤22) SYNTAX score were like those with moderate or high scores (≥22). On the contrary,

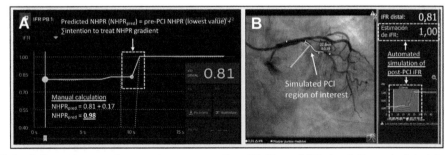

Fig. 4. PCI simulation using non-hyperemic pressure ratios. (*A*) Manual PCI simulation calculated from the formula; predicted NHPR (NHPR$_{pred}$) = pre-PCI NHPR (lowest value) + ∑intention to treat NHPR gradient(s). Distal iFR 0.81, with focal region of pressure loss of 0.17 units. With the addition of the 0.17 units of pressure loss to the distal iFR, a predicted iFR can be calculated of 0.98. (*B*) Automated iFR simulation using the SyncVision (Philips) software system with baseline pre-PCI iFR of 0.81, and after simulated treatment of the lesion the predicted iFR is 1.00.

in FAME III, patients undergoing PCI with an anatomical SYNTAX score of >22 experienced worse outcomes than those with a score of ≤22.

In SYNTAX II, IVUS was used to guide stent implantation in 84.1% of patients (76.4% of the total number of lesions), with subsequent balloon optimization in 30.2%.[3] As identified in the SYNTAX II IVUS substudy, post-procedural minimum lumen area is in an independent predictor of TVR (at 2 years), with a threshold of 5.2 mm^2 (quantified by ROC analysis).[67] It remains plausible that should IVUS have been used in a similar way in FAME III, a substantial reduction in the number of repeat revascularizations might have occurred, as intravascular imaging was used in only 11.7% of cases in FAME III.

An important development in SYNTAX II, compared with SYNTAX, was the management of CTOs by expert operators, whose revascularization rate increased from 50% to 84%. As FAME III did not implement this as part of the study design, it is possible that a lower degree of revascularization completeness had been achieved in patients presenting with a CTO.

Additional aspects of FAME III that merit emphasis also include the following; solely FFR was used to determine the functional significance of a vessel (not NHPR), 39% of the patients presented with acute coronary syndrome (ACS), post-PCI physiology was performed in only 60% of patients with a median residual FFR of 0.88 (the relevance of post-PCI physiology previously discussed), and 18% of patients with high-tertile SYNTAX score underwent PCI where CABG would ordinarily be the guideline-directed treatment of choice.

It is also important to highlight the excellent 1-year clinical results observed in the CABG arm, which is likely related to improvements in surgical technique from the original SYNTAX trial.

In a nutshell, the results of the FAME III trial highlight the importance of implementing a compendium of best practices in revascularization, rather than a single tool such as coronary physiology. Furthermore, this study supports the notion that revascularization strategies should be carefully considered in highly complex disease and therapy should be tailored to reflect the comorbidities of the patient and the pattern of CAD.

SUMMARY

The SYNTAX II trial highlights that the simultaneous use of physiology with other contemporary techniques and technologies are key to perform state-of-the-art PCI, and holistically offer prognostic benefit to patients. Physiology has been one of the key technological advances since the inception of PCI, which has progressively evolved over the last 20 years and can now offer the precise characterization of lesions through longitudinal vessel analysis, support with procedural planning and guidance, and assist with post-PCI optimization.

Also highlighted in this review is the importance of considering intravascular imaging, which can be co-registered with physiology, to guide lesion coverage and to aid in the interrogation of suboptimal post-PCI functional results in cases where residual pressure loss remain after stent deployment.

Although the cornerstone of the state-of-the-art SYNTAX II strategy was the use of physiology to guide the procedure, herein we have also discussed FCA, which is likely to play a significant role in the near future and has already been shown to carry prognostic relevance. Finally, the use of coronary physiology in the simulation of PCI has been mentioned, which is already widespread and especially useful, supporting interventional cardiologists to model plans before embarking on potentially complex procedures.

CLINICS CARE POINTS

- State-of-the-art PCI utilizes physiology, intra-coronary imaging, practical expertise and contemporary technologies to deliver optimal PCI.
- The success of PCI can be improved with the use of physiology and intracoronary imaging through optimization of the final result.
- Simulated PCI allows for accurate prediction and modelling of the final PCI result.
- Functional coronary angiography allows for wire-free assessment of coronary stenoses.

DISCLOSURES

A.P. Banning declares institutional funding for a fellowship from Boston Scientific and speaker fees from Boston Scientific, Medtronic, and Abbott Vascular. P.W. Serruys declares consulting fees from Philips/Volcano, SMT, Xeltis, Novartis, Merillife, Sino Medical, Novartis, and Biosensors. J. Escaned reports speaker and advisory board member for Abbott and Philips, speaker for Abiomed, Boston Scientific and Medis. Dr C. Espejo-Paeres is a recipient of a Rio Hortega grant (CM20/00013) from Instituto de Salud Carlos III (Madrid, Spain).

REFERENCES

1. Neumann FJ, Sousa-Uva M, Ahlsson A, et al. 2018 ESC/EACTS Guidelines on myocardial revascularization. Eur Heart J 2019;40:87–165.
2. Lawton JS, Tamis-Holland JE, Bangalore S, et al. 2021 ACC/AHA/SCAI guideline for coronary artery revascularization: a report of the american college of cardiology/american heart association joint committee on clinical practice guidelines. Circulation 2022;145:e18–114.
3. Escaned J, Collet C, Ryan N, et al. Clinical outcomes of state-of-the-art percutaneous coronary revascularization in patients with de novo three vessel disease: 1-year results of the SYNTAX II study. Eur Heart J 2017;38:3124–34.
4. Escaned J, Banning A, Farooq V, et al. Rationale and design of the SYNTAX II trial evaluating the short to long-term outcomes of state-of-the-art percutaneous coronary revascularisation in patients with de novo three-vessel disease. EuroIntervention 2016;12: e224–34.
5. Serruys PW, Kogame N, Katagiri Y, et al. Clinical outcomes of state-of-the-art percutaneous coronary revascularisation in patients with three-vessel disease: two-year follow-up of the SYNTAX II study. EuroIntervention 2019;15:e244–52.
6. Banning AP, Serruys P, De Maria GL, et al. Five-year outcomes after state-of-the-art percutaneous coronary revascularization in patients with de novo three-vessel disease: final results of the SYNTAX II study. Eur Heart J 2021;43(13):1307–16.
7. Serruys PW, Morice MC, Kappetein AP, et al. Percutaneous coronary intervention versus coronary-artery bypass grafting for severe coronary artery disease. N Engl J Med 2009;360:961–72.
8. Gulati R, Rihal CS, Gersh BJ. The SYNTAX trial: a perspective. Circ Cardiovasc Interv 2009;2:463–7.
9. Cavalcante R, Sotomi Y, Mancone M, et al. Impact of the SYNTAX scores I and II in patients with diabetes and multivessel coronary disease: a pooled analysis of patient level data from the SYNTAX, PRECOMBAT, and BEST trials. Eur Heart J 2017; 38:1969–77.
10. Tonino PA, De Bruyne B, Pijls NH, et al. Fractional flow reserve versus angiography for guiding percutaneous coronary intervention. N Engl J Med 2009; 360:213–24.
11. De Bruyne B, Pijls NH, Kalesan B, et al. Fractional flow reserve-guided PCI versus medical therapy in stable coronary disease. N Engl J Med 2012;367: 991–1001.
12. Zimmermann FM, Ferrara A, Johnson NP, et al. Deferral vs. performance of percutaneous coronary intervention of functionally non-significant coronary stenosis: 15-year follow-up of the DEFER trial. Eur Heart J 2015;36:3182–8.
13. Davies JE, Sen S, Dehbi HM, et al. Use of the instantaneous wave-free ratio or fractional flow reserve in PCI. N Engl J Med 2017;376:1824–34.
14. Gotberg M, Christiansen EH, Gudmundsdottir IJ, et al. Instantaneous wave-free ratio versus fractional flow reserve to guide PCI. N Engl J Med 2017;376: 1813–23.
15. Farooq V, van Klaveren D, Steyerberg EW, et al. Anatomical and clinical characteristics to guide decision-making between coronary artery bypass surgery and percutaneous coronary intervention for individual patients: development and validation of SYNTAX score II. Lancet 2013;381:639–50.
16. Nam CW, Mangiacapra F, Entjes R, et al. Functional SYNTAX score for risk assessment in multivessel coronary artery disease. J Am Coll Cardiol 2011; 58:1211–8.
17. Van Belle E, Rioufol G, Pouillot C, et al. Outcome impact of coronary revascularization strategy reclassification with fractional flow reserve at time of diagnostic angiography: insights from a large French multicenter fractional flow reserve registry. Circulation 2014;129:173–85.
18. Takahashi K, Serruys PW, Fuster V, et al. Redevelopment and validation of the SYNTAX score II to individualise decision-making between percutaneous and surgical revascularisation in patients with complex coronary artery disease: secondary analysis of the multicentre randomised controlled SYNTAXES trial with external cohort validation. Lancet 2020;396:1399–412.
19. Escaned J, Echavarria-Pinto M, Garcia-Garcia HM, et al. Prospective assessment of the diagnostic accuracy of instantaneous wave-free ratio to assess coronary stenosis relevance: results of ADVISE II International, multicenter study (ADenosine Vasodilator Independent Stenosis Evaluation II). JACC Cardiovasc Interv 2015;8:824–33.
20. Kikuta Y, Cook CM, Sharp ASP, et al. Pre-angioplasty instantaneous wave-free ratio pullback predicts hemodynamic outcome in humans with coronary artery disease: primary results of the international multicenter iFR GRADIENT Registry. JACC Cardiovasc Interv 2018;11:757–67.
21. Matsuo A, Kasahara T, Ariyoshi M, et al. Utility of angiography-physiology coregistration maps during percutaneous coronary intervention in clinical practice. Cardiovasc Interv Ther 2021;36:208–18.
22. Collet C, Sonck J, Vandeloo B, et al. Measurement of hyperemic pullback pressure gradients to characterize patterns of coronary atherosclerosis. J Am Coll Cardiol 2019;74:1772–84.
23. Hong SJ, Mintz GS, Ahn CM, et al. Effect of intravascular ultrasound-guided drug-eluting stent implantation: 5-year follow-up of the IVUS-XPL randomized trial. JACC Cardiovasc Interv 2020;13:62–71.
24. Gao XF, Ge Z, Kong XQ, et al. 3-year outcomes of the ULTIMATE trial comparing intravascular

ultrasound versus angiography-guided drug-eluting stent implantation. JACC Cardiovasc Interv 2021;14: 247–57.

25. Hong SJ, Zhang JJ, Mintz GS, et al. Improved 3-year cardiac survival after IVUS-guided long DES implantation: a patient-level analysis from 2 randomized trials. JACC Cardiovasc Interv 2022;15:208–16.

26. Lee SY, Choi KH, Song YB, et al. Use of intravascular ultrasound and long-term cardiac death or myocardial infarction in patients receiving current generation drug-eluting stents. Sci Rep 2022;12: 8237.

27. Bourantas CV, Zhang YJ, Garg S, et al. Prognostic implications of coronary calcification in patients with obstructive coronary artery disease treated by percutaneous coronary intervention: a patient-level pooled analysis of 7 contemporary stent trials. Heart 2014;100:1158–64.

28. Fujino A, Mintz GS, Matsumura M, et al. A new optical coherence tomography-based calcium scoring system to predict stent underexpansion. EuroIntervention 2018;13:e2182–9.

29. Frimerman A, Abu-Fane R, Levi Y, et al. Novel method for real-time coregistration of coronary physiology and angiography by iFR. JACC Cardiovasc Interv 2019;12:692–4.

30. Nijjer SS, Sen S, Petraco R, et al. Pre-angioplasty instantaneous wave-free ratio pullback provides virtual intervention and predicts hemodynamic outcome for serial lesions and diffuse coronary artery disease. JACC Cardiovasc Interv 2014;7:1386–96.

31. Nijjer SS, Sen S, Petraco R, et al. The Instantaneous wave-Free Ratio (iFR) pullback: a novel innovation using baseline physiology to optimise coronary angioplasty in tandem lesions. Cardiovasc Revasc Med 2015;16:167–71.

32. Brilakis ES, Mashayekhi K, Tsuchikane E, et al. Guiding principles for chronic total occlusion percutaneous coronary intervention. Circulation 2019;140: 420–33.

33. Xenogiannis I, Gkargkoulas F, Karmpaliotis D, et al. Temporal trends in chronic total occlusion percutaneous coronary interventions: insights from the PROGRESS-CTO registry. J Invasive Cardiol 2020; 32:153–60.

34. Maeremans J, Walsh S, Knaapen P, et al. The hybrid algorithm for treating chronic total occlusions in europe: the recharge registry. J Am Coll Cardiol 2016; 68:1958–70.

35. Tajti P, Karmpaliotis D, Alaswad K, et al. The Hybrid approach to chronic total occlusion percutaneous coronary intervention: update from the PROGRESS CTO registry. JACC Cardiovasc Interv 2018;11: 1325–35.

36. Ybarra LF, Rinfret S, Brilakis ES, et al. Definitions and clinical trial design principles for coronary artery chronic total occlusion therapies: CTO-ARC consensus recommendations. Circulation 2021; 143:479–500.

37. Galassi AR, Werner GS, Boukhris M, et al. Percutaneous recanalisation of chronic total occlusions: 2019 consensus document from the EuroCTO Club. EuroIntervention 2019;15:198–208.

38. Kereiakes DJ, Windecker S, Jobe RL, et al. Clinical outcomes following implantation of thin-strut, bioabsorbable polymer-coated, everolimus-eluting SYNERGY stents. Circ Cardiovasc Interv 2019;12: e008152.

39. Bangalore S, Toklu B, Patel N, et al. Newer-generation ultrathin strut drug-eluting stents versus older second-generation thicker strut drug-eluting stents for coronary artery disease. Circulation 2018;138: 2216–26.

40. Collet C, Onuma Y, Sonck J, et al. Diagnostic performance of angiography-derived fractional flow reserve: a systematic review and Bayesian meta-analysis. Eur Heart J 2018;39:3314–21.

41. Kogame N, Ono M, Kawashima H, et al. The impact of coronary physiology on contemporary clinical decision-making. JACC Cardiovasc Interv 2020;13: 1617–38.

42. Tu S, Barbato E, Koszegi Z, et al. Fractional flow reserve calculation from 3-dimensional quantitative coronary angiography and TIMI frame count: a fast computer model to quantify the functional significance of moderately obstructed coronary arteries. JACC Cardiovasc Interv 2014;7:768–77.

43. Xu B, Tu S, Song L, et al. Angiographic quantitative flow ratio-guided coronary intervention (FAVOR III China): a multicentre, randomised, sham-controlled trial. Lancet 2021;398:2149–59.

44. Witberg G, De Bruyne B, Fearon WF, et al. Diagnostic performance of angiogram-derived fractional flow reserve: a pooled analysis of 5 prospective cohort studies. JACC Cardiovasc Interv 2020;13: 488–97.

45. Trobs M, Achenbach S, Rother J, et al. Comparison of fractional flow reserve based on computational fluid dynamics modeling using coronary angiographic vessel morphology versus invasively measured fractional flow reserve. Am J Cardiol 2016;117:29–35.

46. Neleman T, Masdjedi K, Van Zandvoort LJC, et al. Extended validation of novel 3D quantitative coronary angiography-based software to calculate vFFR: the FAST EXTEND study. JACC Cardiovasc Imaging 2021;14:504–6.

47. Masdjedi K, Tanaka N, Van Belle E, et al. Vessel fractional flow reserve (vFFR) for the assessment of stenosis severity: the FAST II study. EuroIntervention 2022;17:1498–505.

48. Papafaklis MI, Muramatsu T, Ishibashi Y, et al. Fast virtual functional assessment of intermediate coronary lesions using routine angiographic data and

blood flow simulation in humans: comparison with pressure wire - fractional flow reserve. EuroIntervention 2014;10:574–83.

49. Kim KH, Doh JH, Koo BK, et al. A novel noninvasive technology for treatment planning using virtual coronary stenting and computed tomography-derived computed fractional flow reserve. JACC Cardiovasc Interv 2014;7:72–8.

50. Douglas PS, Pontone G, Hlatky MA, et al. Clinical outcomes of fractional flow reserve by computed tomographic angiography-guided diagnostic strategies vs. usual care in patients with suspected coronary artery disease: the prospective longitudinal trial of FFR(CT): outcome and resource impacts study. Eur Heart J 2015;36:3359–67.

51. Driessen RS, Danad I, Stuijfzand WJ, et al. Comparison of coronary computed tomography angiography, fractional flow reserve, and perfusion imaging for ischemia diagnosis. J Am Coll Cardiol 2019;73:161–73.

52. Tu S, Ding D, Chang Y, et al. Diagnostic accuracy of quantitative flow ratio for assessment of coronary stenosis significance from a single angiographic view: a novel method based on bifurcation fractal law. Catheter Cardiovasc Interv 2021;97(Suppl 2):1040–7.

53. Patel MR, Jeremias A, Maehara A, et al. 1-Year outcomes of blinded physiological assessment of residual ischemia after successful PCI: DEFINE PCI trial. JACC Cardiovasc Interv 2022;15:52–61.

54. van Zandvoort LJC, Ali Z, Kern M, et al. Improving PCI outcomes using postprocedural physiology and intravascular imaging. JACC Cardiovasc Interv 2021;14:2415–30.

55. Kogame N, Takahashi K, Tomaniak M, et al. Clinical implication of quantitative flow ratio after percutaneous coronary intervention for 3-vessel disease. JACC Cardiovasc Interv 2019;12:2064–75.

56. Agarwal SK, Kasula S, Hacioglu Y, et al. Utilizing post-intervention fractional flow reserve to optimize acute results and the relationship to long-term outcomes. JACC Cardiovasc Interv 2016;9:1022–31.

57. Biscaglia S, Tebaldi M, Brugaletta S, et al. Prognostic value of QFR measured immediately after successful stent implantation: the international multicenter prospective HAWKEYE study. JACC Cardiovasc Interv 2019;12:2079–88.

58. Rimac G, Fearon WF, De Bruyne B, et al. Clinical value of post-percutaneous coronary intervention fractional flow reserve value: a systematic review and meta-analysis. Am Heart J 2017;183:1–9.

59. Jeremias A, Davies JE, Maehara A, et al. Blinded physiological assessment of residual ischemia after successful angiographic percutaneous coronary intervention: the DEFINE PCI study. JACC Cardiovasc Interv 2019;12:1991–2001.

60. Collison D, Didagelos M, Aetesam-Ur-Rahman M, et al. Post-stenting fractional flow reserve vs coronary angiography for optimization of percutaneous coronary intervention (TARGET-FFR). Eur Heart J 2021;42:4656–68.

61. Omori H, Kawase Y, Mizukami T, et al. Comparisons of nonhyperemic pressure ratios: predicting functional results of coronary revascularization using longitudinal vessel interrogation. JACC Cardiovasc Interv 2020;13:2688–98.

62. Zhang R, Xu B, Dou K, et al. Post-PCI outcomes predicted by pre-intervention simulation of residual quantitative flow ratio using augmented reality. Int J Cardiol 2022;352:33–9.

63. Modi BN, Sankaran S, Kim HJ, et al. Predicting the physiological effect of revascularization in serially diseased coronary arteries. Circ Cardiovasc Interv 2019;12:e007577.

64. Sonck J, Nagumo S, Norgaard BL, et al. Clinical validation of a virtual planner for coronary interventions based on coronary CT angiography. JACC Cardiovasc Imaging 2022;15:1242–55.

65. Bom MJ, Schumacher SP, Driessen RS, et al. Noninvasive procedural planning using computed tomography-derived fractional flow reserve. Catheter Cardiovasc Interv 2021;97:614–22.

66. Fearon WF, Zimmermann FM, De Bruyne B, et al. Fractional Flow reserve-guided pci as compared with coronary bypass surgery. N Engl J Med 2022;386:128–37.

67. Katagiri Y, De Maria GL, Kogame N, et al. Impact of post-procedural minimal stent area on 2-year clinical outcomes in the SYNTAX II trial. Catheter Cardiovasc Interv 2019;93:E225–34.

68. Pijls NH, Klauss V, Siebert U, et al. Coronary pressure measurement after stenting predicts adverse events at follow-up: a multicenter registry. Circulation 2002;105:2950–4.

69. Klauss V, Erdin P, Rieber J, et al. Fractional flow reserve for the prediction of cardiac events after coronary stent implantation: results of a multivariate analysis. Heart 2005;91:203–6.

70. Nam CW, Hur SH, Cho YK, et al. Relation of fractional flow reserve after drug-eluting stent implantation to one-year outcomes. Am J Cardiol 2011;107:1763–7.

71. Li SJ, Ge Z, Kan J, et al. Cutoff value and long-term prediction of clinical events by ffr measured immediately after implantation of a drug-eluting stent in patients with coronary artery disease: 1- to 3-year results from the DKCRUSH VII registry study. JACC Cardiovasc Interv 2017;10:986–95.

72. Fournier S, Ciccarelli G, Toth GG, et al. Association of improvement in fractional flow reserve with outcomes, including symptomatic relief, after percutaneous coronary intervention. JAMA Cardiol 2019;4:370–4.

73. Hwang D, Lee JM, Lee HJ, et al. Influence of target vessel on prognostic relevance of fractional flow reserve after coronary stenting. EuroIntervention 2019;15:457–64.

Moving?

Make sure your subscription moves with you!

To notify us of your new address, find your **Clinics Account Number** (located on your mailing label above your name), and contact customer service at:

Email: journalscustomerservice-usa@elsevier.com

800-654-2452 (subscribers in the U.S. & Canada)
314-447-8871 (subscribers outside of the U.S. & Canada)

Fax number: 314-447-8029

Elsevier Health Sciences Division
Subscription Customer Service
3251 Riverport Lane
Maryland Heights, MO 63043

*To ensure uninterrupted delivery of your subscription, please notify us at least 4 weeks in advance of move.

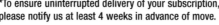

Printed and bound by CPI Group (UK) Ltd, Croydon, CR0 4YY

03/10/2024

01040365-0016